The Effect of Childhood Emotional Maltreatment on Later Intimate Relationships

The Effect of Childhood Emotional Maltreatment on Later Intimate Relationships addresses timely topics on the effect of emotional child abuse and neglect on the formation and maintenance of intimate relationships in adolescence and adulthood. This collection of manuscripts addresses current theory, research and practice pertinent to the difficulties experienced by survivors of childhood emotional maltreatment. Topics addressed in this volume include: attachment theory, interpersonal problems, codependency and self silencing, and relationship violence and sexual aggression. The manuscripts reflect current research regarding the influence of childhood emotional maltreatment on intimate relationships while suggesting directions for future research on this important topic.

This book was previously published as a special issue of the *Journal of Aggression, Maltreatment and Trauma*.

Nancy Dodge Reyome, Ph.D. is currently the Director of Research and Sponsored Programs and an Associate Professor of Psychology at the State University of New York at Potsdam. She received her Ph.D. in Human Development and Family Studies from Cornell University in 1988 and has conducted research on the developmental implications of child abuse and neglect for over 25 years.

The Effect of Childhood Emotional Maltreatment on Later Intimate Relationships

Edited by
Nancy Dodge Reyome

Routledge
Taylor & Francis Group
LONDON AND NEW YORK

First published 2011
by Routledge
4 Park Square, Milton Park, Abingdon, Oxon OX14 4RN
605 Third Avenue, New York, NY 10017

Routledge is an imprint of the Taylor & Francis Group, an informa business

First issued in paperback 2013

This book is a reproduction of the *Journal of Aggression, Maltreatment and Trauma*, vol.19, issue 1-2. The Publisher requests to those authors who may be citing this book to state, also, the bibliographical details of the special issue on which the book was based.

Typeset in Times New Roman by
Taylor & Francis Books

British Library Cataloguing in Publication Data
A catalogue record for this book is available from the British Library

ISBN13: 978-0-415-59369-4 (hbk)
ISBN13: 978-0-415-85107-7 (pbk)

Contents

PART 2

INTRODUCTION TO PART 1

NANCY DODGE REYOME
State University of New York College at Potsdam, Potsdam, New York, USA

Researchers have historically overlooked the influence of childhood emotional abuse on the emerging attachment system and the formation of later intimate relationships in adolescence and adulthood. The purpose of this special issue of the Journal of Aggression, Maltreatment and Trauma is to shed some light on the role of emotional forms of child maltreatment on the development of attachment and provide some insight into how clinicians might overcome attachment difficulties that result from childhood histories of emotional abuse. This introduction provides a brief overview of each article in this special issue.

This issue of the *Journal of Aggression, Maltreatment and Trauma* is the first of two special issues concerned with the influence of childhood emotional maltreatment on the formation and maintenance of intimate relationships in adolescence and adulthood. This special issue focuses on theory and research pertinent to the effect of early emotional maltreatment on the emerging attachment system and later intimate relationships. The influence of childhood maltreatment on the formation of early attachment relationships has been a topic of research for nearly three decades, but very little work has actually been done to tease out the effect of emotional forms of maltreatment on the attachment system (Baer & Martinez, 2006; Carlson, Cicchetti, Barnett, & Braunwald, 1989; Crittenden & Ainsworth, 1989; Egeland & Sroufe, 1981; Morton & Browne, 1998). The content of this issue is a step toward rectifying that oversight. There are four articles in this special issue. The first article provides a theoretical and empirical overview of the topic. The second article explores the influence of emotional maltreatment on attachment in youth who have been placed in foster care. The third article is an empirical report on some of the connections proposed in the first article. The final article presents evidence from the clinical world on the efficacy of particular therapeutic methods in addressing attachment difficulties in survivors of childhood emotional maltreatment.

In the first article, Riggs presents a comprehensive theoretical and empirical overview of the influence of childhood emotional abuse on the developing attachment system. She provides a framework for demonstrating how attachment difficulties experienced by emotionally abused children translate into later problems with intimate relationships for these individuals. Riggs introduces a model based on theory and research that focuses on how childhood emotional abuse influences the development of the attachment system, which subsequently influences socioemotional development and ultimately provides the foundation for the formation of later interpersonal relationships. Through this model she explains that childhood emotional abuse is related to the development of insecure attachment during childhood. Further, Riggs argues that individuals with insecure attachments demonstrate poor emotion regulation, ineffective coping strategies, low self-esteem, deficits in self-understanding, impaired social skills, and poor mental health. Riggs argues that it is through these psychological and social mechanisms that insecure attachment has a deleterious effect on the formation of later intimate and romantic relationships of childhood emotional abuse survivors.

In the second article, Taussig and Culhane explore the influence of emotional abuse on psychological and interpersonal functioning in a study of preadolescent youth in foster placement. The young people in the Taussig and Culhane study were exposed to a myriad of emotionally abusive behaviors, including overall emotional maltreatment, verbal aggression, parentification, abandonment, and violence exposure. Among the outcome variables measured in this study were attachment to caregivers, parents, and peers. For the entire sample studied, the authors discovered that the emotional trauma associated with abandonment was associated with poorer attachment relationships with peers. Interestingly, they found the attachment relationships of males were most affected by a history of emotional maltreatment. Specifically, they found that males who experienced verbal aggression experienced difficulty in attachment relationships with parents and males who experienced overall emotional maltreatment had difficulties in attachments to peers. Although exploratory in nature, this study provides new avenues for further examination as researchers look at the contribution of different forms of emotional maltreatment to the formation of attachment.

Using an attachment theory perspective, Riggs and Kaminski investigated childhood emotional abuse, adult attachment security, and depression as predictors of relational functioning and psychological aggression in the romantic relationships of young adults. Among other things, their study sought to explore the link between childhood emotional abuse and adult attachment quality and the link between childhood emotional abuse and later intimate relationship functioning. The authors conclude that the results of the study uphold the theoretical model introduced in the first Riggs article, linking a history of childhood emotional abuse to insecure attachment in late adolescence and adulthood and determining that insecure attachment style makes a significant contribution to functioning in romantic relationships in later life.

Finally, the Carbone article presents five clinical case studies of individuals with insecure attachment histories attributable to childhood emotional abuse and social rejection from parents and peers. In detailing the experiences of each of the individual cases presented, Carbone discusses how three treatment methods—cognitive behavioral therapy, rational emotive therapy, and eye movement desensitization and reprocessing—were used in each case to assist the individual in overcoming the negative social cognitions and internal working models of relationships associated with a history of childhood emotional abuse and social rejection. This article provides a glimpse into the clinical techniques used to help emotional abuse survivors reprocess and reframe these painful experiences and begin to lead socially productive and satisfying adult lives.

Childhood maltreatment has long been associated with the formation of insecure, disorganized attachment relationships in childhood and adulthood. The content of this issue supports and reinforces this finding while exploring ways that childhood emotional maltreatment has a unique, possibly more devastating effect on the emerging attachment system than other forms of maltreatment. Further, material in this issue provides hope for assisting adult survivors with overcoming the devastating interpersonal effects of childhood emotional trauma by exploring successful clinical interventions for moving survivors forward in their effort to experience healthy, secure adult relationships.

REFERENCES

Baer, J., & Martinez, C. (2006). Child maltreatment and insecure attachment: A meta-analysis. *Journal of Reproductive and Infant Psychology, 24*, 187–197.

Carlson, V., Cicchetti, D., Barnett, D., & Braunwald, D. (1989). Disorganized/disoriented attachment relationships in maltreated infants. *Developmental Psychology, 25*, 525–531.

Crittenden, P., & Ainsworth, M. (1989). Child maltreatment and attachment theory. In D. Cicchetti & V. Carlson (Eds.), *Child maltreatment: Theory and research on the causes and consequences of child abuse and neglect* (pp. 432–463). Cambridge, UK: Cambridge University Press.

Egeland, B., & Sroufe, A. (1981). Attachment and early maltreatment. *Child Development, 52*, 44–52.

Morton, N., & Browne, K. (1998). Theory and observation of attachment and its relation to child maltreatment: An overview. *Child Abuse and Neglect, 22*, 1093–1104.

THEORETICAL ISSUES

Childhood Emotional Abuse and the Attachment System Across the Life Cycle: What Theory and Research Tell Us

SHELLEY A. RIGGS
University of North Texas, Denton, Texas, USA

The purpose of this article is to review the theoretical and empirical literature regarding the normative development of the attachment system from infancy through adulthood, and then discuss deviations from the normal developmental pathways that occur in response to emotionally abusive parenting (e.g., strong rejection, intrusive or controlling, hostile, or frightening behavior). A theoretical model grounded in attachment theory is presented describing the development of maladaptive interaction patterns in adult romantic relationships. The model proposes that early emotional abuse engenders insecure attachment, which impairs emotional regulation, fosters negative views of self and others that support maladaptive coping responses, interferes with social functioning and the capacity for intimate adult attachments, contributes to poor mental health, and consequently shapes the quality of romantic relationships.

A large body of literature documents the harmful effects of physical abuse, sexual abuse, and neglect. Scholarly interest in emotional abuse[1] as a distinct form of maltreatment emerged later and has grown slowly. Although frequently co-occurring, the latest findings indicate that relative to other forms of maltreatment (i.e., physical abuse, sexual abuse, physical neglect), emotional abuse has specific and independent consequences (Briere & Runtz, 1990; Gross & Keller, 1992; Mullen, Martin, Anderson, Romans, & Herbison, 1996; Nicholas & Bieber, 1996) and might, in fact, be the most pervasive and damaging type of abuse (Hart, Binggeli, & Brassard, 1997; McGee & Wolfe, 1991). Despite recent progress in the field, rarely has the extant research been driven by an overarching developmental theory (Wright, 2007). Attachment theory (Bowlby, 1969, 1973, 1980) is uniquely suited to fill this gap because it is built on the salient themes of early parent–child interactions and close interpersonal relationships throughout the life span. Moreover, attachment theory is now one of the most sophisticated and extensively researched theories of human development, which provides a comprehensive account of both normal and abnormal development. The purpose of this article is to examine the phenomenon of childhood emotional abuse from the framework of attachment theory and construct a theoretical model of development that accounts for the impact of childhood emotional abuse on romantic relationship functioning in adulthood.

Figure 1 presents a conceptual model grounded in attachment theory describing the intergenerational cycle of childhood emotional abuse in the absence of intervention. The model proposes that emotional abuse by attachment figures in infancy and early childhood contributes to the development of insecure attachment organization, which impairs emotional regulation and fosters negative internal working models of self and others that initiate and sustain negative coping responses. As the child matures, these deficits create substantial vulnerability for maladaptive interpersonal schemas that interfere with social functioning, contributing to poor peer relations in childhood and adolescence (see Taussig & Culhane, 2010), and later insecurity in the adult romantic attachment system. Maladaptive coping, social problems, and insecure attachment, in turn, are risk factors for psychological distress at all ages (see Riggs & Kaminski, 2010). These pathways of influence culminate in romantic relationship dysfunction that may be characterized by problems with intimacy (see Carbone, 2010; Dodge Reyome, in press; Dodge Reyome, Ward, & Witkiewitz, in press), caregiving and caretaking

---

1 Some scholars have used the terms *psychological abuse* and *emotional abuse* interchangeably (e.g., Thompson & Kaplan, 1996), others have argued that they are distinct constructs (e.g., O'Hagan, 2006), and still others have maintained that emotional abuse is a type of psychological abuse distinguished from psychosocial neglect (e.g., Stein et al., 2000, as cited in Allen, 2001). Although these definitions and distinctions are important, they are beyond the scope of this article, so I have elected to use the term *emotional abuse* broadly to encompass theory and research regarding psychological abuse, emotional abuse, and emotional neglect that occurs in childhood.

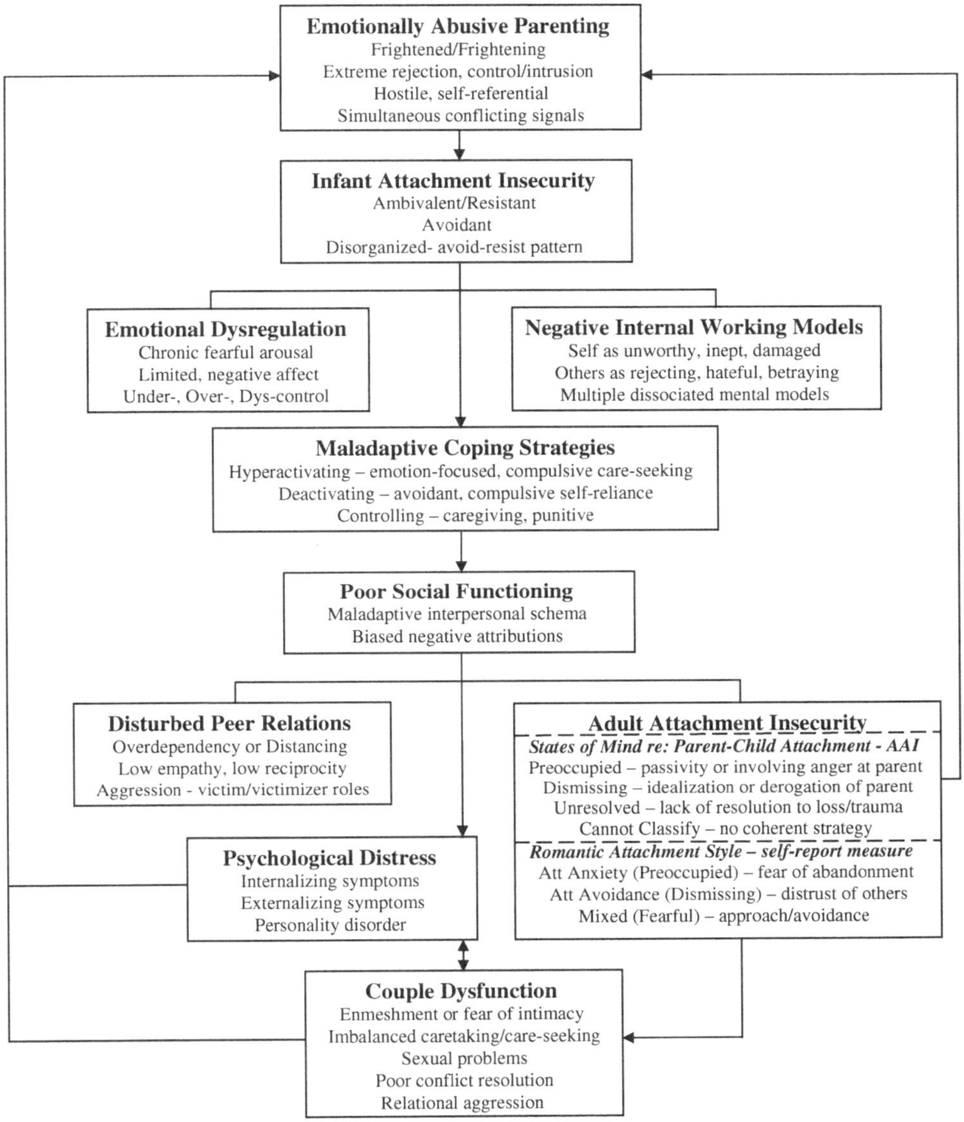

FIGURE 1 Hypothesized hierarchical regression models for relationship adjustment, psychological aggression, and psychological victimization.

(see Dodge Reyome, in press; Dodge Reyome et al., in press), sexual functioning (see Zurbriggen, Gobin, & Freyd, in press), conflict resolution (see Berzenski & Yates, in press; Dodge Reyome, in press), or relational aggression (see Berzenski & Yates, in press; Riggs & Kaminski, 2010). Without intervention at some point, the cycle may repeat itself in the next generation when adult attachment insecurity, emotional disturbance, and poor marital relations negatively affect parenting behavior, potentially resulting in emotionally abusive behavior toward offspring.

This article reviews the theoretical and empirical literature that supports the proposed model, describing the ways childhood emotional abuse can undermine the adaptive development of the attachment system and lead to difficulties in intimate relationships in adulthood. The first major section describes the basic tenets of attachment theory as it applies to early development, reviews attachment research that can inform ongoing efforts to define emotional abuse, and then explores the potential influence of emotional abuse on attachment organization in infancy and toddlerhood. The subsequent section discusses the continuity of the attachment system and examines the effects of emotional abuse in childhood and adolescence. Next, the literature regarding adult attachment and mental health is reviewed and the expected impact of emotional abuse on romantic relationship functioning is described. Finally, the conclusion considers the implications for future research and intervention.

EARLY DEVELOPMENT

Attachment in Infancy

Drawing on biological, evolutionary, and ethological theories, Bowlby (1980, 1982, 1988) postulated the existence of an attachment behavioral control system similar to other physiological systems in its homeostatic organization, but distinct from systems managing other behaviors such as feeding or sexual conduct. The biological function of the attachment bond between a parent and a child is protection because the attainment of proximity to a more powerful other increases the chances of individual survival (Bowlby, 1973). Although not always in evidence, the attachment system actively monitors personal safety and the accessibility of the attachment figure at some level on a continuing basis. Most visible in children when tired, ill, or afraid, the attachment system is activated whenever the individual perceives a threat to security, stimulating behaviors designed to achieve proximity to an attachment figure, especially in stressful circumstances (Bowlby, 1980). In optimal circumstances, attachment behavior is terminated when the attachment figure restores a sense of security through sensitive responding and physical or emotional accessibility.

Attachment relationships are hypothesized to exist not only within a behavioral system governing infant–parent interaction, but also within a conceptual system governing significant social relations throughout the life span. Bowlby (1969, 1973, 1980) theorized that in the last quarter of the first year of life, humans develop *internal working models* (IWMs) to represent the emotions and expectations arising out of early dyadic patterns of communication between infant and caregiver. Unlike simple cognitive schemas,

IWMs are thought to include affective, defensive, and descriptive cognitive components (Bretherton, 1985; Main, Kaplan, & Cassidy, 1985). Parental styles of structuring and guiding interaction direct the general organization and structure of children's memories in a process of dialogic coconstruction in which both partners take an active role (Bretherton, 1993). Optimally, children can freely express both positive and negative affect and receive appropriate caregiver responses, which directly attend to the child's communications by soothing and comforting negative states or sharing and enhancing positive states. In this way, children become aware of their internal emotional experiences and learn to control and manipulate their behavioral responses in interactions with the caregiver. Well-coordinated regulatory patterns derived from these early transactions contribute to the capacity for self-regulation and provide the basis for an integrated sense of self as a coherent whole (E. A. Carlson & Sroufe, 1995; Sroufe & Fleeson, 1986).

Through affective and communicative attunement between caregiver and child, developing processes of perception, cognition, behavior, and language merge with existing patterns of regulating and expressing emotion and maintaining organization (Bretherton, 1985, 1993). Rules for evaluating behavior, thoughts, and feelings eventually come to operate automatically outside of awareness (Bowlby, 1980) and may be associated with the development of neural networks governing the types and degree of stimuli needed to activate (i.e., perceived threat) and deactivate (i.e., felt security) the attachment system (Fraley, Davis, & Shaver, 1998). The consolidation of IWMs forms the basis for conceptual representations of self, others, and the world, which enable individuals to predict and interpret others' behaviors and to plan their own response.

In support of the theoretical link between sensitive and responsive caregiving and the development of secure attachment patterns, research has established that differences in caregivers' behaviors and adult attachment representations measured by the Adult Attachment Interview (AAI; George, Kaplan, & Main, 1985) are associated with discrete patterns of infant attachment behavior in the Strange Situation laboratory procedure (Ainsworth, Blehar, Waters, & Wall, 1978). Table 1 provides a convenient overview of the various infant and adult attachment classifications and related parenting behavior, which are described in the following sections. Adult caregivers classified as secure on the AAI tend to demonstrate sensitive and responsive caregiving and have *secure* infants, who in the lab demonstrate active exploration in the caregiver's presence, normal distress at separation, active greeting, and subsequent calming after the caregiver's return. In contrast, three distinct patterns of insecure adult attachment representations predict three different nonoptimal caregiving styles and three types of insecure attachment in infants (Adam, Gunnar, & Tanaka, 2004; Lyons-Ruth, Bronfman, & Parsons, 1999; Main & Hesse, 1990; Main et al., 1985; van IJzendoorn,

TABLE 1 Features Associated With Attachment Classification

Infant/Adult Classification	Secure/Autonomous	Avoidant/Dismissing	Ambivalent/Preoccupied	Disorganized/Unresolved or Fearful
Infant				
Strange Situation (SS) behavior	Explores readily Expresses distress at departure of caregiver Soothed upon return of parent	Extreme autonomy Avoids closeness and contact Attachment deactivated	Extreme distress in absence of parent Demanding or resistant Attachment overactivated	Disorganized/disoriented No coherent strategy Conflicting, disjointed behavior
Adult				
Adult Attachment Interview (AAI)	Coherent, autonomous, collaborative Few discourse violations	Incoherence: Violates discourse rules Idealization Lack of recall Derogation	Incoherence: Violates discourse rules Involving anger Passivity Confusion	Unresolved: Assigned along with primary classification Lapses in reasoning or discourse re: loss or trauma Lack of resolution to trauma
Parenting behavior (as associated with AAI & SS)	Sensitive, responsive when needed or wanted Maintains contact	Avoids emotional or physical closeness Rejecting	Inconsistently available Role reversal Blurred boundaries	Frightened/frightening Hostile/helpless Maltreatment by some
Self-reported romantic attachment style	Low attachment avoidance and attachment anxiety Positive self and other models	High attachment avoidance: Distrust of others Positive self-model, negative other model	High attachment anxiety: Fear of abandonment Negative self-model, positive other model	Fearful: Not determined by trauma, but empirically related High attachment avoidance and attachment anxiety Negative self and other models
Organizational/relational strategy	Flexible/adaptive Balance between exploration and attachment Healthy connection to others	Minimize emotion and attachment behavior Defensively turn away Overly self-reliant Distant, disengaged	Exaggerate emotion and attachment behavior Internalization Overly dependent on others Enmeshment	Unresolved: Related to underlying primary strategy, but generally disorganized/disoriented Fearful: Approach/avoidance

1995). Presumably, insecure attachment strategies are adopted by infants because they are adaptive in relation to their attachment figure's behavioral responses. For example, caregivers classified as dismissing tend to reject their infants' bids for attention in the home and have infants who show *avoidant* (e.g., indifferent, overly self-reliant) attachment behaviors that are effective in keeping the attachment figure from turning away from the infant. Caregivers classified as preoccupied are either unpredictable or intrusive toward the infant in the home and generally have infants who exhibit *ambivalent* (e.g., clingy, anxious, angry) attachment behaviors that are effective in gaining the caregiver's attention. A fourth infant classification can be assigned in conjunction with one of the three primary categories and is characterized by contradictory infant behaviors with no coherent strategy, but rather a mixture of the other attachment strategies; research evidence indicates that this *disorganized* attachment pattern is associated with child maltreatment, parental lack of resolution to trauma or loss, maternal frightened or frightening behavior, maternal psychopathology, and excessive alcohol use (see Lyons-Ruth & Jacobvitz, 1999, for a review).

Emotionally Abusive Caregiving

Whereas the differentiation among physical, sexual, and emotional abuse is fairly straightforward, it is much more difficult to discriminate among imperfect parenting, parental mistakes, and emotionally abusive parental behavior (Messman-Moore & Coates, 2007; Wright, 2007). Several research groups (e.g., Bifulco, Brown, & Harris, 1994; Hart, Brassard, Binggeli, & Davidson, 2002; Thompson & Kaplan, 1996) have identified a wide range of caregiver behaviors comprising emotional abuse, but the lack of consensus makes it difficult to compare and generalize across research findings. Because parental behavior lies along a continuum, determining where acceptable behavior becomes emotionally abusive is clearly complicated and subject to varied opinions (Messman-Moore & Coates, 2007; Wright, 2007). Attachment theory and research might provide clues regarding how to distinguish emotionally abusive parenting and its effects on children.

The attachment literature identifies insensitive, rejecting, and intrusive and role-reversing parenting as key contributors to insecure attachment (Ainsworth et al., 1978; van IJzendoorn, 1995). However, Collins and Feeney (2004) described avoidant and ambivalent infant attachment patterns as "good enough" strategies to obtain sufficient amounts of security and contact with others. Additionally, although theory and research suggest that insecure attachment creates a vulnerability for psychopathology (see Carlson & Sroufe, 1995, for a review), many insecure children and adults do not demonstrate interpersonal or psychological problems, and avoidant or dismissing individuals have been noted to exhibit an absence of problems (e.g., Riggs & Jacobvitz, 2002). Furthermore, Solomon and George (1999) argued that reparative actions by caregivers (e.g., hugs, apologies, explanations) following negative parenting behaviors will minimize the deleterious effects of these interactions.

Meta-analytic findings indicate parenting that is somewhat inconsistent and self-preoccupied or somewhat rejecting and dismissing is associated with ambivalent and resistant or avoidant infant behavior, but not disorganized attachment behavior (van IJzendoorn, 1995). In laboratory assessments where avoidant and ambivalent infants have established a coherent, albeit nonoptimal strategy for obtaining and maintaining proximity to caregivers, disorganized infants demonstrate disorientation, simultaneous approach avoidance, freezing behaviors, and other odd actions that do not seem to have a clearly identifiable purpose or pattern (Main & Morgan, 1996; Main & Solomon, 1986). Main and Hesse (1990) theorized that this disorganization arises when caregivers display frightening or frightened behaviors, thus presenting their children with the irresolvable paradox of wanting to seek security from their attachment figures when threatened and afraid, but also fearing the attachment figure who is "the source of and solution to their alarm" (p. 163). Evidence linking disorganized infant attachment to physical maltreatment and parental frightened or frightening behavior supports this hypothesis (Carlson, Cicchetti, Barnett, & Braunwald, 1989; Lyons-Ruth, Bronfman, & Parsons, 1999; Lyons-Ruth, Connell, Grunebaum, & Botein, 1990; Schuengel, Bakermans-Kranenburg, & van IJzendoorn, 1999).

Lyons-Ruth and her colleagues (e.g., Lyons-Ruth, Alpern, & Repacholi, 1993; Lyons-Ruth, Bronfman, & Atwood, 1999; Lyons-Ruth, Easterbrooks, & Cibelli, 1997; Lyons-Ruth, Melnick, Bronfman, Sherry, & Llanas, 2004; Lyons-Ruth, Repacholi, McLeod, & Silva, 1991) have conducted a 20+-year longitudinal study with a low-income sample of community and clinical parent–infant dyads, many of them demonstrating disorganized attachment behaviors. Building on earlier work linking parents' frightening and/or frightened behaviors to infant disorganization (Lyons-Ruth, Bronfman, & Parsons, 1999; Main & Hesse, 1990; Schuengel et al., 1999), this research group identified two profiles of problematic parenting that are associated with two subcategories of disorganized infant classification. One parenting profile, called *helpless-fearful regarding attachment,* is characterized by nonhostile and ostensibly responsive behavior with high levels of parental withdrawal, fearfulness, and inhibition. Helpless-fearful parenting is related to a disorganized attachment pattern termed *disorganized-secure* or *disorganized-approach* because infants still approach their parents and achieve physical contact despite demonstrating disorganized behaviors. This pattern is relatively difficult to identify and appears to be more common in low-risk, middle-class samples. The second parenting profile, called *hostile-self-referential regarding attachment,* is characterized by excessive role reversal, frightening and negative and intrusive behavior, as well as behavior that both elicits and rejects the infant's attachment-related emotions and behaviors. Of the five primary parenting scales coded, affective communication errors (e.g., simultaneous conflicting signals, nonresponse, or mismatched response) were the most strongly related to infant disorganization. This contradictory combination of both rejecting and attention-seeking behaviors by parents was associated with a second disorganized pattern in infants called *disorganized-insecure* or *disorganized-avoid-resist* because their disorganized behaviors were mixed with other behaviors resembling the avoidant and ambivalent or resistant groups. Despite clear group differences in behavioral manifestation, the evidence indicates that both subgroups of disorganized infants are at risk for similar negative outcomes, including conflict, apprehension, and dysphoria in reunions with caregivers, as well as highly aggressive behavior with peers by ages 5 and 7 (Lyons-Ruth, 1996; Lyons-Ruth et al., 1993; Lyons-Ruth et al., 1997).

Similar to frightening parenting described in earlier work, the hostile-self-referential parenting pattern appears to fit clearly within the bounds of what typically would be considered emotional abuse in the literature. However, parenting behaviors coded as frightened or helpless-fearful are often subtle and nonabusive (Hesse & Main, 2006; Lyons-Ruth et al., 2004). Consequently, despite similar outcomes, it is less clear where the frightened or helpless patterns fall on the parenting continuum, although they might be a form of emotional neglect in that they deprive children of needed support and positive interactions. Theoretically, in the context of both types of hostile or helpless (or frightened or frightening) relationships, insecurely attached children experience fearful arousal that has no resolution because they receive no comfort or soothing to reduce their anxiety (Hesse & Main, 2006; Lyons-Ruth et al., 2004).

Based on the available theory and research, the proposed model in Figure 1 construes only extreme and relentless rejection (e.g., antipathy, degradation), intrusiveness (e.g., controlling, guilting, role-reversing behavior), or both, which is frightening to the child and not followed by parental efforts to reconcile, as constituting emotional abuse. As suggested by the work of Lyons-Ruth, it might be the incongruous mixture of the two types of extreme parenting, especially simultaneous conflicting signals, that represents the most harmful mode of emotional abuse. The model assumes that emotionally abusive parenting will foster the development of insecure attachment in children. Although all three types of insecure attachment are possible consequences, the more severe the abuse, the more likely it is that the infant will demonstrate a disorganized-avoid-resist pattern.

Early Effects of Emotional Abuse

Figure 1 depicts two primary components of insecure attachment organization that are affected by emotional abuse: the capacity for emotional regulation and IMWs. As a consequence of "fright without solution" (Hesse & Main, 2006) caused by frightened or frightening or hostile or helpless parental behavior, insecure children experience a disregulation of arousal caused by chronic activation of the fight-or-flight mechanisms and consequently do not learn to regulate emotion effectively (Lyons-Ruth et al., 2004). In the earliest stages of development, emotions are diffuse and infants have little control over their behavioral expression, relying instead on the dyadic regulation provided by their caregivers' responses to behavioral signals (Sroufe & Fleeson, 1986). As normal development progresses, diffuse emotions become more and more refined and an increasing number of positive and negative emotions are experienced. In contrast, when children experience emotionally abusive parenting, the inability to regulate more complex emotions sets in motion a series of developmental failures in their emotional growth. O'Hagan (2006) argued that children who suffer emotional abuse experience only a limited number of emotions, which are dominated by negative rather than positive affect. It also seems likely that emotional abuse interferes with children's understanding of emotions such that they have difficulty identifying emotions in themselves or others (i.e., they lack empathy and ability to recognize social cues). As a result, emotional expression may become distorted so that these children often function at the outermost limits of the emotional spectrum (O'Hagan, 2006) and conceivably demonstrate conflicting emotional and behavioral responses consistent with attachment disorganization.

Emotional abuse also profoundly influences children's developing understanding of self and others (Liem & Boudewyn, 1999). In optimal circumstances, infants whose caregivers respond contingently and appropriately to infant signals will develop a secure attachment, characterized by positive IWMs of self as capable of affecting the environment or caregiver and worthy of care, as well as positive IWMs of others as reliable and supportive (Bartholomew & Horowitz, 1991). As a result, secure infants will feel safe enough to explore the environment but will actively seek comfort and protection from attachment figures when they are fatigued, sick, injured, or afraid. Conversely, infants whose caregivers respond in an inconsistent or intrusive manner will likely develop negative self-models as incompetent, unworthy, and powerless (see Dodge Reyome et al., in press). Attachment theory suggests that negative IWMs of self may contribute to self-blame, overdependence on the attachment figure, limited exploration, and subsequent ineffective use of social support. Other infants whose caregivers respond in a rejecting manner are likely to develop negative IWMs of others as unresponsive, inconsiderate, rejecting, or harsh (Liem & Boudewyn, 1999), making it less likely that children will trust other people or turn to others for help.

As depicted in Figure 1, the proposed theoretical model predicts that extreme forms of insecure, emotionally abusive parenting will intensify and strengthen negative internal models of the self (e.g., inept, damaged, contemptible, disgusting) or others (e.g., cruel, betraying, unforgiving, hateful). As a consequence of maltreatment, children lack a "sense of self-efficacy and capacity to manipulate the environment in service of emotional and instrumental coping" (Liem & Boudewyn, 1999, p. 1143). Children who experience a mixture of inconsistency or intrusion and rejection from their parents are likely to be doubly disadvantaged by negative IWMs of both self and others. The model further proposes that emotionally abusive parenting may engender dissociated mental representations that create a high risk for maladaptive social relations and psychopathology (see Carbone, this 2010; Riggs & Kaminski, 2010). According to Bowlby (1973, 1980), defensive exclusion occurs when individuals deactivate or block normal attachment responses or separate attachment information from consciousness to minimize conflict and anxiety. Experiences kept from awareness in this way might include strong rejection or punishment for attachment behaviors and feelings, direct or implied threats of abandonment, more severe abuse, and other events that are too painful to think about or that parents would prefer children not recognize (Bowlby, 1980, 1988). Defensive exclusion processes that are unconsciously activated and closed to environmental feedback may create distortions in IWMs, resulting in dissociation between conscious and unconscious working models and the formation of multiple incompatible belief systems (Bowlby, 1980). Bowlby (1973) suggested that these incongruent representations play a critical role in maladaptive adjustment and psychopathology.

CHILDHOOD AND ADOLESCENCE

Continuity of Attachment

Although the proposed model assumes that emotional abuse begins at birth, there are clearly situations when children might not experience emotional abuse until later ages when parental treatment shifts from acceptable to abusive or a new abusive caregiver enters their lives. The impact of this later emotional abuse will vary, depending to some degree on the children's past attachment experiences, their current attachment network, and other circumstances. Bowlby (1988) and Ainsworth (1989) believed that the attachment pattern formed in early childhood becomes an essential component of a person's overall personality structure with considerable influence on personality traits and individual ways of being and reacting to the world. Several longitudinal studies have demonstrated stability of attachment classification from infancy through 6 years of age and up to adolescence and early adulthood (see Grossmann, Grossmann, & Waters, 2005, for a review of major longitudinal studies following infants into adulthood). Yet, the attachment organization developed in childhood does not predetermine an individual's attachment style in later life, nor does it necessarily forecast a particular prognosis for lifetime adjustment and mental health. Several studies have found lawful discontinuity of attachment from infancy to adolescence through early adulthood in relation to disruptive life events, such as death, divorce, and maltreatment (Allen, McElhaney, Kuperminc, & Jodl, 2004; Cozzarelli, Karafa, Collins, & Tagler, 2003; Waters, Merrick, Treboux, Crowell, & Albersheim, 2000).

Collins and Sroufe (1999) proposed a transactional model whereby early attachment experiences continue to affect children's functioning and later relationships, but children also contribute to their own development and environments by responding and engaging with others according to previous patterns of adaptation and expectations. Specifically, IWMs of self and others formed in childhood influence immediate emotional reactions, the cognitive processes that maintain and amplify or lessen emotional responses, and the resulting behavior. According to the transactional model, experience-based variations in acquiring specific relational skills (e.g., empathy, social perception, communication, negotiation, conflict resolution) and interpersonal cognitions or biases likely mediate the link between early attachments and later relationships.

Theoretically, continuity in attachment patterns can be explained at least partially by the impact of early IWMs on cognitive-affective processes, which direct attention to specific stimuli, create biases in memory encoding and retrieval, guide expectations regarding the availability of others, and influence attributions regarding the behavior of others in ambiguous situations (Cassidy, 2000). For example, research indicates that secure children make realistic or benevolent attributions regarding the intentions of peers, whereas avoidant children showed more unrealistic or hostile and negative biases (Suess, Grossmann, & Sroufe, 1992). These cognitive-affective processes influence the individual's decisions, emotional responses, and behaviors. In particular, secure individuals tend to be open and flexible in emotional expression, but insecure children may either minimize (avoidant) or heighten (ambivalent) the expression of negative emotions, which then elicits the kind of treatment the individual receives from others and typically reinforces the IWMs in a self-perpetuating cycle across new contexts and developmental stages (Cassidy, 1994).

Consistent with this idea, Sroufe and Fleeson (1986) reported findings that avoidant preschoolers appeared to elicit punitive reactions from teachers, whereas ambivalent or resistant children were rated as more emotionally immature by teachers and thus received more nurturance and tolerance from them. Importantly, these researchers noted that in different peer dyads children often displayed opposite or complementary behavior (e.g., child was rejected or conversely rejecting) depending on the attachment strategy of the dyadic partner, suggesting that the whole relationship is internalized and carried forward into new relationships in such a way that the particular role enacted will depend on the other partner's responses. For example, having learned both roles in the victim–victimizer dichotomy, in peer interactions, a maltreated child may assume the role of victimizer, bullying other children who appear weak and easy targets, or conversely the same child may assume the role of victim and be bullied by other children who are more dominant and aggressive.

Effects of Emotional Abuse in Childhood and Adolescence

Yates (2007) conceptualized emotional abuse as a form of chronic relational adversity that disrupts development across social, emotional, self, cognitive, and biological domains. Thus, childhood emotional abuse, like other forms of early maltreatment, poses a serious challenge to the formation and maintenance of secure attachments, causing significant interference with the adaptive development of emotional regulation and IWMs of self and others (Cicchetti & Toth, 2000; Collins, Guichard, Ford, & Feeney, 2004). Although emotional abuse at any age is likely to have detrimental effects, the transactional model of Collins and Sroufe (1999) suggests that emotional abuse in infancy may be more damaging than emotional abuse occurring later in development because early experiences interact with later experiences to determine present-day outcomes. Although a secure attachment established in infancy might somewhat protect children from the full impact of later emotional abuse, insecure infant attachment could create a greater vulnerability to maladaptive responses to emotional abuse occurring at older ages. However, the child's current attachment network is also critical, such that the presence of a secure relationship with a supportive adult might counteract the negative impact of emotional abuse from another caregiver.

Consistent with the proposed model in Figure 1, O'Hagan (2006) described two prototypes of emotionally abused children who possess coping strategies similar to the behaviors expected for the avoidant and ambivalent attachment groups. Specifically, like the behaviors expected of avoidantly attached children, some emotionally abused children might exhibit the extreme of "dominant silent, invisible negative emotion" because they have learned that the natural expression of emotions provokes hostile reactions from the caregiver and strive to inhibit any observable indications of affect. According to O'Hagan, the constant suppression will eventually become automatic and weaken the capacity to feel positive affect, leaving their emotional world ruled by indifference, apathy, dejection, and unspoken hatred. At the other extreme, similar to the exaggerated emotional coping of ambivalently attached children, some emotionally abused children exhibit "dominant audible and visible negative emotions," likely modeled after a caregiver's highly visible emotional displays, which can be loud, aggressive, erratic, unrestrained, and destructive (O'Hagan, 2006).

Although some emotionally abused children might demonstrate ambivalent and avoidant attachment strategies, theoretically, if the abuse begins at birth, it seems likely that these children start out as disorganized infants, who by definition do not demonstrate a predominant, coherent strategy for seeking and maintaining proximity to the attachment figure. However, as noted in Figure 1, by the time they reach school age, disorganized children show more organized coping strategies that have been described as "controlling" toward the parent (Main & Cassidy, 1988; Wartner, Grossmann, Fremmer-Bombik, & Suess, 1994). Rather than seeking comfort and protection for their own needs, this controlling strategy appears to be designed to maintain engagement with the caregiver by gratifying the caregiver's self-preoccupation (Lyons-Ruth, Bronfman, & Parsons, 1999; Main & Cassidy, 1988) and might take the form of caretaking of the parent by the child or a hostile and punitive stance toward the parent. Lyons-Ruth et al. (2004) speculated that these two types of controlling strategies are developmental extensions of the two subcategories of disorganized infant attachment. Cross-sectional studies have reported that both controlling strategies are associated with children's externalizing symptoms (Greenberg, Speltz, DeKlyen, & Endriga, 1991; Moss, Parent, Gosselin, Rousseau, & St-Laurent, 1996; Moss, Rousseau, Parent, St-Laurent, & Saintonge, 1998; Solomon, George, & De Jong, 1995; Speltz, Greenberg, & DeKlyen, 1990). In adolescence, preliminary evidence suggests that behavioral disorders and cognitive distortions are related to controlling behaviors with mothers and disorganized behaviors with fathers (Hilburn-Cobb, 2004).

IWMs of self and others provide the basis for expectations of others and guide responses, thus affecting individual and interpersonal outcomes. Consistent with the idea that emotional abuse negatively impacts IWMs and the ability to regulate affect, research suggests that emotional abuse places children at risk for poor self-concept and disorders of emotional regulation and impulse control. For example, studies with school-age children and adolescents indicate that emotional abuse is associated with low self-esteem and high levels of aggression (see Dodge Reyome et al., in press; Herrenkohl, Egolf, & Herrenkohl, 1997), depression (see Dodge Reyome et al., in press; Kaufman, 1991; Riggs & Kaminski, 2010), depressive attributional style (Cerezo & Frias, 1994), delinquency (Vissing, Straus, Gelles, & Harrop, 1991), emotional instability, and externalizing and internalizing problems (see Dodge Reyome et al., in press; Riggs & Kaminski, 2010; Wenar & Kerig, 2000).

As suggested by evidence linking emotional abuse to children's interpersonal problems with peers (see Taussig & Culhane, 2010; Vissing et al., 1991), the proposed model assumes that the attachment insecurity resulting from emotionally abusive parenting also contributes to poor social functioning. It is in the context of early attachment relationships that children begin to develop the skills needed to build future social relationships, such as self-awareness, empathy, negotiation, and conflict resolution. Across various developmental stages, longitudinal research suggests that security of attachment influences many aspects of interpersonal relationships, including effectiveness in peer groups, reciprocity in relationships, empathy, problem solving and conflict resolution, and establishing close and intimate relationships with peers (see Carlson & Sroufe, 1995, for a review; see also Kestenbaum, Farber, & Sroufe, 1989; Suess et al., 1992). Undoubtedly, emotional abuse in the attachment relationship substantially increases the probability of developing insecure attachment, which is empirically linked to low empathy and reciprocity, hostility or aggression and impulsivity, exploitation or ridicule by peers, social withdrawal or exclusion from group activities, and general patterns of unrelatedness and isolation or complete fusion and dependence where intimacy was achieved at the expense of autonomy (Elicker, Englund, & Sroufe, 1992; Erickson, Egeland, & Sroufe, 1985; Grossmann & Grossmann, 1991; Lewis, Feiring, McGuffog, & Jaskir, 1984; Lyons-Ruth et al., 1993; Renken, Egeland, Marvinney, Sroufe, & Mangelsdorf, 1989; Sroufe, Carlson, & Shulman, 1993; Sroufe & Fleeson, 1986; Troy & Sroufe, 1987; Urban, Carlson, Egeland, & Sroufe, 1991).

ADULT DEVELOPMENT AND FUNCTIONING

Childhood emotional abuse continues to influence individual functioning in adulthood. In retrospective studies, adults who acknowledged emotional abuse in childhood reported low self-esteem, interpersonal sensitivity, hostility, and aggression, as well as symptoms of depression, dissociation, suicidality, and somatization (Bifulco, Moran, Baines, Bunn, & Stanford, 2002; Briere & Runtz, 1988, 1990; Ferguson & Dacey, 1997; Gross & Keller, 1992; Morimoto & Sharma, 2004; Mullen et al., 1996; Nicholas & Bieber, 1996; Spertus, Yehuda, Wong, Halligan, & Seremetis, 2003; Stone, 1993). Moreover, evidence indicates that childhood emotional abuse is significantly related to poor interpersonal skills and relationship dysfunction in adulthood (see Berzenski & Yates, in press; Carbone, 2010; Davis, Petretic-Jackson, & Ting, 2001; Dodge Reyome, in press; Dodge Reyome et al., in press; Messman-Moore & Coates, 2007; Paradis & Boucher, in press; Riggs & Kaminski, this 2010; Varia & Abidin, 1999). The theoretical model presented in Figure 1 proposes that these negative outcomes are largely due to the deleterious impact of emotional abuse on the emergent attachment system, leading to emotional dysregulation, negative IWMs, cognitive biases and distortions, maladaptive coping strategies, and insecure adult attachment style. The model further suggests that all of these factors are likely mediators between early childhood emotional abuse and mental health, which in turn might mediate their associations with romantic relationship quality (DiLillo, Lewis, & Di Loreto-Colgan, 2007; Perry, DiLillo, & Peugh, 2007).

The following two sections review the relevant correlates of adult attachment classifications, with a special emphasis on coping patterns and mental health, then explore the potential impact of childhood emotional abuse on romantic relationship functioning.

Adult Attachment, Coping, and Mental Health

In the late 1980s, two different lines of adult attachment research emerged distinguished by conceptual and methodological differences (see Riggs et al., 2007, for a review). The developmental line of adult attachment research focuses on early childhood experience with parents and its impact on caregiving and infant attachment behavior, and it has generally employed the AAI (George et al., 1985) to assess adults' current mental representations with respect to early parent–child attachments. The social or personality line of adult attachment research studied adult relationships with romantic partners, which are assumed to be outgrowths of early attachment bonds, and typically measures adult romantic attachment using self-report instruments assumed to assess consciously held attitudes regarding close relationships (Bartholomew, 1997; Simpson & Rholes, 2002). Both lines of research identify adult attachment classifications analogous to the infant attachment patterns described in earlier research (Ainsworth et al., 1978; Crittenden, 1985; Main & Solomon, 1986) and are relevant to the proposed model—the latter in association with romantic relationship functioning and the former in relation to the potential for intergenerational transmission of emotionally abusive parenting behaviors. Consequently, both literatures are reviewed here and both forms of adult attachment (self-reported romantic attachment vs. AAI current representations of parent–child attachment) are included in Table 1 and the model depicted in Figure 1.

Conceptually, there are obvious similarities between parent–child attachment and adult romantic attachment, but there are also important differences. Both types of attachment bonds consist of four defining features: secure base, proximity maintenance, safe haven, and separation distress (Hazan & Zeifman, 1999). However, adult romantic relationships generally involve three systems: the attachment system, the caregiving system, and the sexual system (Ainsworth, 1989; Shaver, Hazan, & Bradshaw, 1988). Whereas infant–caregiver attachment is predominately asymmetrical in terms of caregiving, which is exclusively the adult's role, adult romantic attachment is bidirectional and reciprocal because each partner uses the other as a source of security and also serves as a provider of security. According to Hazan and Zeifman (1999), the two types of attachment bonds also differ in terms of distinct motivations for physical contact and evolutionary function; that is, infants seek proximity to reduce distress and promote safety and survival, whereas adults seek proximity initially based on sexual attraction and the propagation of the species, and later for mutual comfort and protection.

Bartholomew (1990; Bartholomew & Horowitz, 1991) theorized that IWMs of self and others formed in childhood are related to the degree of abandonment anxiety, interpersonal avoidance, or both that individuals experience throughout their lives. Having established trust and open communication in past relationships, individuals classified as secure experience low levels of attachment anxiety and avoidance and are likely to remain open and flexible in their interpretation of and response to new information. Consistent with this conceptualization, Main et al. (1985) hypothesized that language provides the means to organize experiences in the form of a coherent life narrative, or secure working model of attachment, which meaningfully integrates self-/other-awareness and contributes to ongoing self-interpretation. In interviews using the AAI, secure attachment manifests in coherent, autonomous, and cooperative discourse regarding childhood attachment experiences and the ability to provide an integrated, credible account of early experiences and their meaning (Main & Goldwyn, 1998).

When the attachment system is activated after a threat is perceived, the positive mindset of secure individuals influences the adaptive mobilization of internal resources and social support during the stress and coping process (Mikulincer & Shaver, 2003). Consequently, a secure attachment organization with positive models of self and others should act as a buffer against maladaptive responses to stress, allowing individuals to pursue and effectively utilize support from friends, family, or mental health practitioners (Riggs & Jacobvitz, 2002). Research findings generally suggest that secure individuals perceive stressors as less threatening, employ more constructive coping methods, and experience higher self-efficacy about coping (see Mikulincer & Florian, 1998, for a review). As a result, secure individuals are less likely to show symptoms of emotional disturbance (e.g., Kobak & Sceery, 1988; Riggs & Jacobvitz, 2002) and are more likely to demonstrate effective coping strategies, such as a healthy degree of self-disclosure and help-seeking (Lopez, Melendez, Sauer, Berger, & Wyssmann, 1998; Mikulincer & Nachshon, 1991; Riggs, Jacobvitz, & Hazen, 2002). Researchers have also reported that secure attachment patterns in adults are associated with personality traits indicative of self-confidence, self-acceptance and self-esteem, identity and integration, psychological well-being and resiliency, empathy, agreeableness, warmth, intimacy and balance in friendships, extroversion, and engagement with the social world (e.g., Bartholomew & Horowitz, 1991; Benoit, Zeanah, & Barton, 1989; Diehl, Elnick, Bourbeau, & Labouvie-Vief, 1998; Onishi, Gjerde, & Block, 2001; Shaver & Brennan, 1992; Treboux, Crowell, & Colon-Downs, 1992).

In contrast, theory and research suggest that insecure individuals are at risk for the development of interpersonal and emotional problems due to significant interference with cognitive or affective aspects of mental representations, which limits their ability to respond flexibly in unfavorable situations (Carlson & Sroufe, 1995). Cognitive distortions triggered by present-day events resembling earlier anxiety-provoking interactions may promote the formation of multiple models, which are inflexible and fairly impermeable to new information (Bowlby, 1980, 1988). Among individuals who were emotionally abused as children, significant life stressors can stimulate high levels of anxious arousal, resulting in an escalation of defenses, maladaptive behaviors, vulnerability to cognitive disorganization and the formation of dissociated contradictory mental models, and ultimately an emotional disorder. Theoretically, the particular manifestation of emotional and behavioral disturbance will depend to a large extent on the predominant attachment strategy previously adopted by the individual.

Among preoccupied individuals who have experienced inconsistent, controlling, or role-reversing parenting, negative beliefs about the self engender anxiety regarding abandonment, but generally positive views of others favor help-seeking (Bartholomew, 1990). In stressful circumstances, uncertainty about the responsiveness of the attachment figure increases anxiety levels and sustains the activity of the attachment system, leading to emotion-focused coping strategies (Mikulincer & Shaver, 2003). Consequently, preoccupied individuals appear to employ a hyperactivating style, whereby they exaggerate emotions and become overinvolved in the availability (or lack thereof) of others (Dozier, Stovall, & Albus, 1999), which might manifest itself in AAI discourse as passive dependence, confusion, or anger toward parental attachment figures (Main & Goldwyn, 1998). Although individuals with preoccupied attachment style might seek social support when threatened, they can exaggerate the danger and demand assistance with very little justification (i.e., their reaction is out of proportion to the stimulus) or exhibit clingy overdependence and ineptitude. Studies have linked AAI preoccupied attachment to increased psychological distress, a high incidence of mood disturbance and anxiety symptoms, and borderline personality disorder (Cole-Detke & Kobak, 1996; Fonagy et al., 1996; Kobak & Sceery, 1988; Patrick, Hobson, Castle, Howard, & Maughan, 1994; Pianta, Egeland, & Adam, 1996; Rosenstein & Horowitz, 1996). Self-reported preoccupied attachment has been empirically associated with negative self-view, high neuroticism, low self-control and tolerance, interpersonal dependence and reliance, as well as histrionic, dependent, and borderline personality traits (Allen, Coyne, & Huntoon, 1998; Bartholomew & Horowitz, 1991; Brennan & Shaver, 1998; Collins & Read, 1990; Diehl et al., 1998; Onishi et al., 2001; Shaver & Brennan, 1992).

Individuals with dismissing attachment strategies are likely to have childhood histories of avoidant attachment marked by parental rejection. As a result, they develop an intra- and interpersonal strategy intended to deactivate or inhibit natural attachment responses with the goals of avoiding negative emotional states and achieving distance, control, and independence (Shaver & Mikulincer, 2002). To maintain IWMs of the self as invulnerable and others as untrustworthy or weak, dismissing individuals tend to use avoidant coping strategies involving denial, externalization, detachment, withdrawal, perfectionism, anger, and possibly narcissism (Bowlby, 1979; Carlson & Sroufe, 1995; Crittenden, 1995; Dozier et al., 1999; Rosenstein & Horowitz, 1996). When threatened, people with dismissing attachment might experience distress and anxiety at a physiological level, but fail to consciously acknowledge these feelings, instead denying the impact of stressors and withdrawing from others to preserve their self-reliance and inhibit any distress-related emotions (Mikulincer & Florian, 1998; Mikulincer & Shaver, 2003; Simpson, Rholes, & Nelligan, 1992). Researchers have consistently reported that the dismissing category is associated with hostility, interpersonal avoidance, loneliness, distrust, low emotional expressiveness, low agreeableness, weak ego resiliency, low levels of self-disclosure and intimacy, and interpersonal difficulty at work (Bartholomew & Horowitz, 1991; N. Collins & Read, 1990; Hazan & Shaver, 1987, 1990; Kobak & Sceery, 1988; Onishi et al., 2001; Shaver & Brennan, 1992). On the AAI, dismissing attachment is associated with a lack of memory for childhood events, and idealization or derogation of attachment figures. With respect to mental disorders, recent studies have provided empirical support linking the AAI dismissing classification to conduct disorder, antisocial personality or criminality, substance abuse, and bipolar disorder in clinical populations (e.g., Allen, Hauser, & Borman-Spurrell, 1996; Cole-Detke & Kobak, 1996; Fonagy et al., 1996; Rosenstein & Horowitz, 1996; Tyrell & Dozier, 1997). Studies utilizing self-report instruments have found that dismissing attachment is associated with somatization and repressive tendencies (Mikulincer, Florian, & Weller, 1993; Onishi et al., 2001).

In the developmental literature utilizing the AAI, a fourth classification is the unresolved category, which parallels and is associated with having an infant classified as disorganized (van IJzendoorn, Schuengel, & Bakermans-Kranenburg, 1999). Unresolved adults typically demonstrate a predominant secure, dismissing, or preoccupied strategy, but by definition, have experienced either a traumatic loss or physical or sexual abuse, which is unintegrated and contributes to lapses in discourse or reasoning during discussions of the trauma (Main & Goldwyn, 1998). The unresolved classification has been empirically linked to emotional distress and substance abuse, psychiatric hospitalization, suicidal ideation, dissociative disorders, posttraumatic stress disorder (PTSD), and borderline and schizotypal personality disorders (Adam, Sheldon-Keller, & West, 1996; Alexander, 1992; Allen et al., 1996; Dozier et al., 1999; Fonagy et al., 1996; Fonagy et al., 1995; Patrick et al., 1994; Riggs & Jacobvitz, 2002; Riggs et al., 2007; Stovall-McClough & Cloitre, 2006; van IJzendoorn & Bakermans-Kranenburg, 1996).

Given that disorganized children might be at greater risk for subsequent loss, trauma, or both (Lyons-Ruth et al., 2004), the theoretical model in Figure 1 suggests that early emotional abuse might contribute indirectly to a lack of resolution of these experiences on the AAI in adulthood. Further, the coding of lapses in reasoning and discourse, which are the hallmark of the AAI unresolved classification, might tap into dissociative mechanisms (Riggs et al., 2007), which have been found to be associated with early emotional abuse (Briere & Runtz, 1988; Ferguson & Dacey, 1997). However, a fifth AAI category called cannot classify is sometimes found in high-risk samples and is associated with a history of psychiatric disorder, marital violence, PTSD symptoms, and sexual or physical abuse (Allen et al., 1996; Holtzworth-Munroe, Stuart, & Hutchinson, 1997; Riggs et al., 2007; Stalker & Davies, 1995). The cannot classify category is characterized by an unusual mixture of secure, preoccupied, and dismissing features and represents a "global breakdown in the organization and maintenance of a singular [attachment] strategy" (Hesse, 1996, p. 4). Although further clarification and refinement of this category is needed, the combination of conflicting attachment strategies associated with the cannot classify category is reminiscent of the hostile-self-referential parenting profile and infant disorganized-avoid-resist pattern, suggesting that emotionally abused children might be at risk for this type of global breakdown in the adult attachment system. Based on empirical associations between parents' AAI attachment classifications and their infants' attachment patterns (van IJzendoorn, 1995), the model presented in Figure 1 proposes that insecure states of mind regarding childhood attachment experiences, especially unresolved and cannot classify states, represent a crucial link connecting adult attachment to emotionally abusive parenting, thus perpetuating the cycle of emotional abuse.

In the social and personality literature, a fourth self-report attachment category labeled fearful is characterized by both negative self and others models (Bartholomew, 1990). This attachment pattern is prevalent among adults reporting a childhood history of physical or sexual trauma (Alexander, 1993; Riggs et al., 2007; Shaver & Clark, 1994) and can also characterize survivors of severe emotional abuse. Simpson and Rholes (2002) theorized that fearful individuals are unable to determine the viability of seeking help from a romantic attachment figure and consequently experience strong internal conflicts that lead to behavioral and emotional disruption. As a result, like disorganized infants and parents with a hostile caregiving profile, fearful adults can exhibit a mixture of preoccupied and dismissing behaviors in their close relationships. These chaotic coping strategies might generate a confusing array of approach and avoidance behaviors (Simpson & Rholes, 2002) or might cause fearful individuals overwhelmed by stress to completely shut down, refuse to take action, and withdraw (Bartholomew & Horowitz, 1991). Similar to preoccupied attachment, fearful individuals lack self-worth but desire and ruminate about close relationships; like dismissing attachment, they distrust others, causing them to avoid intimacy for fear of being hurt.

Not surprisingly, empirical findings suggest that the fearful style is associated with the poorest adjustment of the four self-report prototypes. Studies have documented strong statistical relationships between the fearful style and a variety of maladaptive personality traits, such as distrustful interpersonal distance, anxious self-preoccupation, hostility, and low levels of the following: self-disclosure, intimacy, reliance on others, self-confidence, assertiveness, sociability, empathy, responsibility, and sense of well-being or self-worth (Bartholomew & Horowitz, 1991; Diehl et al., 1998; Onishi et al., 2001). Theoretical predictions that contradictory mental models of self and others contribute to psychopathological symptoms are supported by significant associations between the fearful style and neurotic defenses, depression, anxiety expressed in body symptoms, substance abuse, and dissociation, as well as paranoid, schizoid, schizotypal, avoidant, self-defeating, borderline, narcissistic, and obsessive-compulsive personality traits (Anderson & Alexander, 1996; Brennan & Shaver, 1995, 1998; Brennan, Shaver, & Tobey, 1991; Carnelley, Pietromonaco, & Jaffe, 1994; Diehl et al., 1998; Levy, Meehan, Weber, Reynosa, & Clarkin, 2005; Onishi et al., 2001; Riggs et al., 2007).

Impact of Emotional Abuse on Romantic Relationships

By interfering with the development and functioning of the attachment system, early maltreatment by parents creates deficits in areas of interpersonal functioning, which contribute to poor romantic relationship functioning and marital dissatisfaction (Carbone, 2010; Davis et al., 2001; DiLillo, 2001; DiLillo et al., 2007; Dodge Reyome, in press; Dodge Reyome et al., in press; Paradis & Boucher, in press; Perry et al., 2007). Although there is a small, but growing body of literature on the impact of childhood emotional abuse on adult romantic relationships, and a rather large body of literature on the links between adult attachment style and romantic relationships, relatively little work has been done to integrate these literatures. Other than one study reporting that nonclinical adults who acknowledged childhood emotional abuse were more likely to endorse dismissing or preoccupied attachment styles (Varia & Abidin, 1999), research on direct associations between early emotional abuse and adult attachment is lacking (see Riggs & Kaminski, 2010). Consequently, the following discussion considers preliminary work on childhood emotional abuse and adult relationships, but primarily concentrates on reviewing attachment theory and research that supports the proposed developmental model illustrated in Figure 1.

Although longitudinal evidence has recently emerged linking infant attachment classification to emotional expression and conflict resolution behavior with romantic partners in early adulthood (Roisman, Collins, Sroufe, & Egeland, 2005; Simpson, Collins, Tran, & Haydon, 2007), the bulk of the relevant literature focuses on links between adult attachment and various aspects of romantic relationships. At a general level, there is ample and consistent evidence that compared to insecure attachment, secure adult attachment is related to better marital functioning and satisfaction (e.g., Banse, 2004; Cohn, Cowan, Cowan, & Pearson, 1992; Eiden, Teti, & Corns, 1995; Fuller & Fincham, 1995), as well as healthier emotional regulation and less withdrawal during marital interactions (Paley, Cox, Burchinal, & Payne, 1999). More focused research has demonstrated that adult attachment style is significantly associated with fundamental components of romantic relationships involving multiple behavioral systems that interact to influence dyadic functioning and satisfaction, including the capacity for intimacy, partner caretaking and support, sexual behavior, conflict management, and relational aggression (Collins & Read, 1990; Dutton, Saunders, Starzomski, & Bartholomew, 1994; Senchak & Leonard, 1992; Shi, 2003; Simpson, 1990; Simpson, Rholes, & Phillips, 1996; Simpson, Winterheld, Rholes, & Orina, 2007; Wekerle & Wolfe, 1998). The component features of romantic relationships that are most likely to characterize the relationships of adults with different attachment styles are discussed next and summarized in Table 2.

Intimacy

Retrospective research findings suggest that early emotional abuse impairs the ability to develop intimacy with others later in life (Carbone, 2010; Davis et al., 2001). According to Collins and Sroufe (1999), to achieve intimacy a person must be (a) oriented to value and seek closeness, (b) able to tolerate intense emotions that are inherently involved in close relationships, and (c) capable of self-disclosure, reciprocity, and sensitivity to and concern for others' feelings and well-being. Theoretically, early caregiving relationships contribute to the capacity for intimacy by providing the initial context for learning reciprocity and empathy and also via their influence on IWMs that guide relationship expectations and the development of self-worth and self-efficacy (Collins & Sroufe, 1999). Building on previous attachment experiences, as children venture outside the home, the capacity for intimacy evolves slowly through a series of transformations in peer interactions.

Secure children clearly have an advantage in this developmental sequence because they have developed the social competence and skills that will help them succeed in interpersonal relationships at each developmental stage. For example, research indicates that secure infants later display more empathy than insecure infants (Elicker et al., 1992; Kestenbaum et al., 1989; Sroufe, 1983), and older secure children are more likely to demonstrate the ability to communicate, respond empathically, and resolve conflict (see Collins & Sroufe, 1999, for review; see also Kerns, 1994). Other findings suggest that secure adolescents are more popular with their peers, demonstrate the highest mastery of social skills, have higher self-esteem, and are more oriented toward emotional depth that comes with romantic involvement (see Collins & Sroufe, 1999, for review). As adults, because they tend to have positive cognitions about relational events (e.g., arguments)

TABLE 2 The Adult Attachment System and Romantic Relationship Components

Components	Secure Attachment	Insecure Attachment		
		Preoccupied (High Anxiety)	Fearful (High Anxiety and Avoidance)	Dismissing (High Avoidance)
Intimacy	• Value intimacy, closeness • Balance of intimacy and autonomy • Self-disclosure, reciprocity • Tolerates intense emotions	• Desire intimacy, but anxious regarding abandonment • Enmeshment, dependency • Overdisclosure • Exaggerated emotions (e.g., jealousy)	• Desire but fear of intimacy • Variable fusion and distance • Hypersensitive to rejection • Low disclosure • Unable to tolerate intense emotion	• Distrust, avoid intimacy • Disengagement, compulsive self-reliance • Low disclosure; blame others • Inhibition of emotions, withdrawal
Care				
Careseeking	• Seek support when stressed • Perceive support as helpful	• Excessive seeking of care and reassurance • Feel unlovable, unworthy • Negative support strategies	• Approach/avoidance: Want care, but fear being hurt • Perceive support as harmful • Negative support strategies	• Unlikely to seek support • Perceive support as unhelpful, noncaring
Caregiving	• Availability • Act as secure base • Openness and flexibility • Attunement and responsivity	• Compulsive caregiving • Low reciprocity • Low responsiveness	• Controlling style • Contradictory caregiving: Rejecting, smothering	• Instrumental care • Discomfort and rejection of partner's attachment needs

(Continued)

TABLE 2 *(Continued)*

Components	Secure Attachment	Insecure Attachment		
		Preoccupied (High Anxiety)	Fearful (High Anxiety and Avoidance)	Dismissing (High Avoidance)
Sex	• Later onset • Enjoy physical contact • Prefer normative behaviors • Unlikely to have sex outside of relationship	• Earlier onset with goal of gaining acceptance • More willing to engage in risky sexual behavior • Use sex to seek care	• May seek sex then abruptly withdraw • Averse to intimate touch • Strong negative emotions after sex	• Earlier onset with goal of increasing status and prestige • Unlikely to use touch to express emotion • Casual attitude, promiscuity
Conflict	• Optimistic attributions • Constructive communication • Compromise • Problem-solving strategies	• Self-blame • High obliging, guilt • Hostility, attacking • Controlling: Coercion, threat	• Perceive conflict as threat: Fight–flight activation • Extreme attachment behaviors • Intimacy anger: Anxiety may lead to relational aggression	• Hostile misattributions • Avoidant coping, withdrawal • Low obliging, low compromise • Anger, dominating of partner

and provide optimistic explanations for ambiguous relational events to minimize the potential of negative impact (Collins, 1996; Collins & Feeney, 2004), secure individuals are more likely to achieve high levels of intimacy in their romantic relationships without losing personal autonomy and typically are comfortable with self-disclosure and responsive when their romantic partners self-disclose to them (Collins & Feeney, 2004; Grabill & Kerns, 2000; Mikulincer & Nachshon, 1991).

In contrast, children who experience an emotionally abusive attachment relationship are at a clear disadvantage in interpersonal contexts due to insecure IWMs of attachment and problems with emotional regulation. Abuse-related emotional and cognitive deficits, such as negatively biased information processing or perceptual vigilance, contribute to the development of maladaptive schema and rigid interpersonal beliefs, which repeat throughout life (Carbone, 2010; Rogosch, Cicchetti, & Aber, 1995; Young, Klosko, & Weishaar, 2003). Given the demands for intimacy, trust, and conflict management, romantic relationships are likely to be central contexts for acting out these maladaptive interpersonal schemas (Crawford & Wright, 2007). In particular, experiences of childhood emotional abuse may contribute to schema related to interpersonal disconnection and rejection, which have significant long-term effects because they interfere with the ability to form secure, fulfilling relationships with partners (Messman-Moore & Coates, 2007). Preliminary evidence suggests that early emotional abuse is related to later maladaptive schemas of mistrust and abuse, emotional deprivation, emotional inhibition, self-sacrifice, defectiveness and shame, and abandonment (Cecero, Nelson, & Gillie, 2004; Crawford & Wright, 2007; Dodge Reyome, in press; Dodge Reyome et al., in press; Messman-Moore & Coates, 2007).

Not only do insecure adults experience difficulty managing the powerful emotions activated in close relationships, but the biased interpretations and maladaptive coping strategies associated with negative models of self or others create an imbalance in the search for connection and maintenance of autonomy, which are necessary for a healthy intimate relationship (Blatt & Levy, 2003). For example, preoccupied individuals desire intimacy, but findings suggest they tend to become enmeshed, losing their autonomy in romantic relationships and might self-disclose too easily and too much to gain approval of others (Collins & Feeney, 2004; Shaver, Schachner, & Mikulincer, 2005). A high level of anxiety in relationships and doubt that they can be understood, validated, and loved by a romantic partner (Grabill & Kerns, 2000) can result in relational dissatisfaction, negative attributions for partner's transgressions, and romantic jealousy (Collins, 1996; Collins & Feeney, 2004; Guerrero, 1998). On the other hand, dismissing adults generally avoid intimate relationships and deny need for closeness (Collins & Feeney, 2004; Feeney & Noller, 1990). Research has shown that dismissing individuals use distancing strategies when experiencing relational distress, demonstrate low self-disclosure, and respond negatively when others self-disclose to them (Bradford, Feeney, & Campbell, 2002; Collins & Feeney, 2004; Feeney, 1999; Fraley & Shaver, 1999).

With negative IWMs of both self and others, fearful adults are liable to experience the greatest difficulties in intimate relationships. Initiated in the context of defective or emotionally abusive relationships with parents, high levels of anxiety about abandonment combined with a deep-seated mistrust of others likely engender an intense fear of intimacy (Wood, 2007). Like preoccupied adults, they fervently desire intimacy but feel unworthy of love and are hypersensitive to rejection. Moreover, similar to dismissing adults, fearful individuals view their romantic partners as unreliable and use distancing strategies during times of distress (Brennan, Wu, & Love, 1998; Collins & Feeney, 2004). As a result, their emotional desire for intimacy is usually overridden by their negative cognitions regarding self and others (Collins & Feeney, 2004). If fearful adults do enter into an intimate relationship, theory suggests that emotionally abused individuals whose history is marked by disorganized attachment in infancy and controlling attachment strategies in childhood might demonstrate a controlling and overdominating interpersonal style, which could prompt jealous rages and attempts to isolate romantic partners. In addition, dissociated mental models triggered by painful relational events reminiscent of earlier attachment experiences might initiate the fight-or-flight response, engendering paradoxical approach-avoidance behaviors that confuse and bewilder partners, one minute appearing madly in love and desiring complete enmeshment and the next minute disconnecting from and disparaging the very same partner who was adored moments before.

Caretaking and care-seeking

Relationships with peers and romantic partners are optimally reciprocal, with each partner giving and taking in a balanced fashion. Because they have received inadequate and abusive care from parents, emotionally abused children are likely to develop a warped conception of what a loving and caring relationship entails (see Carbone, 2010; Dodge Reyome et al., in press). On one side of the caregiving relationship is the ability to seek and accept care from others. Research indicates that secure adults are willing to ask their romantic partners for both emotional and instrumental support and believe the caretaking behaviors of their partners are motivated by altruistic rather than selfish concerns (Collins & Feeney, 2004; Knobloch, Solomon, & Cruz, 2001). In contrast, empirical findings suggest that insecure attachment is characterized by either extreme of help-seeking, with dismissing individuals being unlikely to seek support or ineffective in their efforts to do so (Collins & Feeney, 2000; Kunce & Shaver, 1994), and preoccupied individuals demonstrating excessive reassurance seeking (Collins & Feeney, 2004; Shaver et al., 2005). Among preoccupied adults, early strategies of heightening attachment behavior, although adaptive for the purpose of maintaining proximity to the attachment figure in childhood, could become maladaptive at older ages when immature dependency and clinging designed to increase care from others interferes with autonomous exploration and the development of self-efficacy. Simpson and Rholes (2002) theorized that fearful adults are unable to determine the viability of support seeking and consequently experience strong internal conflicts. Contradictory approach-avoidance tendencies might manifest in aborted or disguised bids for care and comfort from relationship partners. Although receipt of a partner's caregiving is usually related to relationship satisfaction (Carnelley, Pietromonaco, & Jaffe, 1996), consistent with previous research indicating that avoidant children tend to interpret the behavior of others more negatively (Suess et al., 1992), Collins and Feeney (2004) found that emerging adults who were dismissing tended to interpret their partners' support as unhelpful and noncaring, whereas fearful participants were likely to view their partners' support attempts as hurtful.

On the flip side, the ability to provide care to others in part develops from the experience of being cared for by an attachment figure. Emotionally abusive parents model "care" to their children in atypical and unacceptable ways, potentially leaving them with a distorted understanding of appropriate caregiving. Cassidy (2000) suggested that "giving care" in adult partnerships involves (a) being available in times of trouble, (b) serving as a secure base and being comfortable with a partner's exploration, (c) demonstrating openness and flexibility, and (d) recognizing when a person needs care (i.e., sensitive attunement) and subsequently providing love, acceptance, and respect (i.e., responsivity). The comfort level and ability to effectively provide these things to partners is related to adult attachment style. Research has shown that secure adults are more likely to provide care and support to their romantic partners (Carnelley et al., 1996; J. Feeney, 1996; Simpson, Rholes, Orina, & Grich, 2002), whereas insecure adults are less likely to be sensitive or supportive to their partners and more likely to be controlling (Feeney & Collins, 2001; Kunce & Shaver, 1994; Simpson et al., 2002). In addition, a high level of attachment avoidance (dismissing and fearful styles) is related to low compulsive caregiving (defensive behavior involving caring for others and prioritizing their needs while simultaneously rejecting care from others), whereas a high level of attachment anxiety (preoccupied and fearful styles) has been linked to poor overall caregiving, characterized by less reciprocity, low responsiveness, negative support strategies, or high levels of compulsive caregiving (Brennan, Wu, et al., 1998; Collins & Feeney, 2000; Feeney & Collins, 2001; Kunce & Shaver, 1994). Fearful adults, in particular, might display compulsive caregiving behaviors to cope with their fears and to compensate for a lack of intimate contact with their romantic partner (Collins & Feeney, 2004) or conversely demonstrate overly controlling and punitive behaviors designed to prevent the feared abandonment by the partner.

Sexual behavior

Early maltreatment has been identified as a risk factor for sexual problems in adulthood (Briere & Runtz, 1990; DiLillo et al., 2007; Mullen et al., 1996; Zurbriggen et al., in press). In particular, emotional abuse by a male parent is especially deleterious to female adult sexuality (Mullen et al., 1996). Despite being identified as one of three key behavioral systems involved in romantic relationships, surprisingly little research has been published about the links between adult attachment organization and the sexual system. However, the available research suggests that secure individuals are likely to become sexually active at later ages, enjoy physical contact that is both intimate and sexual with their partners, prefer "normative" sexual behaviors, experience positive emotions after sexual intercourse, and are unlikely to have sex outside their primary relationships (Brennan, Clark, & Shaver, 1998; Feeney, 1999). Contrariwise, insecure attachment is associated with an earlier age of onset and sexual involvement without commitment (Collins & Sroufe, 1999). Schachner and Shaver (2004) hypothesized that early sexual involvement for adolescents high in attachment avoidance might be motivated by the desire to increase one's status and prestige, whereas those with high levels of attachment anxiety might be motivated to engage in early sexual relations to reduce insecurity and foster intense intimacy lacking in other attachment relationships. Research suggests that dismissing individuals are not likely to use touch to express emotions but endorse more casual attitudes toward sex, including promiscuity, "one-night stands," extra-relationship sex, and pleasurable sex without love (Brennan & Shaver, 1995; Brennan, Wu, et al., 1998; Collins & Feeney, 2004; Feeney, 1999; Feeney, Noller, & Patty, 1993; Hazan & Zeifman, 1994). Preoccupied individuals may be less discriminate about their sexual partners, more willing to engage in risky sexual behavior, and more likely to use sex to seek care and satisfy their needs for closeness and acceptance (Brennan, Wu, et al., 1998; Collins & Feeney, 2004). Findings also suggest that fearful individuals might be averse to intimate touch and experience strong negative emotions after sexual intercourse (Brennan, Wu, et al., 1998). Because fearful adults experience a high level of ambivalence regarding romantic relationships, both craving and fearing intimacy, they might actively seek out sexual relationships but then in response to overwhelming anxiety abruptly withdraw and end contact with the partner to protect themselves from potential pain and rejection.

Conflict resolution and relational aggression

Given the varied coping strategies, it should not be surprising that different attachment styles are associated with distinct conflict resolution approaches in close relationships. Research has demonstrated that during relationship conflict, secure individuals are more likely than insecure individuals to use problem-solving strategies, integrating and compromising behaviors, self-disclosure, mutual discussion, and constructive communication (Carnelley et al., 1994; Corcoran & Mallinckrodt, 2000; J. Feeney, 1994; J. Feeney, Noller, & Callan, 1994; Mikulincer & Nachshon, 1991; Pistole, 1989, 1993). Secure adults are also less likely than insecure adults to engage in withdrawal and verbal aggression (Creasey, Kershaw, & Boston, 1999; Senchak & Leonard, 1992).

In contrast, because insecure individuals suffer from social information processing deficits (e.g., failure to listen carefully, not validating partner's positive messages) related to negative expectations derived from IWMs, they may frequently misinterpret their partners' verbal and nonverbal messages (Creasey et al., 1999). Early maltreatment theoretically contributes to an understanding of close relationships as involving greater conflict and could create a predisposition to interpret even benign or neutral environmental cues as threats, which can then lead to intense emotional responses, distorted perceptions and interpretations of others' behavior, and subsequent preemptive retaliatory behaviors (Bugental, 1993). Consistent with this idea, several studies have demonstrated associations between insecure attachment and attacking or dominating and controlling behaviors, as well as fewer compromising behaviors during conflict with partners (Feeney & Collins, 2001; Marchand, 2004; Shi, 2003). In addition, research has found that dismissing adults tend to avoid or withdraw from conflict, demonstrate low levels of obliging behavior, and are the least likely to use compromising and integrating behavior (Corcoran & Mallinckrodt, 2000; Creasey et al., 1999; Shi, 2003). Preoccupied attachment, on the other hand, is related to high levels of obliging behavior and feelings of hurt and guilt after arguments (Pistole, 1989; Shi, 2003), but also has been linked to a lack of mutual negotiation, greater hostility, and the use of coercion or pressure, blame, threats, and physical and verbal aggression (Corcoran & Mallinckrodt, 2000; Feeney et al., 1994; Simpson et al., 1996). According to Collins and Feeney (2004), fearful adults are likely to interpret conflicts with romantic partners as relationship threatening. As a result, it is conceivable that they could respond to relational conflict with extreme forms of attachment behavior such as intense anger or threats of self-harm.

It is well documented that victims of child abuse are more likely to demonstrate relational aggression and perpetrate intimate partner violence in adolescence and adulthood (Berzenski & Yates, in press; Dodge Reyome, in press; Fang & Corso, 2007; Riggs & Kaminski, 2010; Wekerle & Wolfe, 1998; Zurbriggen et al., in press). Recent evidence specifically suggests that childhood emotional abuse contributes to higher interpersonal conflict, hostility, aggression, and partner victimization in later life (Crawford & Wright, 2007; Messman-Moore & Coates, 2007; Nicholas & Bieber, 1996; Wekerle et al., 2001). Cicchetti and Toth (1995, 2000) suggested that abuse-related schemas formed in childhood and activated in later intimate relationships place individuals at risk for continued abuse by a partner or for perpetrating abuse on a partner. Insecure attachment creates an inherent risk for relationship problems, but early abuse introduces the expectation of abusive or violent interactions with significant power differentials between the victim and victimizer roles (Cicchetti & Howes, 1991; Crittenden & Ainsworth, 1989; Dodge, Pettit, & Bates, 1997). In particular, IWMs of the self as bad, unworthy, or incapable might create a greater likelihood of tolerating poor treatment by others, whereas IWMs of others as abusive, hostile, or rejecting can decrease the likelihood of considering relational aggression and violence outside the range of normal human experience (Liem & Boudewyn, 1999). Once again, because of negative models of both self and others, fearful adults are likely to be the most vulnerable to highly conflictual and potentially abusive intimate relationships.

Attachment theorists have proposed that IWMs are self-perpetuating and persist because individuals tend to selectively enter relationships or caregiving environments that confirm their beliefs about self and others and for which their learned attachment strategies are most suitable (Bowlby, 1969, 1973; Collins & Feeney, 2004; Collins & Sroufe, 1999). This idea is supported by empirical findings indicating that secure children appear to be more attracted to other children with secure histories, whereas insecure children spend more time in isolation or interacting with adults or other insecure children (Elicker et al., 1992; Sroufe et al., 1993; Urban et al., 1991). In addition, when avoidant children were paired with another insecure child (either avoidant or ambivalent), there was a tendency for victimization to occur (Troy & Sroufe, 1987). Similarly, studies have also reported that secure adults tend to more often become romantically involved with other secure adults, whereas insecure adults more often become involved with other insecure adults (Collins & Read, 1990; Kirkpatrick & Davis, 1994). However, insecure men and women do not tend to pair with partners who share their attachment insecurities, but rather complement those insecurities and confirm their expectations. Pistole (1994) theorized that the common couple combination of dismissing and preoccupied attachment styles might contribute to the development of a negative pursuit-distance pattern when an avoidant partner's discomfort with closeness and distancing strategies trigger the preoccupied partner's fear of abandonment and subsequent frantic pursuit of connection, which in turn actually intensifies the dismissing partner's distancing reaction. Taking into account the notion that individuals internalize the whole relationship and can enact complementary roles (Collins & Sroufe, 1999; Sroufe & Fleeson, 1986), theory and research both suggest that individuals who have been emotionally abused in childhood might unconsciously look for romantic partners whose behaviors match their negative expectations and ultimately repeat the pattern of abuse by either perpetrating abuse on their partner or being victimized by their partner. Preliminary support for this hypothesis emerged in a recent study reporting that female college students who reported psychological aggression in their adult relationships were more likely to demonstrate high levels of attachment anxiety and report a preference for dating men with characteristics common to perpetrators of partner psychological aggression (Zayas & Shoda, 2007).

Dutton et al. (1994) proposed a model of intimate partner violence grounded in attachment theory. Dutton et al. conceptualized *intimacy anger* as a form of protest behavior directed at a romantic partner when a person anticipates separation or abandonment by the partner. In contrast to secure and dismissing adults, who have positive self-models and thus tend not to consciously experience insecurity in relationships, preoccupied and fearful adults have negative self-models that make them chronically anxious about abandonment and rejection, and consequently are likely to experience high levels of anger, jealousy, and emotional instability in relationships, which have been found to be strongly associated with verbal and physical abuse in romantic relationships (Dutton, 1994; Dutton & Starzomski, 1993). Dutton et al. proposed that the fearful classification might be most strongly associated with intimacy anger because the combination of negative IWMs of both self and others would lead to avoidance of intimacy despite an intense desire for closeness, resulting in chronic frustration of attachment needs followed by intense anger. Their findings with a sample of men in treatment for spousal assault supported this hypothesis, showing strong associations of fearful attachment with self-reported anger, jealousy, symptoms of trauma, and borderline personality disorder, as well wives' reports of their husbands' verbal abuse (i.e., dominance and isolation, psychological aggression). Similar, but weaker associations were reported for preoccupied attachment. Dutton et al. speculated that partner relational aggression develops as a consequence of attachment rage and subsequent efforts to dominate or isolate partners might be an attempt to minimize anxiety about abandonment. "The yoked dysphoric modes—anger and anxiety—thus may have a common origin in insecure attachment and operate to generate both abusing and controlling behaviors" (p. 1382).

CONCLUSION

Current theory and research suggest that emotional abuse in early caregiving relationships has a profound impact on the attachment system, which affects individual development at every phase of life and might reach further into the next generation. As depicted in Figure 1, the presented model proposes that childhood emotional abuse initially interferes with the ability to regulate emotions and contributes to insecure attachment characterized by negative IWMs of self, others, or both. In particular, hostile-self-referential parenting is associated with disorganized-avoid-resist infant attachment patterns and possibly later controlling strategies among school-age children and adolescents. These children demonstrate both internalizing and externalizing problems, as well as perceptual biases and social deficits in peer relationships, which interfere with the adaptive development of interpersonal competencies. By adulthood, insecure internal models of attachment comprise multiple maladaptive interpersonal schemas and are manifested in hyperactivating or deactivating coping patterns that create a vulnerability for emotional disruption and psychological disorder. For instance, the approach-avoidance paradox experienced by disorganized infants is likely to be repeated in adult attachment relationships that trigger early maladaptive interpersonal schema related to abusive experiences.

Theoretically, early emotional abuse contributes indirectly via these cognitive-affective factors to high levels of attachment anxiety and avoidance, the combination of which produces a fearful romantic attachment style, which is associated with the most severe forms of psychological disturbance and dysfunction in romantic relationships. In addition, adults who were emotionally abused as children might not be able to resolve early experiences of maltreatment from parents and consequently might demonstrate the lapses of reasoning and discourse that characterize unresolved attachment on the AAI. Lack of resolution to trauma, in turn, has been related to dissociation and other serious psychopathology, as well as frightened-frightening or hostile-helpless parenting, both of which are associated with disorganized attachment in the next generation of infants. Thus, the AAI unresolved classification could contribute directly and the self-report fearful attachment style could contribute more indirectly via romantic dysfunction or psychopathology to another cycle of disturbed parenting in a process of intergenerational transmission of emotional abuse.

More research is needed to provide empirical support for the proposed model. Attachment theory might provide a useful theoretical foundation to guide future studies investigating the long-term impact of childhood maltreatment, and to identify the differential effects of emotional abuse versus other types of child abuse and neglect. The recent research on distinct parenting profiles associated with different manifestations of disorganized infant attachment potentially can inform ongoing efforts to define childhood emotional abuse and possibly distinguish it from emotional neglect. Studies are sorely needed to examine connections between early emotional abuse and attachment organization at all levels of development and to clarify how the effects of emotional abuse differ from other forms of maltreatment, particularly in relation to later personality traits, as well as psychological and relational functioning. In particular, research testing the proposed model's pathways of influence might identify mediators or moderators in the relationship between childhood emotional abuse and romantic relationship functioning. Although retrospective studies are informative, confirmation for a true causal model must await data from longitudinal studies following emotionally abused infants and children into adulthood.

On a more positive note, the available evidence indicates that attachment patterns can shift in response to alterations in the environment affecting the caregiving relationship, making flexibility rather than determinism the general rule of attachment development (Erickson et al., 1985; Thompson, 1991). By tracing the developmental sequelae of childhood emotional abuse that culminates in dysfunctional interaction patterns in adult romantic relationships, it might be possible to identify specific areas to focus on for intervention at various stages of development. Fortin and Chamberland (1995) recommended that intervention efforts target (a) the alleviation of socioeconomic stress and provision of better opportunities; (b) reduction of family dysfunction by modifying parents' unrealistic expectations of child behavior, satisfying parents' psychological and social needs, and eliminating maladaptive behavioral patterns within the family; (c) promotion of the development of skills, awareness, and positive self-concept in parents and children; and (d) facilitation of social support from the extended family network, peers, and community members.

Clearly, the best hope for children goes beyond parenting skills training to include broader ecological considerations as well as more in-depth restructuring of parents' IWMs of attachment. Yet, IWMs function largely outside of awareness, and therefore are resistant to change unless a conflict between the model and reality becomes extremely apparent (Bretherton, Ridgeway, & Cassidy, 1990). Only repeated interactions that explicitly highlight a contradiction with established working models, such as those encountered in a secure relationship with an adult partner (Egeland, Jacobvitz, & Sroufe, 1988) or an insightful therapist (Bowlby, 1979; Bretherton, 1990), can provide opportunities for integrating dissociated mental models and fundamentally changing attachment patterns. In addition to intensive individual therapy, adults with a history of emotional abuse who report relationship problems might benefit from couples counseling that takes an attachment-based approach, such as emotion-focused therapy for couples, which has been adapted specifically for work with couples where one or both partners report a history of attachment trauma (Carbone, 2010; Johnson, 2002). Thus, although emotional abuse in childhood can jeopardize the functioning of the attachment system, it does not necessarily condemn someone permanently to unhappy romantic relationships. With appropriate support and intervention, it is possible to overcome this unfortunate historical disadvantage and find happiness and contentment with a loving partner.

REFERENCES

Adam, E. K., Gunnar, M. R., & Tanaka, A. (2004). Adult attachment, parent emotion, and observed parenting behavior: Mediator and moderator models. *Child Development, 75*, 110–122.

Adam, K., Sheldon-Keller, A., & West, M. (1996). Attachment organization and history of suicidal behavior in clinical adolescents. *Journal of Consulting and Clinical Psychology, 64*, 264–272.

Ainsworth, M. (1989). Attachments beyond infancy. *American Psychologist, 44*, 709–716.

Ainsworth, M. D. S., Blehar, M. C., Waters, E., & Wall, S. (1978). *Patterns of attachment: A psychological study of the strange situation.* Oxford, UK: Lawrence Erlbaum Associates.

Alexander, P. (1992). Application of attachment theory to the study of sexual abuse. *Journal of Consulting and Clinical Psychology, 60*, 185–195.

Alexander, P. C. (1993). The differential effects of abuse characteristics and attachment in the prediction of long-term effects of sexual abuse. *Journal of Interpersonal Violence, 9*, 346–362.

Allen, J. A. (2001). *Traumatic relationships and serious mental disorders*. Chichester, UK: Wiley.

Allen, J., Coyne, L., & Huntoon, J. (1998). Complex posttraumatic stress disorder in women from a psychometric perspective. *Journal of Personality Assessment, 70*, 277–298.

Allen, J., Hauser, S., & Borman-Spurrell, E. (1996). Attachment theory as a framework for understanding sequelae of severe adolescent psychopathology: An 11-year follow-up study. *Journal of Consulting and Clinical Psychology, 6*, 254–263.

Allen, J., McElhaney, K., Kuperminc, G., & Jodl, K. (2004). Stability and change in attachment security across adolescence. *Child Development, 75*, 1792–1805.

Anderson, C. L., & Alexander, P. C. (1996). The relationship between attachment and dissociation in adult survivors of incest. *Psychiatry, 59*, 240–254.

Banse, R. (2004). Adult attachment and marital satisfaction: Evidence for dyadic configuration effects. *Journal of Social and Personal Relationships, 21*, 273–282.

Bartholomew, K. (1990). Avoidance of intimacy: An attachment perspective. *Journal of Social and Personal Relationships, 7*, 147–178.

Bartholomew, K. (1997). Adult attachment processes: Individual and couple perspectives. *British Journal of Medical Psychology, 70*, 249–263.

Bartholomew, K., & Horowitz, L. M. (1991). Attachment styles among young adults: A test of four-category model. *Journal of Personality and Social Psychology, 61*, 226–244.

Benoit, D., Zeanah, C., & Barton, M. (1989). Maternal attachment disturbances in failure to thrive. *Infant Mental Health Journal, 10*, 185–202.

Berzenski, S. R., & Yates, T. M. (in press). A developmental process analysis of the contribution of childhood emotional abuse to relationship violence. *Journal of Aggression, Maltreatment and Trauma.*

Bifulco, A., Brown, G., & Harris, T. (1994). Childhood Experience of Care and Abuse (CECA): A retrospective interview measure. *Journal of Child Psychology and Psychiatry, 35*, 1419–1435.

Bifulco, A., Moran, P. J., Baines, R., Bunn, A., & Stanford, K. (2002). Exploring psychological abuse in childhood: II. Association with other abuse and adult clinical depression. *Bulletin of the Menninger Clinic, 66*, 241–258.

Blatt, S. J., & Levy, K. N. (2003). Attachment theory, psychoanalysis, personality development and psychopathology. *Psychoanalytic Inquiry, 23*, 102–150.

Bowlby, J. (1969). *Attachment and loss: Vol. 1. Attachment.* New York: Basic Books

Bowlby, J. (1973). *Attachment and loss: Vol. 2. Separation.* New York: Basic Books.

Bowlby, J. (1979). *The making and breaking of affectional bonds.* New York: Tavistock.

Bowlby, J. (1980). *Attachment and loss: Vol. 3. Loss.* New York: Basic Books.

Bowlby, J. (1982). Attachment and loss: Retrospect and prospect. *American Journal of Orthopsychiatry, 52*, 664–678.

Bowlby, J. (1988). Developmental psychiatry comes of age. *American Journal of Psychiatry, 145*, 1–10.

Bradford, S., Feeney, J., & Campbell, L. (2002). Links between attachment orientations and dispositional and diary-based measures of disclosures in dating couples: A study of actor and partner effects. *Personal Relationships, 9*, 491–506.

Brennan, K. A., Clark, C. L., & Shaver, P. R. (1998). Self-report measurement of adult attachment: An integrative overview. In J. A. Simpson & W. S. Rholes (Eds.), *Attachment theory and close relationships* (pp. 46–76). New York: Guilford.

Brennan, K. A., & Shaver, P. R. (1995). Dimensions of adult attachment, affect regulation, and romantic relationship functioning. *Personality & Social Psychology Bulletin, 21*, 267–283.

Brennan, K. A., & Shaver, P. R. (1998). Attachment styles and personality disorders: Their connections to each other and to parental divorce, parental death, and perceptions of parental caregiving. *Journal of Personality, 66*, 835–878.

Brennan, K. A., Shaver, P. R., & Tobey, A. E. (1991). Attachment styles, gender, and parental problem drinking. *Journal of Social and Personality Relationships, 8*, 451–466.

Brennan, K., Wu, S., & Love, J. (1998). Adult romantic attachment and individual differences in attitudes toward physical contact in the context of adult romantic relationships. In J. A. Simpson & W. S. Rholes (Eds.), *Attachment theory and close relationships* (pp. 394–428). New York: Guilford.

Bretherton, I. (1985). Attachment theory: Retrospect and prospect. In I. Bretherton & E. Waters (Eds.), *Growing points of attachment theory and research* (pp. 66–104). *Monographs of the Society for Research in Child Development, 50*(1–2, Serial No. 129).

Bretherton, I. (1990). Communication patterns, internal working models, and the intergenerational transmission of attachment relationships. *Infant Mental Health Journal, 11*, 237–252.

Bretherton, I. (1993). From dialogue to IWMs: The co-construction of self in relationships. In C. A. Nelson (Ed.), *Minnesota Symposium on Child Psychology: Vol. 26. Memory and affect in development* (pp. 237–263). Hillsdale, NJ: Lawrence Erlbaum Associates.

Bretherton, I., Ridgeway, D., & Cassidy, J. (1990). Assessing internal working models of the attachment relationship: An attachment story completion task for 3-year-olds. In M. T. Greenberg, D. Cicchetti, & E. M. Cummings (Eds.), *Attachment in the preschool years* (pp. 273–308). Chicago: University of Chicago Press.

Briere, J., & Runtz, M. (1988). Multivariate correlates of childhood psychological and physical maltreatment among university women. *Child Abuse & Neglect, 12*, 331–341.

Briere, J., & Runtz, M. (1990). Differential adult symptomatology associated with three types of child abuse histories. *Child Abuse & Neglect, 14*, 257–364.

Bugental, D. (1993). Communication in abusive relationships: Cognitive constructions of interpersonal power. *American Behavioral Scientist, 36*, 288–308.

Carbone, D. J. (2010). Using cognitive therapies to treat unstable attachment patterns in adults with childhood histories of social rejection. *Journal of Aggression, Maltreatment and Trauma, 19*(1), 105–134.

Carlson, E. A., & Sroufe, L. A. (1995). Contributions of attachment theory to developmental psychopathology. In E. Cicchetti & D. J. Cohen (Eds.), *Developmental psychopathology* (Vol. 1, pp. 581–617). New York: Wiley.

Carlson, V., Cicchetti, D., Barnett, D., & Braunwald, K. (1989). Disorganized/disoriented attachment relationships in maltreated infants. *Developmental Psychology, 25*, 525–531.

Carnelley, K., Pietromonaco, P., & Jaffe, K. (1994). Depression, working models of others, and relationship functioning. *Journal of Personality and Social Psychology, 66*, 127–140.

Carnelley, K., Pietromonaco, P., & Jaffe, K. (1996). Attachment, caregiving, and relationship functioning in couples: Effects of self and partner. *Personal Relationships, 3*, 257–277.

Cassidy, J. (1994). Emotion regulation: Influences of attachment relationships. *Monographs of the Society for Research in Child Development, 59*(2), 228–283.

Cassidy, J. (2000). Adult romantic attachments: A developmental perspective on individual differences. *Review of General Psychology, 4*, 111–131.

Cecero, J. J., Nelson, J. D., & Gillie, J. M. (2004). Tools and tenets of schema therapy: Toward the construct validity of the Early Maladaptive Schema Questionnaire–Research version (EMSQ–R). *Clinical Psychology and Psychotherapy, 11*, 344–357.

Cerezo, M. A., & Frias, D. (1994). Emotional and cognitive adjustment in abused children. *Child Abuse & Neglect, 18*, 923–932.

Cicchetti, D., & Howes, P. (1991). Developmental psychopathology in the context of the family: Illustrations from the study of child maltreatment. *Canadian Journal of Behavioural Science/Revue canadienne des sciences du comportement, 23*, 257–281.

Cicchetti, D., & Toth, S. L. (1995). Child maltreatment and attachment organization: Implications for intervention. In S. Goldberg, R. Muir, & J. Kerr (Eds.), *Attachment theory: Social, developmental, and clinical perspectives* (pp. 279–308). Hillsdale, NJ: Analytic Press.

Cicchetti, D., & Toth, S. (2000). Developmental processes in maltreated children. In D. J. Hansen (Ed.), *Nebraska Symposium on Motivation: Vol. 46. Motivation and child maltreatment* (pp. 85–160). Lincoln: University of Nebraska Press.

Cohn, D. A., Cowan, P. A., Cowan, C. P., & Pearson, J. (1992). Mothers' and fathers' working models of childhood attachment relationships, parenting styles, and child behavior. *Development and Psychopathology, 4*, 417–431.

Cole-Detke, H., & Kobak, R. (1996). Attachment processes in eating disorder and depression. *Journal of Consulting and Clinical Psychology, 64*, 282–290.

Collins, N. (1996). Working models of attachment: Implications for explanations, emotion, and behavior. *Journal of Personality and Social Psychology, 71*, 810–832.

Collins, N., & Feeney, B. (2000). A safe haven: An attachment theory perspective on support seeking and caregiving in intimate relationships. *Journal of Personality and Social Psychology, 78*, 1053–1073.

Collins, N., & Feeney, B. (2004). An attachment theory perspective on closeness and intimacy. In D. Mashek & A. Aron (Eds.), *Handbook of closeness and intimacy* (pp. 163–187). Mahwah, NJ: Lawrence Erlbaum Associates.

Collins, N. L., Guichard, A. C., Ford, M. B., & Feeney, B. C. (2004). Working models of attachment: New developments and emerging themes. In W. S. Rholes & J. A. Simpson (Eds.), *Adult attachment: Theory, research, and clinical implications* (pp. 196–239). New York: Guilford.

Collins, N., & Read, S. (1990). Adult attachment relationships, working models, and relationship quality in dating couples. *Journal of Personality and Social Psychology, 58*, 644–683.

Collins, W. A., & Sroufe, L. A. (1999). Capacity for intimate relationships: A developmental construction. In W. Furman, B. B. Brown, & C. Feiring (Eds.), *The development of romantic relationships in adolescence* (pp. 125–147). New York: Cambridge University Press.

Corcoran, K., & Mallinckrodt, B. (2000). Adult attachment, self-efficacy, perspective taking, and conflict resolution. *Journal of Counseling & Development, 78*, 473–483.

Cozzarelli, C., Karafa, J., Collins, N., & Tagler, M (2003). Stability and change in adult attachment styles: Associations with personal vulnerabilities, life events, and global construals of self and others. *Journal of Social and Clinical Psychology, 22*, 315–346.

Crawford, E., & Wright, M. O. (2007). The impact of childhood psychological maltreatment on interpersonal schemas and subsequent experiences of relationship aggression. *Journal of Emotional Abuse, 7*, 93–116.

Creasey, G., Kershaw, K., & Boston, A. (1999). Conflict management with friends and romantic partners: The role of attachment and negative mood regulation expectancies. *Journal of Youth and Adolescence, 28*, 523–543.

Crittenden, P. M. (1985). Maltreated infants: Vulnerability and resiliency. *Journal of Child Psychology and Psychiatry, 26*, 85–96.

Crittenden, P. M. (1995). Attachment and psychopathology. In S. Goldberg, R. Muir, & J. Kerr (Eds.), *Attachment theory: Social, developmental, and clinical perspectives* (pp. 367–406). Hillsdale, NJ: Analytic Press.

Crittenden, P. M., & Ainsworth, M. (1989). Attachment and child abuse. In D. Cicchetti & V. Carlson (Eds.), *Child maltreatment: Theory and research on the causes and consequences of child abuse and neglect* (pp. 432–463). New York: Cambridge University Press.

Davis, J. L., Petretic-Jackson, P. A., & Ting, L. (2001). Intimacy dysfunction and trauma symptomatology: Long-term correlates of different types of child abuse. *Journal of Traumatic Stress, 14*, 63–79.

Diehl, M., Elnick, A., Bourbeau, L., & Labouvie-Vief, G. (1998). Adult attachment styles: Their relations to family context and personality. *Journal of Personality and Social Psychology, 74*, 1656–1669.

DiLillo, D. (2001). Interpersonal functioning among women reporting a history of childhood sexual abuse: Empirical findings and methodological issues. *Clinical Psychology Review, 21*, 553–576.

DiLillo, D., Lewis, T., & Di Loreto-Colgan, A. (2007). Child maltreatment history and subsequent romantic relationships: Exploring a psychological route to dyadic difficulties. *Journal of Aggression, Maltreatment and Trauma, 15*, 19–36.

Dodge, K. A., Pettit, G. S., & Bates, J. E. (1997). How the experience of early physical abuse leads children to become chronically aggressive. In D. Cicchetti & S. Toth (Eds.), *Rochester Symposium on Development Psychopathology: Vol. 8. The effects of trauma on the developmental process* (pp. 263–268). Rochester, NY: University of Rochester Press.

Dodge Reyome, N. (in press). Childhood emotional maltreatment and later intimate relationships: Themes from the empirical literature. *Journal of Aggression, Maltreatment and Trauma.*

Dodge Reyome, N., Ward, K. S., & Witkiewitz, K. (in press). Psychosocial variables as mediators of the relationship between childhood emotional maltreatment, codependency, and self silencing. *Journal of Aggression, Maltreatment and Trauma.*

Dozier, M., Stovall, C., & Albus, K. (1999). Attachment and psychopathology in adulthood. In J. Cassidy & P. Shaver (Eds.), *Handbook of attachment: Theory, research, and clinical applications* (pp. 497–519). New York: Guilford.

Dutton, D. G. (1994). Behavioral and affective correlates of Borderline Personality Organization in wife assaulters. *International Journal of Criminal Justice and Behavior, 17*(3), 26–38.

Dutton, D. G., Saunders, K., Starzomski, A., & Bartholomew, K. A. (1994). Intimacy-anger and insecure attachment as precursors of abuse in intimate relationships. *Journal of Applied Social Psychology, 24*, 1367–1386.

Dutton, D. G., & Starzomski, A. (1993). Perpetrator characteristics associated with women's reports of psychological and physical abuse. *Violence and Victims, 8*, 326–335.

Egeland, B., Jacobvitz, D., & Sroufe, L. A. (1988). Breaking the cycle of abuse. *Child Development, 59*, 1080–1088.

Eiden, R. D., Teti, D. M., & Corns, K. M. (1995). Maternal working models of attachment, marital adjustment, and the parent–child relationship. *Child Development, 66*, 1504–1518.

Elicker, J., Englund, M., & Sroufe, L. A. (1992). Predicting peer competence and peer relationships in childhood from early parent–child relationships. In R. Parke & G. Ladd (Eds.), *Family-peer relationships: Modes of linkage* (pp. 77–106). Hillsdale, NJ: Lawrence Erlbaum Associates.

Erickson, M. F., Egeland, B., & Sroufe, L. A. (1985). The relationship between quality of attachment and behavior problems in preschool in a high-risk sample. In I. Bretherton & E. Waters (Eds.), *Growing points of attachment theory and research* (pp. 147–186). *Monographs of the Society for Research in Child Development, 50*(1–2, Serial No. 209).

Fang, X., & Corso, P. S. (2007). Child maltreatment, youth violence, and intimate partner violence: Developmental relationships. *American Journal of Preventive Medicine, 33*, 281–290.

Feeney, B., & Collins, N. (2001). Predictors of caregiving in adult intimate relationships: An attachment theoretical perspective. *Journal of Personality and Social Psychology, 80*, 972–994.

Feeney, J. (1994). Attachment style, communication patterns and satisfaction across the life cycle of marriage. *Personal Relationships, 1*, 333–348.

Feeney, J. (1996). Attachment, caregiving, and marital satisfaction. *Personal Relationships, 3*, 401–416.

Feeney, J. A. (1999). Adult attachment, emotional control, and marital satisfaction. *Personal Relationships, 6*, 169–185.

Feeney, J. A., & Noller, P. (1990). Attachment style as a predictor of adult romantic relationships. *Journal of Personality and Social Psychology, 58*, 281–291.

Feeney, J., Noller, P., & Callan, V. (1994). Attachment style, communication and satisfaction in the early years of marriage. In K. Bartholomew & D. Perlman (Eds.), *Attachment processes in adulthood* (pp. 269–308). London: Jessica Kingsley.

Feeney, J., Noller, P., & Patty, J. (1993). Adolescents' interactions with the opposite sex: Influence of attachment style and gender. *Journal of Adolescence, 16*, 169–186.

Ferguson, K., & Dacey, C. (1997). Anxiety, depression and dissociation in women health care providers reporting a history of childhood psychological abuse. *Child Abuse & Neglect, 21*, 941–952.

Fonagy, P., Leigh, T., Steele, M., Steele, H., Kennedy, R., Mattoon, G., et al. (1996). The relation of attachment status, psychiatric classification, and response to psychotherapy. *Journal of Consulting and Clinical Psychology, 64*, 22–31.

Fonagy, P., Steele, M., Steele, H., Leigh, T., Kennedy, R., Mattoon, G., et al. (1995). Attachment, the reflective self, and borderline states: The predictive specificity of the Adult Attachment Interview and pathological emotional development. In S. Goldberg, R. Muir, & J. Kerr (Eds.), *Attachment theory: Social, developmental, and clinical perspectives* (pp. 233–277). Hillsdale, NJ: Analytic Press.

Fortin, A., & Chamberland, C. (1995). Preventing the psychological maltreatment of children. *Journal of Interpersonal Violence, 10*, 275–295.

Fraley, R. C., Davis, K. E., & Shaver, P. R. (1998). Dismissing-avoidance and the defensive organization of emotion, cognition, and behavior. In J. A. Simpson & W. S. Rholes (Eds.), *Attachment theory and close relationships* (pp. 249–279). New York: Guilford.

Fraley, R., & Shaver, P. (1999). Loss and bereavement: Attachment theory and recent controversies concerning "grief work" and the nature of detachment. *Handbook of attachment: Theory, research, and clinical applications* (pp. 735–759). New York: Guilford.

Fuller, T. L., & Fincham, F. D. (1995). Attachment style in married couples: Relation to current marital functioning, stability over time, and method of assessment. *Personal Relationships, 2*, 17–34.

George, C., Kaplan, N., & Main, M. (1985). *The Berkeley Adult Attachment Interview*. Unpublished protocol, University of California at Berkeley, Berkeley, CA.

Grabill, C., & Kerns, K. (2000). Attachment style and intimacy in friendships. *Personal Relationships, 7*, 363–378.

Greenberg, M., Speltz, M., DeKlyen, M., & Endriga, M. (1991). Attachment security in preschoolers with and without externalizing behavior problems: A replication. *Development and Psychopathology, 3*, 413–430.

Gross, A. B., & Keller, H. R. (1992). Long-term consequences of childhood physical and psychological maltreatment. *Aggressive Behavior, 18*, 171–185.

Grossmann, K. E., & Grossmann, K. (1991). Attachment quality as an organizer of emotional and behavioral responses in a longitudinal perspective. In C. M. Parkes, J. Stevenson-Hinde, & P. Marris (Eds.), *Attachment across the life cycle* (pp. 93–114). London: Tavistock/Routledge.

Grossmann, K., Grossmann, K., & Waters, E. (2005). *Attachment from infancy to adulthood: The major longitudinal studies*. New York: Guilford.

Guerrero, L. (1998). Attachment-style differences in the experience and expression of romantic jealousy. *Personal Relationships, 5*, 273–291.

Hart, S., Binggeli, N., & Brassard, M. (1997). Evidence for the effects of psychological maltreatment. *Journal of Emotional Abuse, 1*(1), 27–58.

Hart, S. N., Brassard, M. R., Binggeli, N. J., & Davidson, H. A. (2002). Psychological maltreatment. In J. E. B. Myers, L. Berliner, J. Brier, C. T. Hendrix, C. Jenny, & T. A. Reid (Eds.), *The APSAC handbook on child maltreatment* (2nd ed.) (pp. 79–103). Thousand Oaks, CA: Sage.

Hazan, C., & Shaver, P. (1987). Romantic love conceptualized as an attachment process. *Journal of Personality and Social Psychology, 52*, 511–524.

Hazan, C., & Shaver, P. (1990). Love and work: An attachment-theoretical perspective. *Journal of Personality and Social Psychology, 59*, 270–280.

Hazan, C., & Zeifman, D. (1994). Sex and the psychological tether. In K. Bartholomew & D. Perlman (Eds.), *Attachment processes in adulthood* (pp. 151–178). London: Jessica Kingsley.

Hazan, C., & Zeifman, D. (1999). Pair bonds as attachments: Evaluating the evidence. In J. Cassidy & P. Shaver (Eds.), *Handbook of attachment: Theory, research, and clinical applications* (pp. 336–354). New York: Guilford.

Herrenkohl, R., Egolf, B., & Herrenkohl, E. (1997). Preschool antecedents of adolescent assaultive behavior: A longitudinal study. *American Journal of Orthopsychiatry, 67*, 422–432.

Hesse, E. (1996). Discourse, memory, and the Adult Attachment Interview: A note with emphasis on the emerging cannot classify category. *Infant Mental Health Journal, 17*, 4–11.

Hesse, E., & Main, M. (2006). Frightened, threatening, and dissociative parental behavior in low-risk samples: Description, discussion, and interpretations. *Development and Psychopathology, 18*, 309–343.

Hilburn-Cobb, C. (2004). Adolescent psychopathology in terms of multiple behavioral systems: The role of attachment and controlling strategies and frankly disorganized behavior. In L. Atkinson & S. Goldberg (Eds.), *Attachment issues in psychopathology and intervention* (pp. 95–135). Mahwah, NJ: Lawrence Erlbaum Associates.

Holtzworth-Munroe, A., Stuart, G., & Hutchinson, G. (1997). Violent versus nonviolent husbands: Differences in attachment patterns, dependency, and jealousy. *Journal of Family Psychology, 11*, 314–331.

Johnson, S. M. (2002). *Emotionally focused couple therapy with trauma survivors: Strengthening attachment bonds*. New York: Guilford.

Kaufman, J. (1991). Depressive disorders in maltreated children. *Journal of the American Academy of Child & Adolescent Psychiatry, 30*, 257–265.

Kerns, K. (1994). A longitudinal examination of links between mother–child attachment and children's friendships in early childhood. *Journal of Social and Personal Relationships, 11*, 379–381.

Kestenbaum, R., Farber, E., & Sroufe, L. A. (1989). Individual differences in empathy among preschoolers' concurrent and predictive validity. In N. Eisenberg (Ed.), *Empathy and related emotional responses: New directions for child development* (pp. 51–56). San Francisco: Jossey-Bass.

Kirkpatrick, L., & Davis, K. (1994). Attachment style, gender, and relationship stability: A longitudinal analysis. *Journal of Personality and Social Psychology, 66*, 502–512.

Knobloch, L., Solomon, D., & Cruz, M. (2001). The role of relationship development and attachment in the experience of romantic jealousy. *Personal Relationships, 8*, 205–224.

Kobak, R. R., & Sceery, A. (1988). Attachment in later adolescence: Working models, affect regulation, and perceptions of self and others. *Child Development, 59*, 135–146.

Kunce, L. J., & Shaver, P. R. (1994). An attachment-theoretical approach to caregiving in romantic relationships. In K. Bartholomew & D. Perlman (Eds.), *Advances in personal relationships: Vol. 5. Attachment processes in adulthood* (pp. 205–237). London: Jessica Kingsley.

Levy, K. N., Meehan, K. B., Weber, M., Reynosa, J., & Clarkin, J. F. (2005). Attachment and borderline personality disorder: Implications for psychotherapy. *Psychopathology, 38*, 64–74.

Lewis, M., Feiring, C., McGuffog, C., & Jaskir, J. (1984). Predicting psychopathology in six-year-olds from early social relations. *Child Development, 55*, 123–136.

Liem, J. H., & Boudewyn, A. C. (1999). Contextualizing the effects of childhood sexual abuse on adult self- and social functioning: An attachment theory perspective. *Child Abuse & Neglect, 23*, 1141–1157.

Lopez, F., Melendez, M., Sauer, E., Berger, E., & Wyssmann, J. (1998). IWMs, self-reported problems, and help-seeking attitudes among college students. *Journal of Counseling Psychology, 45*, 79–83.

Lyons-Ruth, K. (1996). Attachment relationships among children with aggressive behavior problems: The role of disorganized early attachment patterns. *Journal of Consulting and Clinical Psychology, 64*, 64–73.

Lyons-Ruth, K., Alpern, L., & Repacholi, B. (1993). Disorganized infant attachment classification and maternal psychosocial problems as predictors of hostile-aggressive behavior in the preschool classroom. *Child Development, 64*, 572–585.

Lyons-Ruth, K., Bronfman, E., & Atwood, G. (1999). A relational diathesis model of hostile-helpless states of mind: Expressions in mother–infant interaction. In J. Solomon & C. George (Eds.), *Attachment disorganization* (pp. 33–70). New York: Guilford.

Lyons-Ruth, K., Bronfman, E., & Parsons, E. (1999). Atypical maternal behavior and disorganized infant attachment strategies: Frightened, frightening, or atypical maternal behavior and disorganized infant attachment strategies. In J. Vondra & D. Barnett (Eds.), *Atypical patterns of infant attachment: Theory research, and current directions* (pp. 67–96). *Monographs of the Society for Research in Child Development, 64*(3, Serial No. 258).

Lyons-Ruth, K., Connell, D., Grunebaum, H., & Botein, S. (1990). Infants at social risk: Maternal depression and family support services as mediators of infant development and security of attachment. *Child Development, 61*, 85–98.

Lyons-Ruth, K., Easterbrooks, M. A., & Cibelli, C. D. (1997). Infant attachment strategies, infant mental lag, and maternal depressive symptoms: Predictors of internalizing and externalizing problems at age 7. *Developmental Psychology, 33*, 681–692.

Lyons-Ruth, K., & Jacobvitz, D. (1999). Attachment disorganization: Unresolved loss, relational violence, and lapses in behavioral and intentional strategies. In J. Cassidy & P. R. Shaver (Eds.), *Handbook of attachment theory and research* (pp. 520–554). New York: Guilford.

Lyons-Ruth, K., Melnick, S., Bronfman, E., Sherry, S., & Llanas, L. (2004). Hostile-helpless relational models and disorganized attachment patterns between parents and their young children: Review of research and implications for clinical work. In L. Atkinson & S. Goldberg (Eds.), *Attachment issues in psychopathology and intervention* (pp. 65–94). Mahwah, NJ: Lawrence Erlbaum Associates.

Lyons-Ruth, K., Repacholi, B., McLeod, S., & Silva, E. (1991). Disorganized attachment behavior in infancy: Short-term stability, maternal and infant correlates, and risk-related subtypes. *Development and Psychopathology, 3*, 377–396.

Main, M., & Cassidy, J. (1988). Categories of response to reunion with the parent at age six: Predicted from attachment classifications and stable over a one-month period. *Developmental Psychology, 24*, 415–426.

Main, M., & Goldwyn, R. (1998). *Adult attachment scoring and classification system.* Unpublished manuscript, University of California at Berkeley, Berkeley, CA.

Main, M., & Hesse, E. (1990). Parents' unresolved traumatic experiences are related to infant disorganized attachment status: Is frightened and/or frightening parental behavior the linking mechanism? In M. T. Greenberg, D. Cicchetti, & E. M. Cummings (Eds.), *Attachment in the preschool years* (pp. 161–182). Chicago: University of Chicago Press.

Main, M., Kaplan, N., & Cassidy, J. (1985). Security in infancy, childhood and adulthood: A move to the level of representation. In I. Bretherton & E. Waters (Eds.), *Growing points of attachment theory and research* (pp. 66–104). *Monographs of the Society for Research in Child Development, 50*(1–2, Serial No. 209).

Main, M., & Morgan, H. (1996). Disorganization and disorientation in infant strange situation behavior: Phenotypic resemblance to dissociative states? In L. K. Michelson & W. J. Ray (Eds.), *Handbook of dissociation: Theoretical, empirical, and clinical perspectives* (pp. 107–138). New York: Plenum.

Main, M., & Solomon, J. (1986). Discovery of a new, insecure-disorganized/disoriented attachment pattern. In T. B. Brazelton & M. Yogman (Eds.), *Affective development in infancy* (pp. 95–124). Westport, CT: Ablex.

Marchand, J. (2004). Husbands' and wives' marital quality: The role of adult attachment orientations, depressive symptoms, and conflict resolution behaviors. *Attachment & Human Development, 6*, 99–112.

McGee, R. A., & Wolfe, D. A. (1991). Psychological maltreatment: Toward an operational definition. *Development and Psychopathology, 2*, 425–444.

Messman-Moore, T. L., & Coates, A. A. (2007). The impact of childhood psychological abuse on adult interpersonal conflict: The role of early maladaptive schemas and patterns of interpersonal behavior. *Journal of Emotional Abuse, 7*, 75–92.

Mikulincer, M., & Florian, V. (1998). The relationship between adult attachment styles and emotional and cognitive reactions to stressful events. In J. A. Simpson & W. S. Rholes (Eds.), *Attachment theory and close relationships* (pp. 143–165). New York: Guilford.

Mikulincer, M., Florian, V., & Weller, A. (1993). Attachment styles, coping strategies, and posttraumatic psychological distress: The impact of the Gulf War in Israel. *Journal of Personality and Social Psychology, 58*, 273–280.

Mikulincer, M., & Nachshon, O. (1991). Attachment styles and patterns of self-disclosure. *Journal of Personality and Social Psychology, 61*, 321–331.

Mikulincer, M., & Shaver, P. (2003). The attachment behavioral system in adulthood: Activation, psychodynamics, and interpersonal processes. In N. P. Zanna (Ed.), *Advances in experimental social psychology: Vol. 35* (pp. 53–152). San Diego, CA: Academic.

Morimoto, Y., & Sharma, A. (2004). Long-term outcomes of verbal aggression: The role of protective factors. *Journal of Emotional Abuse, 4*, 71–99.

Moss, E., Parent, S., Gosselin, C., Rousseau, D., & St-Laurent, D. (1996). Attachment and teacher-reported behavior problems during the preschool and early school-age period. *Development and Psychopathology, 8*, 511–526.

Moss, E., Rousseau, D., Parent, S., St-Laurent, D., & Saintonge, J. (1998). Correlates of attachment at school-age: Maternal-reported stress, mother–child interaction and behavior problems. *Child Development, 69*, 1390–1405.

Mullen, P. E., Martin, J. L., Anderson, J. C., Romans, S. E., & Herbison, G. P. (1996). The long-term impact of the physical, emotional, and sexual abuse of children: A community study. *Child Abuse & Neglect, 20*, 7–21.

Nicholas, K. B., & Bieber, S. L. (1996). Parental abusive versus supportive behaviors and their relation to hostility and aggression in young adults. *Child Abuse & Neglect, 20*, 1195–1211.

O'Hagan, K. (2006). *Identifying emotional and psychological abuse: A guide for childcare professionals*. Berkshire, UK: Open University Press.

Onishi, M., Gjerde, P. F., & Block, J. (2001). Personality implications of romantic attachment patterns in young adults: A multi-method, multi-informant study. *Personality and Social Psychology Bulletin, 27*, 1097–1110.

Paley, B., Cox, M. J., Burchinal, M. R., & Payne, C. C. (1999). Attachment and marital functioning: Comparison of spouses with continuous-secure, earned-secure, dismissing, and preoccupied attachment stances. *Journal of Family Psychology, 13*, 580–597.

Paradis, A., & Boucher, S. (in press). Child maltreatment history and interpersonal problems in adult couple relationships. *Journal of Aggression, Maltreatment and Trauma*.

Patrick, M., Hobson, R., Castle, D., Howard, R., & Maughan, B. (1994). Personality disorder and the mental representation of early social experience. *Development and Psychopathology, 6*, 375–388.

Perry, A., DiLillo, D., & Peugh, J. (2007). Childhood psychological maltreatment and quality of marriage: The mediating role of psychological distress. *Journal of Emotional Abuse, 7*, 117–142.

Pianta, R., Egeland, B., & Adam, E. (1996). Adult attachment classification and self-reported psychiatric symptomatology as assessed by the Minnesota Multiphasic

Personality Inventory-2. *Journal of Consulting and Clinical Psychology, 64*, 273–281.

Pistole, M. C. (1989). Attachment: Implications for counselors. *Journal of Counseling and Development, 68*, 190–193.

Pistole, M. (1993). Attachment relationships: Self-disclosure and trust. *Journal of Mental Health Counseling, 15*, 94–106.

Pistole, M. (1994). Adult attachment styles: Some thoughts on closeness-distance struggles. *Family Process, 33*, 147–159.

Renken, B., Egeland, B., Marvinney, D., Sroufe, L. A., & Mangelsdorf, S. (1989). Early childhood antecedents of aggression and passive-withdrawal in early elementary school. *Journal of Personality, 57*, 257–281.

Riggs, S. A., & Jacobvitz, D. (2002). Expectant parents' representations of early attachment relationships: Associations with mental health and family history. *Journal of Consulting and Clinical Psychology, 70*, 195–204.

Riggs, S. A., Jacobvitz, D., & Hazen, N. (2002). Adult attachment and history of psychotherapy in a normative sample. *Psychotherapy, 39*, 344–353.

Riggs, S. A., & Kaminski, P. (2010). Childhood emotional abuse, adult attachment, and depression as predictors of relational adjustment and psychological aggression. *Journal of Aggression, Maltreatment and Trauma, 19*(1), 75–104.

Riggs, S. A., Paulson, A., Tunnel, E., Sahl, G., Atkison, H., & Ross, C. A. (2007). Attachment, personality and psychopathology among adult inpatients: Self-reported romantic attachment style vs. AAI states of mind. *Development and Psychopathology, 19*, 263–291.

Rogosch, F., Cicchetti, D., & Aber, J. (1995). The role of child maltreatment in early deviations in cognitive and affective processing abilities and later peer relationship problems. *Development and Psychopathology, 7*, 591–609.

Roisman, G. I., Collins, W. A., Sroufe, L. A., & Egeland, B. (2005). Predictors of young adults' security in their current romantic relationship: A prospective test of the prototype hypothesis. *Attachment and Human Development, 7*, 105–121.

Rosenstein, D. H., & Horowitz, H. A. (1996). Adolescent attachment and psychopathology. *Journal of Consulting and Clinical Psychology, 64*, 244–253.

Schachner, D., & Shaver, P. (2004). Attachment dimensions and sexual motives. *Personal Relationships, 11*, 179–195.

Schuengel, C., Bakermans-Kranenburg, M. J., & van IJzendoorn, M. H. (1999). Frightening maternal behavior linking unresolved loss and disorganized infant attachment. *Journal of Consulting and Clinical Psychology, 67*, 54–63.

Senchak, M., & Leonard, K. E. (1992). Attachment styles and marital adjustment among newlywed couples. *Journal of Social and Personal Relationships, 9*, 51–64.

Shaver, P. R., & Brennan, K. (1992). Attachment styles and the "Big Five" personality traits: Their connections with each other and with romantic relationship outcomes. *Personality and Social Psychology Bulletin, 18*, 536–545.

Shaver, P. R., & Clark, C. L. (1994). The psychodynamics of adult romantic attachment. In J. M. Masling & R. F. Bornstein (Eds.), *Empirical perspectives on object relations theories* (pp. 105–156). Washington, DC: American Psychological Association.

Shaver, P., Hazan, C., & Bradshaw, D. (1988). Love as attachment. In R. J. Sternberg & M. L. Barnes (Eds.), *The psychology of love* (pp. 68–99). New Haven, CT: Yale University Press.

Shaver, P. R., & Mikulincer, M. (2002). Attachment-related psychodynamics. *Attachment and Human Development, 4*, 133–161.

Shaver, P., Schachner, D., & Mikulincer, M. (2005). Attachment style, excessive reassurance seeking, relationship processes, and depression. *Personality and Social Psychology Bulletin, 31*, 343–359.

Shi, L. (2003). The association between adult attachment styles and conflict resolution in romantic relationships. *The American Journal of Family Therapy, 31*, 143–157.

Simpson, J. A. (1990). Influence of attachment styles on romantic relationships. *Journal of Personality and Social Psychology, 59*, 971–980.

Simpson, J., Collins, W., Tran, S., & Haydon, K. (2007). Attachment and the experience and expression of emotions in romantic relationships: A developmental perspective. *Journal of Personality and Social Psychology, 92*, 355–367.

Simpson, J. A., & Rholes, W. S. (2002). Fearful-avoidance, disorganization, and multiple working models: Some directions for future theory and research. *Attachment and Human Development, 4*, 223–229.

Simpson, J. A., Rholes, W., & Nelligan, J. (1992). Support seeking and support giving within couples in anxiety-provoking situations: The role of attachment styles. *Journal of Personality and Social Psychology, 62*, 434–446.

Simpson, J. A., Rholes, W. S., Orina, M., & Grich, J. (2002). Working models of attachment, support giving, and support seeking in a stressful situation. *Personality and Social Psychology Bulletin, 28*, 598–608.

Simpson, J. A., Rholes, W. S., & Phillips, D. (1996). Conflict in close relationships: An attachment perspective. *Journal of Personality and Social Psychology, 71*, 899–914.

Simpson, J. A., Winterheld, H. A., Rholes, W. S., & Orina, M. M. (2007). Working models of attachment and reactions to different forms of caregiving from romantic partners. *Journal of Personality and Social Psychology, 93*, 466–477.

Solomon, J., & George, C., (1999). The place of disorganization in attachment theory: Linking classic observations with contemporary findings. In J. Solomon & C. George (Eds.), *Attachment disorganization* (pp. 3–32). New York: Guilford.

Solomon, J., George, C., & De Jong, A. (1995). Children classified as controlling at age six: Evidence of disorganized representational strategies and aggression at home and at school. *Development and Psychopathology, 7*, 447–463.

Speltz, M., Greenberg, M., & DeKlyen, M. (1990). Attachment in preschoolers with disruptive behavior: A comparison of clinic-referred and nonproblem children. *Development and Psychopathology, 2*, 31–46.

Spertus, I. L., Yehuda, R., Wong, C. M., Halligan, S., & Seremetis, S. V. (2003). Childhood emotional abuse and neglect as predictors of psychological and physical symptoms in women presenting to a primary care practice. *Child Abuse & Neglect, 27*, 1247–1258.

Sroufe, L. A. (1983). Infant–caregiver attachment and patterns of adaptation in preschool: The roots of maladaptation and competence. In M. Perlmutter (Ed.), *Minnesota Symposia in Child Psychology: Vol. 16* (pp. 41–83). Hillsdale, NJ: Lawrence Erlbaum Associates.

Sroufe, L. A., Carlson, E., & Shulman, S. (1993). The development of individuals in relationships: From infancy through adolescence. In D. C. Funder, R. Parke, C. Tomlinson-Keesey, & K. Widaman (Eds.), *Studying lives through time: Approaches to personality and development* (pp. 315–342). Washington, DC: American Psychological Association.

Sroufe, L. A., & Fleeson, J. (1986). Attachment and the construction of relationships. In W. Hartup & Z. Rubin (Eds.), *Relationships and development* (pp. 51–72). Hillsdale, NJ: Lawrence Erlbaum Associates.

Stalker, C. A., & Davies, F. (1995). Attachment organization and adaptation in sexually abused women. *Canadian Journal of Psychiatry, 40*, 234–240.

Stone, N. (1993). Parental abuse as a precursor to childhood onset depression and suicidality. *Child Psychiatry & Human Development, 24*, 13–24.

Stovall-McClough, K. C., & Cloitre, M. (2006). Unresolved attachment, PTSD, and dissociation in women with childhood abuse histories. *Journal of Consulting and Clinical Psychology, 74*, 219–228.

Suess, G. J., Grossmann, K. E., & Sroufe, L. A. (1992). Effects of infant attachment to mother and father on quality of adaptation in preschool: From dyadic to individual organization of self. *International Journal of Behavioral Development, 15*, 43–66.

Taussig, H. N., & Culhane, S. E. (2010). Emotional maltreatment and psychosocial functioning in preadolescent youth placed in out-of-home care. *Journal of Aggression, Maltreatment and Trauma, 19*(1), 52–74.

Thompson, A., & Kaplan, C. (1996). Childhood emotional abuse. *British Journal of Psychiatry, 168*, 143–148.

Thompson, R. A. (1991). Attachment theory and research. In M. Lewis (Ed.), *Child and adolescent psychiatry: A comprehensive textbook* (pp. 100–108). Baltimore: Williams & Wilkins.

Treboux, D., Crowell, J., & Colon-Downs, C. (1992, March). *Self-concept and identity in late adolescence: Relation to working models of attachment*. Paper presented at the biennial meeting of the Society for Research in Adolescence, Washington, DC.

Troy, M., & Sroufe, L. A. (1987). Victimization among preschoolers: The role of attachment relationship history. *Journal of the American Academy of Child and Adolescent Psychiatry, 26*, 166–172.

Tyrell, C., & Dozier, M. (1997, April). *The role of attachment in therapeutic process and outcome for adults with serious psychiatric disorders*. Paper presented at the biennial meeting of Society for Research in Child Development, Washington, DC.

Urban, J., Carlson, E., Egeland, B., & Sroufe, L. A. (1991). Patterns of individual adaptation across childhood. *Development and Psychopathology, 3*, 445–460.

van IJzendoorn, M. H. (1995). Adult attachment representations, parental responsiveness, and infant attachment: A meta-analysis on the predictive validity of the Adult Attachment Interview. *Psychological Bulletin, 117*, 387–403.

van IJzendoorn, M. H., & Bakermans-Kranenburg, M. J. (1996). Attachment representations in mothers, fathers, adolescents, and clinical groups: A meta-analytic search for normative data. *Journal of Consulting and Clinical Psychology, 64*, 8–21.

van IJzendoorn, M., Schuengel, C., & Bakermans-Kranenburg, M. J. (1999). Disorganized attachment in early childhood: Meta-analysis of precursors, concomitants, and sequelae. *Development and Psychopathology, 11*, 225–249.

Varia, R., & Abidin, R. R. (1999). The minimizing style: Perceptions of psychological abuse and quality of past and current relationships. *Child Abuse & Neglect, 23*, 1041–1055.

Vissing,Y. M., Straus, M. A., Gelles, R. J., & Harrop, J. W. (1991). Verbal aggression by parents and psychosocial problems of children. *Child Abuse & Neglect, 15*, 223–238.

Wartner, U. G., Grossmann, K., Fremmer-Bombik, E., & Suess, G. (1994). Attachment patterns at age six in south Germany: Predictability from infancy and implications for pre-school behavior. *Child Development, 65*, 1014–1027.

Waters, E., Merrick, S. K., Treboux, D., Crowell, J., & Albersheim, L. (2000). Attachment security from infancy to early adulthood: A 20-year longitudinal study. *Child Development, 71*, 684–689.

Wekerle, C., & Wolfe, D. A. (1998). The role of child maltreatment and attachment style in adolescent relationship violence. *Development and Psychopathology, 10*, 571–586.

Wekerle, C., Wolfe, D., Hawkins, D., Pittman, A., Glickman, A., & Lovald, B. (2001). Childhood maltreatment, posttraumatic stress symptomatology, and adolescent dating violence: Considering the value of adolescent perceptions of abuse and a trauma mediational model. *Development and Psychopathology, 13*, 847–871.

Wenar, C., & Kerig, P. (2000). *Developmental psychopathology: From infancy through adolescence* (4th ed.). New York: McGraw-Hill.

Wood, E. (2007). *Parental bonding, adult romantic attachment, fear of intimacy, and cognitive distortions among child molesters* (Unpublished doctoral dissertation). University of North Texas, Denton, TX.

Wright, M. O. (2007). The long-term impact of emotional abuse in childhood: Identifying mediating and moderating processes. *Journal of Emotional Abuse, 7*, 1–8.

Yates, T. (2007). The developmental consequences of child emotional abuse: A neurodevelopmental perspective. *Journal of Emotional Abuse, 7*(2), 19–34.

Young, J. E., Klosko, J. S., & Weishaar, J. E. (2003). *Schema therapy: A practitioners' guide*. New York: Guilford.

Zayas, V., & Shoda, Y. (2007). Predicting preferences for dating partners from past experiences of psychological abuse: Identifying psychological ingredients of situations. *Personality and Social Psychology Bulletin, 22*, 123–138.

Zurbriggen, E. L., Gobin, R., & Freyd, J. J. (in press). Childhood emotional abuse and late adolescent sexual aggression perpetration and victimization. *Journal of Aggression, Maltreatment and Trauma*.

CURRENT RESEARCH

Emotional Maltreatment and Psychosocial Functioning in Preadolescent Youth Placed in Out-of-Home Care

HEATHER N. TAUSSIG and SARA E. CULHANE

Kempe Center for the Prevention and Treatment of Child Abuse and Neglect; and the University of Colorado School of Medicine, Aurora, Colorado, USA

This article examines the impact of emotional maltreatment on the psychosocial functioning of youth placed in out-of-home care as a result of maltreatment. Participants included 243 children participating in a randomized controlled trial of a preventive intervention for preadolescent youth placed in out-of-home care. This study analyzed baseline data collected prerandomization from interviews with children and their out-of-home caregivers and data from child welfare records. Bivariate and regression analyses were used to explore the relationships between emotional maltreatment and interpersonal functioning, self-perception, mental health, and behavioral problems for the total sample and by gender. Findings suggest that subtypes of emotional maltreatment are associated with different outcomes and that males are more negatively impacted by emotional maltreatment than are females.

This project was supported by grants from the National Institute of Mental Health (1 R21 MH067618, and 1 R01 MH076919–03, H. Taussig, Principal Investigator) and the Kempe Foundation, Pioneer Fund, and Daniels Fund. The content is solely the responsibility of the authors and does not necessarily represent the official views of the National Institute of Mental Health or the National Institutes of Health. We thank Edward Garrido and Tali Raviv for their review of this article, and Laura Mann, Jennifer Hughes, and Tabitha Webster for their invaluable support in the preparation of the article. We also thank the Denver, Adams, Arapahoe, and Jefferson County Departments of Social Services for their partnership in our research efforts. Finally, we wish to express our appreciation to the children and families who made this research possible.

Although emotional maltreatment has been studied less frequently than physical and sexual abuse, evidence suggests that emotional maltreatment is associated with long-term deleterious consequences in adulthood. In studies with adult samples that rely on retrospective self-reports of maltreatment, a childhood history of emotional maltreatment is associated with low self-esteem, depression, anxiety, trauma symptoms, and the perpetration of or victimization from interpersonal violence (Berzenski & Yates, in press; Briere & Runtz, 1990; Crawford & Wright, 2007; Gibb, Chelminski, & Zimmerman, 2007; Dodge Reyome, in press; Dodge Reyome, Ward, & Witkiewitz, in press; Higgins & McCabe, 2000; Lewis et al., 2006; Mullen, Martin, Anderson, Romans, & Herbison, 1996; Riggs & Kaminski, 2010; Sachs-Ericsson, Verona, Joiner, & Preacher, 2006; Spertus, Yehuda, Wong, Halligan, & Seremetis, 2003; Zurbriggen, Gobin, & Freyd, in press). In many of these retrospective studies, emotional maltreatment serves as a reliable predictor of outcomes over and above the effects of physical abuse, sexual abuse, or both (Crawford & Wright, 2007; Higgins & McCabe, 2000; Sachs-Ericsson et al., 2006; Spertus et al., 2003). As many have noted, however, the reliance on retrospective self-reports is problematic as it raises the possibility that the association between maltreatment and outcomes is attributable to shared method variance, response bias, or both. Two studies that estimated the association between maltreatment and outcomes found that these associations differed depending on whether maltreatment was measured retrospectively or prospectively (Raphael, Widom, & Lange, 2001; Widom, Weiler, & Cottler, 1999).

A small number of prospective and cross-sectional studies have examined the relationships between emotional maltreatment and psychosocial development in childhood and adolescence using teacher reports (Gracia, 1995), parent reports (Vissing, Straus, Gelles, & Harrop, 1991), case worker reports (Chamberland et al., 2005), child welfare records (Crittenden, Claussen, & Sugarman, 1994; Kim & Cicchetti, 2006; Manly, Kim, Rogosch, & Cicchetti, 2001), and observational data (Linder & Collins, 2005) to measure maltreatment experiences. These studies, which reduce the risk of shared method variance and response bias, suggest that emotional maltreatment is associated with significant deviations from normative socioemotional development among children and adolescents. In these studies, emotional maltreatment was associated with internalizing symptoms, externalizing behavior problems, low self-esteem, and interpersonal problems (Chamberland et al., 2005; Crittenden et al., 1994; Gracia, 1995; Kim & Cicchetti, 2006; Linder & Collins, 2005; Manly et al., 2001; Vissing et al., 1991). Cross-sectional (Gibb & Abela, 2008; Solomon & Serres, 1999) and longitudinal (Stuewig &

McCloskey, 2005) studies that use youth self-reports to assess maltreatment also suggest that emotional maltreatment is associated with maladaptive developmental trajectories such as delinquency and depression.

Some studies suggest that emotional maltreatment might have more negative effects on development than do other types of abuse (Crittenden et al., 1994; McGee, Wolfe, & Wilson, 1997). For example, in their study of 160 adolescents randomly selected from the open caseload of a child protection agency, McGee et al. (1997) found that self-report severity ratings of emotional maltreatment were associated with self-reported internalizing and externalizing symptoms, even after controlling for self-reported severity ratings on four other types of maltreatment (physical abuse, sexual abuse, neglect, and family violence). Among the other types of maltreatment, only physical abuse was associated with self-reported symptoms, and it was correlated only with externalizing and not internalizing symptoms.

Although the aforementioned research suggests that the association between emotional maltreatment and adverse outcomes is robust, the interpretation of these findings is complicated by the fact that there is no universally used, operational definition of emotional maltreatment. The terms *emotional abuse, psychological abuse, verbal abuse, emotional maltreatment,* and *psychological maltreatment* have been used interchangeably to describe a wide variety of parenting behaviors believed to be psychologically damaging. In one study, emotional maltreatment might be defined as marital violence, harsh parenting, and parental rejection. In another study, emotional maltreatment might be measured solely by verbal aggression, and in yet another study, emotional maltreatment might include abandonment and exploitation. Furthermore, such studies rarely assess the differential effects of these subtypes of emotional maltreatment. To gain a clear understanding of the impact of emotional maltreatment on psychosocial development and adult adjustment, it is important to understand which subtypes of maltreatment are associated with which outcomes.

As a first step, a clear delineation of those behaviors that are universally accepted as forms of emotional maltreatment is needed. Several authors have proposed different typologies for categorizing emotional maltreatment (Garbarino, Guttman, & Seeley, 1986; Hart, Brassard, & Karlson, 1996; McGee & Wolfe, 1991). In their system for coding maltreatment types, Barnett, Manly, and Cicchetti (1993) provided a definition of emotional maltreatment that includes the following: (a) verbal abuse that thwarts self-esteem and belittles or blames a child, (b) intimidation or threats to a child, (c) acts that prevent age-appropriate autonomy, (d) acts that put children in inappropriate roles or provide them with inappropriate levels of responsibility, (e) abandonment, or (f) exposure to violence. These typologies provide a starting place for studies designed to identify the differential effects of emotional maltreatment subtypes on outcomes.

A few recent studies have begun to explore the possibility that subtypes of maltreatment might differentially predict outcomes (Allen, 2008; Linder & Collins, 2005; Schneider, Ross, Graham, & Zielinski, 2005; Stuewig & McCloskey, 2005). For example, in a retrospective study using a college sample, Allen (2008) used simultaneous regression to explore the differential effects of several parent behaviors: acts designed to terrorize children, acts that ignored children, acts that degraded children, and acts that exposed children to domestic violence. After controlling for physical abuse and all other emotional maltreatment subtypes, terrorizing behaviors predicted anxiety and somatic complaints, ignoring predicted depression and features of personality disorders, degrading behaviors predicted features of personality disorders, and exposure to domestic violence did not predict any of the dependent variables.

This study is designed to expand on this early research in several ways. First, it provides descriptive information on and estimates the differential effects of an overall measure of emotional maltreatment and four subtypes of emotional maltreatment, using data collected from a sample of 243 preadolescent youth placed in foster care as a result of abuse or neglect. Second, this study estimates the relationships between each of these emotional maltreatment classifications and several indexes of psychosocial functioning (social functioning, self-perception, mental health functioning, life satisfaction), as reported by both youth and their current caregivers.

METHOD

Participants

Participants in this study included youth and their current caregivers who were recruited for a randomized controlled trial of a preventive intervention for preadolescent youth placed in out-of-home care. This preventive intervention is known as the Fostering Healthy Futures prevention program and is described elsewhere (Taussig, Culhane, & Hettleman, 2007). Children ages 9 to 11 were eligible for the randomized controlled trial if the following criteria were met: (a) they had been placed in out-of-home care by court order in one of four participating counties within the preceding year, (b) placement was ordered due to maltreatment, and (c) they still resided in out-of-home care at the time of the baseline interview. Ninety-three percent of those meeting eligibility requirements were enrolled. This study analyzed baseline data that were collected prerandomization from interviews with children and their out-of-home caregivers. Although 286 children were interviewed at baseline, the sample for this study includes only 243 children. Data from 4 children were excluded because they were not sufficiently proficient in English to understand the study questions, data from 11 children were excluded because their scores on achievement and intelligence tests indicated significant cognitive impairment, and data from 28 children were excluded because they were siblings of others included in the sample (when siblings were interviewed, one of the siblings was chosen at random to be included in the study's analyses).

The final sample of 243 children was 48.1% female, with a mean age of 10.4 (*SD* = .91). The racial and ethnic distribution of children (nonexclusive categories) was 46.9% Hispanic, 48.6% Caucasian, and 28.0% African American. The sample of caregivers was primarily female (89%). The majority of youth participants were placed in foster (47.3%) or kinship (46.9%) care, with the remaining 5.8% residing in shelters, group homes, and residential treatment centers. About half (49.0%) of the youth were removed from their mothers only, 7.4% from their fathers only, 33.7% from a two-parent household, and the remaining 9.9% from another caregiver(s). The average length of time youth had been in out-of-home care at the time of the interview was 6.4 months (*SD* = 3.7). Children had to be living with their current caregivers for at least 3 weeks prior to being interviewed. The children in our study had been living in their current placement for an average of 5.3 months (*SD* = 3.8) at the time of the interview.

Procedure

This study was approved by the local institutional review board, and informed consent and assent were obtained from all participants. Youth and their current caregivers were interviewed by separate interviewers, typically at the child's residence. Structured youth interviews took between 3 and 4 hr and were typically completed over two sessions. Structured caregiver interviews took approximately 2 hr and were typically completed in one session. Children and caregivers were each paid $40 for their participation.

Measures of Independent Variables

Maltreatment

Trained research assistants coded each child's legal petition and social history (child welfare records' narrative of the history and events preceding the legal filing that led to the child's removal from the home) using the Maltreatment Classification System (MCS; Barnett et al., 1993). The developers of the rating system report adequate estimates of interrater agreement, with kappas ranging from .60 to 1.0 (Manly, Cicchetti, & Barnett, 1994). In this study, emotional maltreatment, physical abuse, sexual abuse, failure to provide, and lack of supervision were coded as present or absent for each participating child. Only maltreatment that occurred within the previous 2 years was coded because of concerns that not all case workers would reliably include information about past history of abuse. The relationship of the perpetrator to the victim and the severity of each maltreatment type were coded using the MCS. Also coded was the presence or absence of maternal history for criminal behavior, alcohol abuse or dependence, other substance use, mental illness, and history of being abused or neglected as a child. Maternal characteristics were coded because most youth (88.8%) had been removed from their biological mother. All records were consensus coded by at least two trained staff and discrepancies were resolved through consultation with one of the senior investigators.

Emotional maltreatment

In our sample of 243 children, 160 (65.8%) were coded as having been emotionally maltreated based on the MCS. Perpetrators of emotional maltreatment were predominantly mothers (54.3%), followed by both parents or caregivers (27.6%), other caregivers (10.6%), and fathers (7.5%).

The legal petitions and social histories of the 160 youth who were coded for emotional maltreatment were recoded for the presence or absence of each of the following, more specific, subtypes of emotional maltreatment (all of which were included in the broader Emotional Maltreatment coding of the MCS): (a) verbal abuse, thwarts self-esteem, or blames child (n = 37); (b) intimidation or threats to child (n = 21); (c) age-inappropriate autonomy (n = 5); (d) inappropriate level of responsibility or parentification (n = 49); (e) abandonment (n = 48); (f) exposure to parental suicide gestures or attempts (n = 8); (g) exposure to violence (n = 69); (h) physical abuse with an emotional maltreatment component (e.g., binding, smothering; n = 10); (i) failure to protect child from a known sexual perpetrator or sexual abuse with emotional component (n = 29); and (j) extreme, unpredictable, or inappropriate behaviors (n = 28). These codes were nonexclusive, and of the 160 children who were recoded, the majority (n = 80) had one subtype code, 36 had two subtype codes, 30 had three subtype codes, and in one extreme case, a child had eight subtype codes.

Some of the newly created emotional maltreatment subtype categories did not have a large enough n (i.e., age-inappropriate autonomy, exposure to parental suicide gestures or attempts, physical abuse with an emotional maltreatment component) or were conceptually unclear (i.e., failure to protect child from a known sexual perpetrator or sexual abuse with emotional component and extreme, unpredictable, or inappropriate behaviors), and therefore were excluded from future analyses. Also, replicating what others have found (Allen, 2008; Linder & Collins, 2005), the data of this study suggested that those children who were coded as being emotionally maltreated solely due to their exposure to violence (n = 25) were faring better on self-reports of functioning. These children, therefore, were removed from the overall emotional maltreatment group before analyses were conducted (although they were retained in the violence exposure category). Finally, because the first two subtypes (i.e., verbal abuse and intimidation or threats) seemed conceptually similar and are often reported together as verbal aggression, we combined these subtypes into a verbal aggression category for subsequent analyses.

Consequently, five different categories of emotional maltreatment were used in all subsequent analyses: (a) overall emotional maltreatment (n = 135, excluding those who were coded as emotionally maltreated due solely to violence exposure), (b) verbal aggression (n = 48), (c) inappropriate level of responsibility or parentification (n = 49), (d) abandonment (n = 48), and (e) violence exposure (n = 69).

Measures of Dependent Variables

With the exception of the measure of life satisfaction, which was modified for use in this study, all of the dependent measures have demonstrated validity and reliability with racially and ethnically diverse samples.

Attachment to substitute caregivers, parents, and peers

Attachment to caregivers, parents, and peers was assessed using a short form of the People in My Life measure (PML; Gifford-Smith, 2000). The PML is a 30-item, self-report measure that was derived from a longer version of the measure (Cook, Greenberg, & Kusche, 1995). It includes two subscales, one measuring attachment to parents (which was used to measure attachment to substitute caregivers as well as parents in this study) and one measuring attachment to peers. The short form has demonstrated high internal consistency (α = .80–.83) and its subscales reliably discriminate between samples of high-risk and normative youth. Sample PML items include questions asking youth to rate whether their caregivers, parents, and peers "help me with my problems," "care about me," "listen to me," "accept me," and "are proud of me." Sample items also include questions asking whether youth "share thoughts and feelings" with caregivers, parents, or friends and "feel angry" with caregivers, parents, or friends. Mean scores range from 1 (*not true*) to 3 (*often true*), with higher scores indicating greater perceived attachment.

Social acceptance and self-esteem

Social acceptance and self-esteem were assessed using the Social Acceptance and Global Self Worth subscales of the Self-Perception Profile for Children (SPPC; Harter, 1982, 1985). The SPPC is a widely used self-report measure of perceived self-competence for third through eighth graders that assesses self-esteem in six domains. All subscales have demonstrated adequate reliability and validity (Harter, 1985). Estimates of internal consistency for both the Social Acceptance (α = .75–.80) and Global Self Worth (α = .78–.84) scales are acceptable, and the two scales are moderately correlated with each other and with the other subscales measuring athletic competence, physical appearance, behavioral conduct, and scholastic competence (r = .20–.73). Mean scores on the Social Acceptance and Global Self Worth scales range from 1 to 4, with higher scores indicating greater perceived social acceptance and self-worth.

Anxiety

Anxiety was assessed using the Total Anxiety score from the Revised Children's Manifest Anxiety Scale (RCMAS; Reynolds & Paget, 1981; Reynolds & Richmond, 1978, 1979, 2000, 2008). The RCMAS is a self-report measure of anxiety that has demonstrated good reliability and validity. It is normed for male and female youth aged 6 to 19. Standardized scores are T scores, having a mean of 50 and a standard deviation of 10.

Posttraumatic stress

Posttraumatic stress symptoms were assessed using the Posttraumatic Stress subscale of the Trauma Symptom Checklist for Children (TSCC; Briere, 1996). The TSCC is a 54-item, six-scale, self-report measure of posttraumatic stress and related symptomatology, which includes normative data on 3,008 children ages 8 to 16 sampled from the general population. All of the TSCC subscales, including the Posttraumatic Stress subscale, have demonstrated adequate reliability (α = .77–.89) and subscale scores covary in the predicted directions with a number of other measures sharing similar content. As with RCMAS scores, standardized scores on the TSCC are T scores.

Life satisfaction

Life satisfaction was assessed using a modified version of the Delighted-Terrible Scale (Andrews & Withey, 1976). The 11-item self-report scale asks respondents to rate their satisfaction in several different domains (e.g., school, home, health, friendships, leisure activities). The items have good internal consistency and construct validity (Andrews & Withey, 1976). Mean scores range from 1 to 3, with higher scores indicating greater life satisfaction.

Social, emotional, and behavioral problems

Social, emotional, and behavioral problems were assessed with the Social Problems and Total Problems subscales of the Child Behavior Checklist

(CBCL; Achenbach & Rescorla, 2001). The CBCL is a widely used caregiver-report measure of child behavior problems. Caregivers rate 113 items on a 3-point scale to yield data on a variety of childhood behavior problems. The CBCL has been standardized separately for males and females in different age groups using a national probability sample that is racially and ethnically diverse. Standardized scores are t scores, which have a mean of 50 and a standard deviation of 10.

Data Analysis Plan

Because little is known about the subtypes of emotional maltreatment, a series of analyses was first run to determine whether the prevalence of distinct subtypes differed by demographic characteristics, other subtypes of emotional abuse, maternal characteristics, or other types of maltreatment. Differences were identified using *t* tests and chi-square statistics. Next, *t* tests were used to estimate the bivariate relationships between each of the emotional maltreatment types and the 10 dependent variables. These bivariate analyses were run for the total sample and for each gender separately. Finally, when the bivariate analysis suggested that an emotional maltreatment type was associated with a dependent variable, multiple regression was used to estimate the effect of the emotional maltreatment type on the dependent variable after controlling for the other four types of maltreatment (sexual abuse, physical abuse, failure to provide, and lack of supervision). All analyses were conducted using the SPSS statistical program, version 16 (SPSS, 2006).

RESULTS

Emotional Maltreatment Types and Demographic Characteristics

There were no age or racial and ethnic differences as a function of any type of emotional maltreatment. Males, however, were more likely to be abandoned, χ^2 (1, N = 243) = 3.88, p = .049, and there was a trend suggesting that males were more often exposed to violence, χ^2 (1, N = 243) = 3.14, p = .076.

Overlap Between Emotional Abuse Subtypes

As shown in Table 1, children who experienced verbal abuse were more likely to have experienced abandonment, χ^2 (1, N = 243) = 9.3, p = .002. Children who experienced inappropriate levels of responsibility were also more likely to have been exposed to violence, χ^2 (1, N = 243) = 6.31, p = .012, and there was a trend suggesting that these children were also more likely to have experienced abandonment, χ^2 (1, N = 243) = 3.01 p = .083.

TABLE 1 Overlap Between Subtypes of Emotional Maltreatment

Type of Maltreatment	Inappropriate responsibility (%)		Abandonment (%)		Violence exposure (%)	
	No	Yes	No	Yes	No	Yes
Verbal abuse	20.6	16.3	15.9	35.4*	17.8	24.6
Inappropriate responsibility			17.9	29.2**	16.1	30.4*
Abandonment					18.4	23.2

*$p \le .05$. **$p \le .10$.

Emotional Maltreatment Types and Maternal Characteristics

As summarized in Table 2, our findings suggest that emotional maltreatment types are, for the most part, not related to maternal characteristics including criminal history, alcohol or substance use problems, mental illness, or maltreatment history. There were only two exceptions. Youth who were identified as emotionally maltreated were less likely to have mothers with a maltreatment history, χ^2 (1, N = 243) = 4.69, p = .030, and youth who were forced to assume inappropriate levels of responsibility were more likely to have mothers with substance abuse problems, χ^2 (1, N = 243) = 3.99, p = .046.

TABLE 2 Maternal Characteristics and Other Maltreatment Types by Emotional Maltreatment Types

	EA (%)		VA (%)		IR (%)		A (%)		VE (%)	
	No	Yes	No	Yes	No	Yes	No	Yes	No	Yes
Maternal characteristics										
Criminal history	51.9	52.2	52.6	50.0	50.8	57.1	52.6	50.0	49.7	58.0
Alcohol abuse	35.2	30.4	33.8	27.1	33.5	28.6	33.3	29.2	29.9	39.1
Substance abuse	68.5	63.0	67.7	56.2	62.4	77.6*	65.6	64.6	67.8	59.4
Mental illness	34.3	32.6	32.8	35.4	34.5	28.6	32.8	35.4	35.1	29.0
Maltreatment history	26.9	15.6*	22.6	12.5	22.7	12.2	22.6	12.5	22.4	15.9
Other maltreatment types										
Physical abuse	20.4	36.3*	20.0	66.7*	31.4	20.4	27.2	37.5	27.6	33.3
Sexual abuse	4.6	15.6*	8.7	18.8*	12.4	4.1**	12.3	4.2**	10.9	10.1
Failure to provide	54.6	49.6	55.4	37.5*	49.0	63.3**	50.8	56.2	51.1	53.6
Lack of supervision	74.1	79.3	80.0	64.6*	73.3	89.8*	76.9	77.1	75.9	79.7

Note: EA = emotional maltreatment; VA = verbal aggression; IR = inappropriate responsibility; A = abandonment; VE = violence exposure.
*$p \le .05$. **$p \le .10$.

Emotional Maltreatment Types and Other Types of Maltreatment

The findings in Table 2 suggest that there are significant associations between emotional maltreatment types and other types of maltreatment. Youth who were identified as emotionally maltreated were more likely to have been physically abused, χ^2 (1, N = 243) = 7.36, p = .007, and sexually abused, χ^2 (1, N = 243) = 7.50, p = .006. Youth who were identified as victims of verbal aggression were more likely to have been physically abused, χ^2 (1, N = 243) = 40.56, p = .000, and sexually abused, χ^2 (1, N = 243) = 4.06, p = .044, but less likely to have been coded for failure to provide, χ^2 (1, N = 243) = 4.94, p = .026, or lack of supervision, χ^2 (1, N = 243) = 5.16, p = .023. Youth who were forced to assume inappropriate levels of responsibility were more likely to have been coded for lack of supervision, χ^2 (1, N = 243) = 5.71, p = .017, and there were trends suggesting that they were less likely to be sexually abused, χ^2 (1, N = 243) = 2.81, p = .093, and more likely to have experienced failure to provide, χ^2 (1, N = 243) = 3.20, p = .074. There was a third trend suggesting that youth who had been abandoned were less likely to have been sexually abused, χ^2 (1, N = 243) = 2.67, p = .102. Finally, exposure to violence was unrelated to the other types of maltreatment.

Bivariate Associations Between Emotional Maltreatment Types and Dependent Variables

Table 3 summarizes the bivariate associations between the five emotional maltreatment types and each of the 10 dependent variables for the total sample and for each gender separately.

Total sample

In the total sample of maltreated children, emotional maltreatment was associated with higher levels of self-reported posttraumatic stress symptoms, $t(241)$ = 2.68, p = .008, but was not associated with any of the other dependent variables. Verbal aggression was associated with lower levels of self-reported social acceptance $t(239)$ = –2.22, p = .027, and self-esteem, $t(239)$ = –2.91, p = .004, and with higher levels of self-reported posttraumatic stress symptoms, $t(241)$ = 2.27, p = .024, but was not associated with the caregiver-report measures of internalizing and externalizing symptoms. There was also a trend suggesting that verbal aggression might be associated with higher levels of self-reported anxiety, $t(241)$ = 1.71, p = .089. Inappropriate responsibility was associated with fewer caregiver-reported social problems, $t(240)$ = –2.18, p = .030, but was not associated with any of the other dependent variables. Abandonment was associated with lower levels of attachment to peers, $t(240)$ = –1.66, p = .098, lower life satisfaction, $t(240)$ = –1.67, p = .096, and higher levels of self-reported

TABLE 1 Bivariate Associations Between Emotional Maltreatment Types and Dependent Variables

	EA				VA				IR				A				VE			
	No		Yes		No		Yes		No		Yes		No		Yes		No		Yes	
	M	*SD*	*M*	*SD*	*M*	*SD*	*M*	*SD*	*M*	*SD*	*M*	*SD*	*M*	*SD*	*M*	*SD*	*M*	*SD*	*M*	*SD*
Attachment to caregivers																				
Total sample	2.6	.38	2.6	.32	2.6	.35	2.5	.34	2.5	.36	2.6	.28	2.6	.35	2.5	.34	2.6	.35	2.5	.35
Females	2.6	.42	2.6	.28	2.6	.35	2.6	.31	2.6	.36	2.7	.29	2.6	.35	2.7	.27	2.6	.36	2.6	.29
Males	2.5	.36	2.5	.34	2.5	.35	2.4	.37	2.5	.37	2.5	.26	2.5	.35	2.4	.34	2.5	.34	2.5	.37
Attachment to parents																				
Total sample	2.6	.45	2.5	.50	2.6	.48	2.5	.47	2.6	.49	2.6	.45	2.6	.46	2.5	.54	2.6	.50	2.6	.44
Females	2.6	.44	2.5	.57	2.5	.55	2.6	.43	2.6	.53	2.6	.52	2.5	.51	2.6	.62	2.5	.56	2.6	.41
Males	2.6	.45	2.6	.42	2.6	.41	2.4*	.52	2.6	.45	2.6	.37	2.6	.41	2.5	.50	2.6	.42	2.6	.45
Attachment to peers																				
Total sample	2.5	.37	2.4	.41	2.5	.39	2.5	.41	2.5	.41	2.4	.33	2.5	.36	2.4*	.50	2.5	.41	2.5	.33
Females	2.5	.40	2.5	.41	2.5	.40	2.5	.43	2.5	.43	2.5	.32	2.5	.35	2.4	.63	2.5	.43	2.5	.28
Males	2.5	.35	2.4*	.40	2.5	.38	2.5	.40	2.5	.39	2.4	.33	2.5	.36	2.4	.43	2.5	.39	2.5	.36
Social acc.																				
Total sample	3.1	.76	3.0	.80	3.1	.75	2.8*	.87	3.0	.77	2.9	.82	3.1	.75	2.9	.90	3.0	.82	3.0	.68
Females	3.0	.74	3.0	.84	3.1	.75	2.8	.91	3.0	.80	3.0	.81	3.0	.74	2.8	1.1	3.0	.84	3.1	.63
Males	3.1	.79	3.0	.76	3.1	.75	2.8**	.84	3.1	.75	2.9	.86	3.1	.77	3.0	.79	3.0	.80	3.0	.72
Self-esteem																				
Total sample	3.4	.67	3.3	.63	3.4	.62	3.1*	.71	3.4	.65	3.3	.64	3.4	.66	3.3	.61	3.4	.66	3.3	.63
Females	3.4	.74	3.4	.62	3.4	.66	3.3	.70	3.4	.67	3.3	.67	3.4	.66	3.2	.72	3.4	.64	3.2	.76
Males	3.4	.62	3.3	.64	3.4	.59	2.9*	.67	3.3	.64	3.3	.63	3.3	.66	3.3	.56	3.3	.67	3.4	.54

(Continued)

TABLE 1 (*Continued*)

	EA				VA				IR				A				VE			
	No		Yes		No		Yes		No		Yes		No		Yes		No		Yes	
	M	*SD*	*M*	*SD*	*M*	*SD*	*M*	*SD*	*M*	*SD*	*M*	*SD*	*M*	*SD*	*M*	*SD*	*M*	*SD*	*M*	*SD*
Anxiety																				
Total sample	50.8	10.4	52.7	10.6	51.3	10.6	54.2**	10.2	51.9	10.5	51.7	10.5	51.1	10.4	54.7*	10.4	52.6	10.4	49.9**	10.7
Females	52.2	11.7	53.2	11.4	52.4	11.5	53.9	11.6	52.6	11.7	53.4	10.8	52.3	11.3	55.5	12.7	53.7	11.0	49.5**	12.5
Males	49.7	9.3	52.2	9.6	50.4	9.7	54.5**	8.1	51.3	9.4	49.8	10.1	50.0	9.4	54.3**	9.2	51.4	9.6	50.2	9.4
Posttraumatic stress																				
Females	47.2	9.2	50.5**	10.7	48.3	10.0	51.9	10.6	49.0	10.5	50.1	9.3	49.2	10.2	49.3	10.6	49.8	10.1	47.0	10.4
Males	47.1	8.4	50.5*	10.5	48.3	9.0	52.0	12.4	48.7	9.4	50.0	10.6	48.3	9.8	50.7	8.9	49.8	10.00	47.0	8.7
Life satisfaction																				
Total sample	2.7	.27	2.7	.27	2.7	.27	2.7	.28	2.7	.26	2.7	.30	2.7	.26	2.6*	.30	2.7	.27	2.7	.28
Females	2.7	.31	2.7	.27	2.7	.27	2.6	.33	2.7	.30	2.7	.25	2.7	.28	2.7	.33	2.7	.30	2.8	.25
Males	2.8	.22	2.7*	.28	2.7	.27	2.7	.19	2.7	.23	2.6	.35	2.7	.24	2.6**	.29	2.7	.24	2.7	.29
Social problems (CBCL)																				
Total sample	61.7	9.5	61.7	9.1	61.5	9.1	62.2	10.3	62.3	9.6	59.1*	7.2	61.8	9.3	61.0	9.2	61.7	9.5	61.6	8.7
Females	63.7	10.9	61.5	10.2	62.8	10.3	61.2	11.1	63.6	10.9	57.7*	6.8	62.6	10.3	61.1	11.6	63.1	10.6	60.1	10.1
Males	60.1	8.0	61.9	8.0	60.5	7.8	63.8**	9.1	61.2	8.2	60.5	7.4	61.0	8.2	61.0	7.8	60.2	8.1	62.6	7.7
Emotional and behavioral problems (CBCL)																				
Total sample	62.7	11.7	62.1	11.6	62.2	11.4	62.9	12.4	63.2	11.5	59.1	11.7	62.8	11.3	60.6	12.6	62.2	11.7	62.7	11.4
Females	63.5	11.6	60.6	11.3	62.0	11.1	60.9	12.5	63.0	11.6	57.0*	9.8	62.5	10.9	57.3**	13.6	62.4	11.2	59.8	12.1
Males	62.1	11.8	63.7	11.8	62.4	11.7	65.7	12.1	63.3	11.5	61.1	13.2	63.1	11.8	62.5	11.8	62.1	12.3	64.6	10.6

Note: EA = emotional maltreatment; VA = verbal aggression; IR = inappropriate responsibility; A = abandonment; VE = violence exposure; CBCL = Child Behavior Checklist.
*$p \leq .05$. **$p \leq .10$.

anxiety, $t(241) = 2.11$, $p = .036$. Violence exposure was associated with lower levels of self-reported posttraumatic stress symptoms, $t(241) = -1.99$, $p = .048$. In addition, there was a trend suggesting that violence exposure might also be associated with fewer self-reported symptoms of anxiety, $t(241) = -1.79$, $p = .074$.

Female sample

In the female sample, there were few associations between emotional maltreatment types and dependent variables. Among females, there was a trend suggesting that emotional maltreatment might be associated with higher levels of self-reported posttraumatic stress symptoms, $t(115) = 1.75$, $p = .083$, and inappropriate responsibility was significantly associated with lower levels of social problems, $t(114) = -2.54$, $p = .012$. There was also a trend suggesting that females' exposure to violence was associated with fewer self-reported symptoms of anxiety, $t(115) = -1.69$, $p = .094$. These findings were consistent with findings from analyses using the total sample. A finding not replicated with the total sample suggests that when females were forced to assume inappropriate levels of responsibility, they had fewer emotional and behavioral problems as indexed by caregiver report, $t(114) = -2.34$, $p = .021$. Finally, a trend suggested that females who were abandoned might also have fewer emotional and behavioral problems, $t(114) = -1.76$, $p = .081$.

Male sample

There were many more associations between the emotional maltreatment types and dependent variables for males, suggesting that emotional maltreatment might have more of an impact on the psychosocial development of males. In the male sample, as with the total sample, emotional maltreatment was associated with more self-reported symptoms of posttraumatic stress, $t(124) = 2.01$, $p = .046$. Abandonment was associated with higher levels of self-reported anxiety, $t(124) = 2.22$, $p = .028$, and there was a trend suggesting that abandonment was also associated with lower levels of life satisfaction, $t(124) = -1.91$, $p = .058$. Verbal aggression was associated with lower levels of self-esteem, $t(123) = -3.69$, $p = .000$, and there were trends suggesting that it was associated with higher levels of self-reported anxiety, $t(124) = 1.80$, $p = .074$, and lower levels of social acceptance, $t(123) = -1.66$, $p = .100$. Findings not replicated with the total sample suggest that emotionally maltreated males reported lower levels of attachment to peers, $t(124) = -2.22$, $p = .028$, and lower life satisfaction, $t(124) = -2.11$, $p = .037$, and that males who were subjected to verbal aggression reported lower levels of attachment to parents, $t(121) = -1.96$, $p = .052$.

Multiple Regression Analyses Measuring the Unique Effects of Emotional Maltreatment

When bivariate analyses suggested that there was an association between an emotional maltreatment type and a dependent variable, multiple regression was used to estimate that relationship controlling for physical abuse, sexual abuse, failure to provide, and lack of supervision.

Total sample

After controlling for the other four abuse types, emotional maltreatment was associated with higher self-reported posttraumatic stress symptoms, $\beta = .149$, $p = .024$. There was a trend suggesting that verbal aggression was associated with lower levels of social acceptance, $\beta = -.122$, $p = .083$, and with lower self-esteem, $\beta = -.123$, $p = .076$, after controlling for the other maltreatment types. However, verbal aggression was no longer associated with self-reported anxiety or with self-reported posttraumatic stress symptoms. A trend suggested that inappropriate responsibility was associated with fewer social problems, $\beta = -.125$, $p = .055$, after controlling for other types of maltreatment. There were also trends suggesting that abandonment was associated with lower levels of life satisfaction, $\beta = -.108$, $p = .094$, and with higher self-reported anxiety, $\beta = .121$, $p = .062$. However, after controlling for other maltreatment types, abandonment was no longer associated with attachment to friends. Violence exposure was associated with lower levels of posttraumatic stress symptoms, $\beta = -.129$, $p = .045$, and a trend suggested that it was also associated with lower levels of self-reported anxiety symptoms, $\beta = -.122$, $p = .057$.

Female sample

In the female sample, inappropriate responsibility was associated with fewer caregiver-reported social problems after controlling for other types of maltreatment, $\beta = -.236$, $p = .014$. There were trends suggesting that inappropriate responsibility, $\beta = -.184$, $p = .057$, and abandonment, $\beta = -.186$, $p = .056$, were associated with fewer emotional and behavioral problems after controlling for other maltreatment types. Emotional maltreatment was no longer associated with self-reported posttraumatic stress symptoms, and violence exposure was no longer associated with self-reported anxiety when controlling for other types of maltreatment.

Male sample

In the male sample, after controlling for other maltreatment, emotional maltreatment was associated with higher self-reported posttraumatic symptoms,

$\beta = .171$, $p = .054$, lower life satisfaction, $\beta = -.186$, $p = .040$, and lower levels of attachment to friends, $\beta = -.198$, $p = .029$. Verbal aggression was associated with lower self-esteem, $\beta = -.257$, $p = .008$, and lower levels of attachment to parents, $\beta = -.195$, $p = .052$. Verbal aggression was no longer associated with social acceptance or with self-reported anxiety after controlling for the other types of maltreatment. Abandonment was associated with lower life satisfaction, $\beta = -.192$, $p = .032$, and higher levels of self-reported anxiety, $\beta = .195$, $p = .031$.

DISCUSSION

This study extends our knowledge about the effects of childhood emotional maltreatment in several ways. First, using a prospective design, the impact of emotional maltreatment was analyzed in a representative sample of maltreated children with a recent entry into out-of-home care. Second, the focus of this study was not only on the relationships between emotional maltreatment and mental health symptoms, but also on the relationships between emotional maltreatment and interpersonal functioning, employing both youth self-report and caregiver reports of functioning. The use of subtypes to describe emotional maltreatment and its associations with functioning also broadens the knowledge base of the field, as most previous research has examined emotional maltreatment as a homogeneous construct.

The descriptive analyses that were conducted suggest that males and females were equally likely to experience emotional maltreatment of any type (including verbal abuse, inappropriate responsibility, and violence exposure), except that males were more likely to be abandoned. There was some overlap among the emotional abuse subtypes, most notably between verbal abuse and abandonment and between inappropriate responsibility and violence exposure. There was no evidence of an association between age and emotional maltreatment or emotional maltreatment subtypes, but our failure to find an effect might be attributable to the fact that our sample had a limited age range (9–11-year-old children). Future studies should examine the rate of emotional maltreatment across the age spectrum, as differences in prevalence by age would have implications for prevention efforts.

In informing prevention efforts, it is important to identify those risk factors associated with the perpetration of emotional maltreatment. In this study, the associations between maternal characteristics (as coded from child welfare records) and perpetration of emotional maltreatment were examined. Maternal characteristics were targeted because the majority of the emotional maltreatment perpetrators in this study were mothers and most children were removed from their mothers. In general, maternal characteristics, which included criminal history, alcohol and substance use problems, mental illness, and maltreatment history, were not related to emotional maltreatment perpetration. Future studies should examine the associations between maternal characteristics and emotional maltreatment with a sample that is restricted to those children who have been emotionally maltreated by their mothers. Preliminarily, however, these analyses suggest that one cannot identify which children are at risk for emotional maltreatment based on their mothers' risk factors. This differs from other studies, which find that maternal characteristics predict perpetration of emotional maltreatment (Chamberland et al., 2005; Mullen et al., 1996). Finally, the overlap between emotional maltreatment and other types of maltreatment was examined. As other studies have found (Chamberland et al., 2005; Crittenden et al., 1994; McGee et al., 1997; Rodgers et al., 2004; Wolfe & McGee, 1994), there was a great deal of overlap between emotional maltreatment types and other types of maltreatment, although there was less overlap between abandonment and violence exposure and other types of maltreatment.

After examining the descriptive characteristics, bivariate and multivariate analyses were conducted to examine the impact of emotional maltreatment and subtypes of emotional maltreatment on social and related functioning. Regression results, after controlling for other types of maltreatment, suggest that it is important to evaluate the effects of emotional maltreatment subtypes. An exclusive focus on the effects of an overall measure of emotional maltreatment would have masked some key subtype differences. For example, it was found that verbal aggression was related to lower perceived social acceptance and self-esteem, but overall emotional maltreatment was not. This theoretically makes sense as verbal aggression, which often belittles children, might make children feel bad about themselves and feel that others do not like them. Abandonment was related to greater anxiety and less life satisfaction, whereas overall emotional maltreatment was not. Similarly, inappropriate responsibility was related to fewer social problems as reported by current caregivers, but overall emotional maltreatment was not. Children who have been forced to care for other children and to maintain household functioning might display parentified behaviors that are viewed by other caregivers as helpful or mature. Finally, exposure to violence was associated with fewer self-reported posttraumatic stress symptoms. Although this might seem counterintuitive, it is important to remember that in this sample, all children had experienced maltreatment. Those children who were coded as having been emotionally maltreated solely because they had been exposed to violence displayed the fewest problems. Thus, witnessing violence might be less traumatic than being the subject of violence, whether verbal, physical, or sexual. These findings are similar to those observed in other studies that compare children who have been exposed to domestic violence with children who have been abused or neglected (Allen, 2008; Chamberland et al., 2005; Lewis et al., 2006; Linder & Collins, 2005).

As the findings of this study suggest, some emotional maltreatment subtypes (e.g., verbal aggression, abandonment) are positively associated with psychosocial problems, whereas others (e.g., inappropriate responsibility, violence exposure) are negatively associated with such problems, relative to other types of maltreatment. The examination of a global category of emotional maltreatment, therefore, might hide critical findings. It is also important to examine a range of outcomes from multiple reporters (McGee et al., 1997; Morimoto & Sharma, 2004), as some important, yet subtle differences were found in this study. Finally, given the overlap between emotional maltreatment and other types of maltreatment, it is critical to control for the impact of other types of maltreatment to isolate the unique effects of emotional maltreatment (Berzenski & Yates, in press; Sachs-Ericsson et al., 2006; Vissing et al., 1991; Zurbriggen et al., in press).

Studies should also examine outcomes by gender, as previous research has found inconsistent results with regard to gender differences concerning the impact of emotional maltreatment (Kim & Cicchetti, 2006; McGee et al., 1997; Morimoto & Sharma, 2004; Vissing et al., 1991; Wolfe & McGee, 1994). In this study, females who had been emotionally maltreated were faring better on some indexes of mental health and social functioning than maltreated females who experienced other types of maltreatment. On the other hand, males who were emotionally maltreated endorsed more posttraumatic stress and anxiety symptoms and reported lower levels of life satisfaction, less attachment to friends, lower self-esteem, and less attachment to their biological parents than did maltreated males who experienced other types of maltreatment. In an effort to understand why males might be more negatively impacted by emotional maltreatment than females, a closer examination of the data revealed that the males in our sample experienced a greater severity of emotional maltreatment than did females, $t(132) = 2.58$, $p = .011$. A recent study found that the association between emotional abuse and adolescent competence was mediated by social withdrawal, but only for males (Shaffer, Yates, & Egeland, 2009). Future studies should examine gender by emotional maltreatment interactions while controlling for severity of emotional maltreatment. In addition, an examination of the relationship between the gender of the perpetrator (mother, father) and the gender of the victim might illuminate any differential impact of emotional abuse.

One of the limitations of this study is that each of the subtypes of emotional maltreatment was not coded for severity. These data would have been helpful in understanding the topography of emotional maltreatment and for analyzing the data to better understand the impact of different subtypes. It is recommended that a standardized method for coding emotional maltreatment subtypes and associated severity be developed because emotional maltreatment, as currently defined in the literature, is a very heterogeneous construct and is often operationalized differently in each study. This would enhance researchers' ability to compare findings across studies and to examine the impact of subtypes within a developmental framework.

Another limitation of this study was that multiple analyses were conducted and the level of significance was not adjusted, thereby increasing the possibility that our findings could be attributable to chance. The significance levels were not adjusted because of the exploratory nature of this study and because the associations between emotional maltreatment and psychosocial functioning have not been previously studied with a sample of preadolescent youth placed in out-of-home care. For this reason, trends were also noted in the tables and accompanying text. Another limitation was the use of caregivers as informants, as the length of time that they knew the child was variable. In addition, the generalizability of these findings is limited by the fact that the sample only included youth within a limited age range and those who were living in out-of-home care as a result of court order.

Finally, this study did not include a control group of nonmaltreated children who were matched on other, important sociodemographic variables. It would have been helpful to compare three groups of children: those who experienced emotional maltreatment, those who were maltreated but did not experience emotional maltreatment, and a nonmaltreated group. This might have better clarified the unique impact of emotional maltreatment on psychosocial outcomes for youth. A strength of the current design, however, was its ability to control for other types of maltreatment, as only 8 children (3% of the sample) experienced solely emotional maltreatment.

The results of this study suggest that emotional maltreatment might impair psychosocial functioning and related outcomes. Adult reports of the impact of childhood emotional maltreatment suggest that problems experienced by youth who are emotionally maltreated will not resolve on their own (see Carbone, 2010; Dodge Reyome, in press; Riggs, 2010; Riggs & Kaminski, 2010). Longitudinal studies are needed to examine not only the impact of emotional maltreatment over time, but salient risk and protective factors developmentally. Analyses of mediation and moderation (e.g., Morimoto & Sharma, 2004; Sachs-Ericsson et al., 2006; Wright, 2007), as well as analyses evaluating the impact of preventive interventions, should help to identify key mechanisms in the development of healthy social functioning for children whose lives have been impacted by grossly inappropriate parenting.

REFERENCES

Achenbach, T. M., & Rescorla, L. A. (2001). *Manual for the ASEBA School-Age Forms and Profiles*. Burlington: University of Vermont, Research Center for Children, Youth, & Families.

Allen, B. (2008). An analysis of the impact of diverse forms of childhood psychological maltreatment on emotional adjustment in early adulthood. *Child Maltreatment, 13*, 307–312.

Andrews, F. M., & Withey, S. B. (1976). *Social indicators of American's perceptions of life quality*. New York: Plenum.

Barnett, D., Manly, J. T., & Cicchetti, D. (1993). Defining child maltreatment: The interface between policy and research. In D. Cicchetti & S. L. Toth (Eds.), *Child abuse, child development, and social policy* (pp. 7–74). Norwood, NJ: Ablex.

Berzenski, S. R., & Yates, T. M. (in press). A developmental process analysis of the contribution of childhood emotional abuse to relationship violence. *Journal of Aggression, Maltreatment and Trauma*.

Briere, J. (1996). *Trauma Symptom Checklist for Children—Professional manual*. Odessa, FL: Psychological Assessment Resources.

Briere, J., & Runtz, M. (1990). Differential adult symptomatology associated with three types of child abuse histories. *Child Abuse & Neglect, 14*, 357–364.

Carbone, D. J. (2010). Using cognitive therapies to treat unstable attachment patterns in adults with childhood histories of social rejection. *Journal of Aggression, Maltreatment and Trauma, 19*(1), 105–134.

Chamberland, C., Laporte, L., Lavergne, C., Tourigny, M., Mayer, M., Wright, J., et al. (2005). Psychological maltreatment of children reported to youth protection services: A situation of grave concern. *Journal of Emotional Abuse, 5*(1), 65–94.

Cook, E., Greenberg, M., & Kusche, C. (1995, March). *People in My Life: Attachment relationships in middle childhood*. Presented at the biennial meeting of the Society for Research in Child Development, Indianapolis, IN.

Crawford, E., & Wright, M. O. (2007). The impact of childhood psychological maltreatment on interpersonal schemas and subsequent experiences of relationship aggression. *Journal of Emotional Abuse, 7*(2), 93–116.

Crittenden, P. M., Claussen, A. H., & Sugarman, D. B. (1994). Physical and psychological maltreatment in middle childhood and adolescence. *Development and Psychopathology, 6*, 145–164.

Dodge Reyome, N. (in press). Childhood emotional maltreatment and later intimate relationships: Themes from the empirical literature. *Journal of Aggression, Maltreatment and Trauma*.

Dodge Reyome, N., Ward, K. S., & Witkiewitz, K. (in press). Psychosocial variables as mediators of the relationship between childhood emotional maltreatment, codependency, and self silencing. *Journal of Aggression, Maltreatment and Trauma*.

Garbarino, J., Guttmann, E., & Seeley, J. W. (1986). *The psychologically battered child*. San Francisco: Jossey-Bass.

Gibb, B. E., & Abela, J. R. (2008). Emotional abuse, verbal victimization, and the development of children's negative inferential styles and depressive symptoms. *Cognitive Therapy and Research*, 32, 161–176.

Gibb, B. E., Chelminski, I., & Zimmerman, M. (2007). Childhood emotional, physical, and sexual abuse, and diagnoses of depressive and anxiety disorders in adult psychiatric outpatients. *Depression and Anxiety, 24*, 256–263.

Gifford-Smith, M. (2000). *People in My Life: Grade 4, Year 5.* Retrieved January 1, 2009, from http://www.childandfamilypolicy.duke.edu/fasttrack/techrept/p/pml/pm15tech.pdf

Gracia, E. (1995). Visible but unreported: A case for the "not serious enough" cases of child maltreatment. *Child Abuse & Neglect, 19*, 1083–1093.

Hart, S. N., Brassard, M. R., & Karlson, H. C. (1996). Psychological maltreatment. In J. Briere, L. Berliner, J. A. Bulkley, C. Jenny, & T. Reid (Eds.), *The APSAC handbook on child maltreatment* (pp. 72–89). Thousand Oaks, CA: Sage.

Harter, S. (1982). The Perceived Competence Scale for Children. *Child Development*, 53, 87–97.

Harter, S. (1985). *Manual for the Self-Perception Profile for Children.* Denver, CO: University of Denver.

Higgins, D. J., & McCabe, M. P. (2000). Relationships between different types of maltreatment during childhood and adjustment in adulthood. *Child Maltreatment, 5*, 261–272.

Kim, J., & Cicchetti, D. (2006). Longitudinal trajectories of self-system processes and depressive symptoms among maltreated and nonmaltreated children. *Child Development, 77*, 624–639.

Lewis, C. S., Jospitre, T., Griffing, S., Chu, M., Sage, R. E., Madry, L., et al. (2006). Childhood maltreatment, familial violence, and retraumatization: Assessing inner-city battered women. *Journal of Emotional Abuse, 6*(4), 47–67.

Linder, J. R., & Collins, W. A. (2005). Parent and peer predictors of physical aggression and conflict management in romantic relationships in early adulthood. *Journal of Family Psychology, 19*, 252–262.

Manly, J. T., Cicchetti, D., & Barnett, D. (1994). The impact of subtype, frequency, chronicity, and severity of child maltreatment on social competence and behavior problems. *Development and Psychopathology, 6*, 121–143.

Manly, J. T., Kim, J. E., Rogosch, F. A., & Cicchetti, D. (2001). Dimensions of child maltreatment and children's adjustment: Contributions of developmental timing and subtype. *Development and Psychopathology, 13*, 759–782.

McGee, R. A., & Wolfe, D. A. (1991). Psychological maltreatment: Toward an operational definition. *Development and Psychopathology, 3*, 3–18.

McGee, R. A., Wolfe, D. A., & Wilson, S. K. (1997). Multiple maltreatment experiences and adolescent behavior problems: Adolescents' perspectives. *Development and Psychopathology, 9*, 131–149.

Morimoto, Y., & Sharma, A. (2004). Long-term outcomes of verbal aggression: The role of protective factors. *Journal of Emotional Abuse, 4*(2), 71–99.

Mullen, P. E., Martin, J. L., Anderson, J. C., Romans, S. E., & Herbison, G. P. (1996). The long-term impact of the physical, emotional, and sexual abuse of children: A community study. *Child Abuse & Neglect, 20*, 7–21.

Raphael, K. G., Widom, C. S., & Lange, G. (2001). Childhood victimization and pain in adulthood: A prospective investigation. *Pain, 92*, 283–293.

Reynolds, C. R., & Paget, K. D. (1981). Factor analysis of the Revised Children's Manifest Anxiety scale for Blacks, Whites, males and females with a national normative sample. *Journal of Consulting and Clinical Psychology, 49*, 352–359.

Reynolds, C. R., & Richmond, O. B. (1978). What I Think and Feel: A revised measure of children's manifest anxiety. *Journal of Abnormal Child Psychology, 6*, 271–280.

Reynolds, C. R., & Richmond, O. B. (1979). What I Think and Feel: A revised measure of children's manifest anxiety. *Journal of Personality Assessment, 43*, 281–283.

Reynolds, C. R., & Richmond, O. B. (2000). *Revised Children's Manifest Anxiety Scale (RCMAS) manual*. Los Angeles: Western Psychological Services.

Reynolds, C. R., & Richmond, O. B. (2008). *Revised Children's Manifest Anxiety Scale (RCMAS) manual* (2nd ed.). Los Angeles: Western Psychological Services.

Riggs, S. A. (2010). Childhood emotional abuse and the attachment system across the life cycle: What theory and research tell us. *Journal of Aggression, Maltreatment and Trauma, 19*(1), 5–51.

Riggs, S. A., & Kaminski, P. (2010). Childhood emotional abuse, adult attachment, and depression as predictors of relational adjustment and psychological aggression. *Journal of Aggression, Maltreatment and Trauma, 19*(1), 75–104.

Rodgers, C. S., Lang, A. J., Laffaye, C., Satz, L. E., Dresselhaus, T. R., & Stein, M. B. (2004). The impact of individual forms of childhood maltreatment on health behavior. *Child Abuse & Neglect, 28*, 575–586.

Sachs-Ericsson, N., Verona, E., Joiner, T., & Preacher, K. J. (2006). Parental verbal abuse and the mediating role of self-criticism in adult internalizing disorders. *Journal of Affective Disorders, 93*, 71–78.

Schneider, M. W., Ross, A., Graham, J. C., & Zielinski, A. (2005). Do allegations of emotional maltreatment predict developmental outcomes beyond that of other forms of maltreatment? *Child Abuse & Neglect, 29*, 513–532.

Shaffer, A., Yates, T. M., & Egeland, B. R. (2009). The relation of emotional maltreatment to early adolescent competence: Developmental processes in a prospective study. *Child Abuse & Neglect, 33*, 36–44.

Solomon, C. R., & Serres, F. (1999). Effects of parental verbal aggression on children's self-esteem and school marks. *Child Abuse & Neglect, 23*, 339–351.

Spertus, I. L., Yehuda, R., Wong, C. M., Halligan, S., & Seremetis, S. V. (2003). Childhood emotional abuse and neglect as predictors of psychological symptoms in women presenting to a primary care practice. *Child Abuse & Neglect, 27*, 1247–1258.

SPSS, Inc. (2006). SPSS for Windows, Rel. 16.0. Chicago: Author.

Stuewig, J., & McCloskey, L. A. (2005). The relation of child maltreatment to shame and guilt among adolescents: Psychological routes to depression and delinquency. *Child Maltreatment, 10*, 324–336.

Taussig, H. N., Culhane, S. E., & Hettleman, D. (2007). Fostering Healthy Futures: An innovative preventive intervention for preadolescent youth in out-of-home care. *Child Welfare Journal, 86*(5), 113–131.

Vissing, Y. M., Straus, M. A., Gelles, R. J., & Harrop, J. W. (1991). Verbal aggression by parents and psychosocial problems of children. *Child Abuse & Neglect, 15*, 223–238.

Widom, C. S., Weiler, B. L., & Cottler, L. B. (1999). Childhood victimization and drug abuse: A comparison of prospective and retrospective findings. *Journal of Consulting and Clinical Psychology, 67*, 867–880.

Wolfe, D. A., & McGee, R. (1994). Dimensions of child maltreatment and their relationship to adolescent adjustment. *Development and Psychopathology, 6*, 165–181.

Wright, M. O. (2007). Introduction: The long term impact of emotional abuse in childhood: Identifying mediating and moderating processes. *The Journal of Emotional Abuse, 7*(2), 1–8.

Zurbriggen, E. L., Gobin, R., & Freyd, J. J. (in press). Childhood emotional abuse and late adolescent sexual aggression perpetration and victimization. *Journal of Aggression, Maltreatment and Trauma*.

Childhood Emotional Abuse, Adult Attachment, and Depression as Predictors of Relational Adjustment and Psychological Aggression

SHELLEY A. RIGGS and PATRICIA KAMINSKI
University of North Texas, Denton, Texas, USA

This study examined the theoretically expected contributions of early emotional abuse, adult attachment, and depression to several aspects of romantic relationship functioning. College students in dating relationships (N = 285) completed an online survey, including measures of childhood emotional maltreatment, adult attachment style, psychological distress, and romantic relationships. Results indicated that childhood emotional maltreatment directly predicted insecure adult attachment. In the full models, emotional maltreatment contributed to dyadic adjustment, but was not a significant predictor of psychological aggression or victimization. In contrast, depression accounted for the largest proportion of variance in the models for reported psychological aggression and victimization, but was nonsignificant for dyadic adjustment. Adult attachment style emerged as an important predictor of all 3 relationship constructs.

A vast body of empirical literature supports the association between most forms of childhood maltreatment and a variety of deleterious outcomes in adolescence and adulthood. One exception, however, is that much less is

We wish to thank all the participants for their cooperation. We also acknowledge Mike Devine for his assistance with the online data collection procedures, as well as Zane Dodd and Sara Pollard for data management support.

known about the specific effect of parents' emotional maltreatment of their children and rarely has the available research been guided by an overarching theory of development (Crawford & Wright, 2007). This gap in the literature is especially problematic given that clinicians working with traumatized children identify emotional maltreatment by a parent figure as the most common type of maltreatment that children endure (Garbarino, Guttman, & Seely, 1986).

There are many reasons why emotional maltreatment remains understudied as well as underreported. First, the phenomenon is difficult to operationally define because it lies along the same continuum as ubiquitous parenting mistakes such as not meeting a child's needs for attention or raising one's voice in a manner that frightens a child (McGee & Wolfe, 1991; Rosen & Martin, 1996). Moreover, the problem of defining maltreatment is likely complicated by differences in parenting norms across cultures as well as individual differences in children's perceptions (e.g., what is considered "yelling" in one family or by one child might not be perceived similarly in another family or by another child). This difficulty in defining emotional maltreatment is even apparent in the U.S. legal system, where definitions vary widely across states and not all states include emotional maltreatment in their child protection statutes (U.S. Department of Health and Human Services, 2007). Finally, because emotional maltreatment tends to co-occur and overlap with other forms of maltreatment (McCloskey, 2001; Ney, Fung, & Wickett, 1994; Rosen & Martin, 1996; Scher, Forde, McQuaid, & Stein, 2004), much of the early literature on child abuse did not examine the independent effects of physical, sexual, and emotional abuse. Recent evidence, however, does indeed document differential outcomes of different forms of maltreatment (Berzenski & Yates, in press; Briere & Runtz, 1990; Gross & Keller, 1992; Nicholas & Bieber, 1996; Zurbriggen, Gobin, & Freyd, in press), suggesting that these constructs and their effects are unique and should be examined independently.

OUTCOMES OF CHILDHOOD EMOTIONAL ABUSE

Despite these barriers to scientific investigation, the notion that emotional abuse harms children is unequivocal. In fact, it is widely regarded as the "core component" of all forms of child abuse (Navarre, 1987). That is, violating a child's physical or sexual boundaries is likely to be experienced as degrading, frightening, exploiting, or some combination of these, thus meeting one definition of emotional abuse (Bernstein, 2002; Hart, Brassard, Binggeli, & Davidson, 2002). Actively rejecting and verbally berating a child are also forms of emotional maltreatment and might be more detrimental to a child's self-esteem than even physical abuse because they constitute a direct threat to a child's developing self-worth (Ney, 1987; Solomon &

Serres, 1999). Indeed, there is empirical evidence to suggest that adults who endured physical abuse as children but also perceived their caregivers to be generally supportive and accepting are at lower risk for depression and low self-esteem in adulthood than nonphysically abused children who did not experience adequate parental warmth (e.g., Wind & Silvern, 1994).

Although there are factors that have slowed and complicated the development of the literature on the longer term effects of emotional maltreatment on children, enough work has been conducted so that certain patterns are evident. For example, children who are subjected to emotional maltreatment are at higher risk for certain problems in adolescence and adulthood, including depression (e.g., Briere & Runtz, 1988; Clemmons, 2005; Dodge Reyome, Ward, & Witkiewitz, in press; Gross & Keller, 1992; Kaufman, 1991; Morimoto & Sharma, 2004; Stuewig & McCloskey, 2005), interpersonal sensitivity (Briere & Runtz, 1988; Morimoto & Sharma, 2004), and relationship difficulties (e.g., Berzenski & Yates, in press; Carbone, 2010; Dodge Reyome, in press; Gauthier, Stollak, Messe, & Aronoff, 1996; Nicholas & Bieber, 1996; Paradis & Boucher, in press; Wekerle & Wolfe, 1998; Zurbriggen et al., in press), which can be as severe as or worse than the sequelae of other types of childhood victimization (Tutty, 1999; Wind & Silvern, 1994).

Whereas chronic emotional maltreatment in childhood is a clear risk factor for certain negative outcomes, researchers have also identified variables that can act as protective factors and promote resilience among individuals with histories of emotional maltreatment. For example, child protective factors that fall into the category of intrapersonal variables include an easy temperament and high IQ (Garmezy, 1987; Losel & Bliesener, 1994; Masten, Morison, Pellegrini, & Tellegen, 1990). Of more interest in this study are those intervening factors between childhood emotional abuse and later outcomes that can be manipulated to minimize the negative impact of maltreatment. For example, increased levels of family cohesion (McGee & Wolfe, 1991; Morimoto & Sharma, 2004) and the development of secure attachments with secondary attachment figures (e.g., other nurturing adults, siblings, later romantic partners; Cicchetti & Rizley, 1981; McGee & Wolfe, 1991) have been shown to moderate the negative impact of emotional abuse and neglect in childhood.

THE ATTACHMENT SYSTEM

To date, the research on childhood emotional abuse has lacked a theoretical foundation to guide questions regarding the intervening processes that influence adult outcomes (Wright, 2007). This study is grounded in attachment theory (Bowlby, 1969, 1973, 1980), which provides a rich empirical and theoretical literature regarding the impact of early parent–child interactions on individual development and interpersonal relationships throughout the life cycle. According to attachment theory, the caregiver's provision of a "secure base" (Ainsworth, Blehar, Waters, & Wall, 1978) from which to explore the environment with minimal anxiety is critical to the development of optimal functioning characterized by a balance between interpersonal connection and autonomous exploration. Ainsworth et al. (1978) identified parental availability and sensitive responsiveness as key ingredients to the development of secure parent–child attachment, which is characterized by positive expectations of self and others that will promote adaptive functioning throughout the life span (Bartholomew & Horowitz, 1991). However, when children are neglected, rejected, and treated harshly or in an inconsistent and intrusive or controlling manner by their attachment figures, they develop negative mental representations of themselves, others, and relationships that are consistent with such treatment (Bowlby, 1969, 1973, 1980; Thompson, 1991) and contribute to maladaptive strategies for regulating emotion and interacting with others (Ainsworth et al., 1978; Carlson & Sroufe, 1995; reviewed in DeWolff & van IJzendoorn, 1997). Thus, early interactions with caregivers that are insensitive, unresponsive, or emotionally abusive will create a risk for insecure adult romantic attachment style, psychological difficulties, and relationship dysfunction possibly marked by emotional mistreatment (Carlson & Sroufe, 1995; Davis, Petretic-Jackson, & Ting, 2001; DiLillo, 2001; DiLillo, Lewis, & Di Lareto-Colgan, 2007; Riggs, 2010).

Whereas individuals with a childhood history of sensitive and responsive caregiving will likely develop secure adult attachment style characterized by a sense of self-efficacy and trust in others, perceptions of parental behavior as largely unavailable and nonsupportive, particularly when marked by a history of maltreatment or abuse, are consistently related to adult attachment insecurity (e.g., Brennan & Shaver, 1998; Lyons-Ruth & Block, 1996; Mickelson, Kessler, & Shaver, 1997; Riggs, 2010; Riggs & Jacobvitz, 2002). Insecure mental representations are associated with two broad dimensions: (a) *attachment anxiety,* which is characterized by a belief that the self is unworthy and preoccupation regarding abandonment by attachment figures, and (b) *attachment avoidance,* which is characterized by a belief that others are unreliable and the tendency to dismiss the importance of emotions and close relationships (Bartholomew & Horowitz, 1991; Blatt & Levy, 2003; Brennan, Clark, & Shaver, 1998). Adults with high levels of attachment anxiety might appear clingy, dependent, and demanding of their attachment figures; conversely, adults with high levels of attachment avoidance can appear aloof and distant due to constricted emotions and distrust in close relationships. Individuals who experience early abuse or trauma appear to have more difficulty developing a coherent attachment strategy and may exhibit inconsistent attachment behaviors marked by high levels of both attachment anxiety and avoidance (see Riggs, 2010).

Evidence supporting Bowlby's (1973) theoretical proposition, that insecure internal working models generate dysfunctional biases in the interpretation and response to stress, has been found in studies showing systematic attachment style differences in adults' affective responses to stress (Mikulincer & Florian, 1998). Research suggests that secure persons perceive and seek more support than insecure persons do (Lopez, Melendez, Sauer, Berger, & Wyssmann, 1998; Riggs, Jacobvitz, & Hazen, 2002). In contrast, insecure persons are less flexible and prone to cognitive distortion and maladaptive responses in the face of life stressors (Bowlby, 1980; Carlson & Sroufe, 1995). High attachment anxiety is associated with a hyperactivating response, which perpetuates distress by exaggerating emotions and care-seeking, whereas high attachment avoidance is associated with a deactivating response, which increases vulnerability by suppressing negative affect and decreasing support-seeking (Mikulincer & Florian, 1998). Individuals with high levels of both attachment anxiety and avoidance appear to be unable to determine the wisdom of help-seeking or the most effective means of gaining assistance, and thus might exhibit a combination of hyperactivating and deactivating strategies that manifest in confusing approach-avoidance tendencies (Simpson & Rholes, 2002).

Due to the associated negative mental representations of the self and other and maladaptive coping strategies, insecure attachment has been identified as a significant risk factor for behavior problems, poor social skills, low self-esteem, and many different forms of emotional disturbance in childhood, adolescence, and adulthood (reviewed in Dozier, Stovall, & Albus, 1999; Greenberg, 1999; see also Diehl, Elnick, Bourbeau, & Labouvie-Vief, 1998; Mickelson et al., 1997; Onishi, Gjerde, & Block, 2001; Riggs & Jacobvitz, 2002; Rosenstein & Horowitz, 1996). In particular, insecure individuals are susceptible to depression due to a circular tendency to re-create negative experiences and the development of a self-image as helpless and hopeless in the face of inescapable adversity (Bemporad & Romano, 1992; Rholes & Simpson, 2004). Research has demonstrated that anxious and preoccupied attachment with its negative model of self is associated with both anxious and depressive symptoms (Cole-Detke & Kobak, 1996; Eng, Heimberg, Hart, Schneier, & Liebowitz, 2001; Williams & Riskind, 2004). Evidence regarding a link between attachment avoidance and depression is mixed, with some studies indicating no relation (Cole-Detke & Kobak, 1996; Williams & Riskind, 2004), whereas others report significant associations (Carnelley, Peitromonaco, & Jaffe, 1994; Mickelson et al., 1997).

A long-lived idea in the developmental literature is the notion that early experiences with parents affect adults' capacity for intimate relationships (Collins & Sroufe, 1999). Research support for this idea comes from studies showing that adverse caregiving experiences and traumatic abuse in childhood are related to insecure adult attachment (Lyons-Ruth & Block, 1996; Riggs, 2010; Riggs & Jacobvitz, 2002) and marital difficulties in adulthood

(Caspi & Elder, 1988; Dodge Reyome, in press; Gilbert, El-Bassel, Schilling, & Friedman, 1997; Whitfield, Anda, Dube, & Felitti, 2003). Studies have reported that attachment security is related to better marital functioning (e.g., Cohn, Cowan, Cowan, & Pearson, 1992; Eiden, Teti, & Corns, 1995), as well as healthier emotional regulation and less withdrawal during marital interactions (Paley, Cox, Burchinal, & Payne, 1999). Other research has demonstrated that adult attachment style is significantly associated with marital cohesion, sexual behavior, partner caretaking, marital adjustment and satisfaction, partner support, conflict management, and relationship stability and termination (Collins & Read, 1990; Dutton, Saunders, Starzomski, & Bartholomew, 1994; Florian, Mikulincer, & Burcholtz, 1995; Senchak & Leonard, 1992; Simpson, Rholes, Orina, & Grich, 2002; Simpson, Rholes, & Phillips, 1996). Given the links between adult attachment style and mental health, it is not surprising that depression also is strongly related to romantic relationship functioning. For example, marital dissatisfaction or distress has repeatedly been found to be associated with depression (e.g., Christian, O'Leary, & Vivian, 1994; Schmaling & Jacobson, 1990), whereas having a partner as a confidante is a protective factor against depression (Brown & Harris, 1978).

Finally, it is likely that adult attachment and psychopathology together contribute to psychological aggression and victimization in romantic relationships. In the domestic violence literature, it is now widely accepted that psychological abuse among partners commonly occurs in the absence of violence and adversely affects victims as much or more than physical abuse (Arias & Pape, 1999; Follingstad, Rutledge, Berg, Hause, & Polek, 1990; Sackett & Saunders, 1999). Although research in the area of partner psychological abuse is recent and scarce, studies have provided some evidence of associations between individual psychological factors and relationship distress. For example, a history of childhood maltreatment or abuse (Berzenski & Yates, in press; Dodge Reyome, in press; Gilbert et al., 1997; Messman-Moore & Coates, 2007; Whitfield et al., 2003; Zurbriggen et al., in press) and insecure romantic attachment style (Dutton et al., 1994) are related to the likelihood of involvement in a physical or psychologically abusive partner relationship. In addition, being psychologically abused by a partner is also associated with mental health problems, such as problem drinking, depression, and posttraumatic stress (Arias & Pape, 1999; Foran & O'Leary, 2008; Sackett & Saunders, 1999).

THIS STUDY

The primary purpose of this study was to explore the associations between emotional maltreatment in childhood and later adult relational outcomes. Theoretically, childhood emotional abuse is believed to have a profound and long-term impact on the attachment system, which in turn is related to individual and couple functioning. This study empirically tested this theoretical model by examining the direct association of emotional abuse to adult attachment style, then using hierarchical regression procedures to assess the contributions of emotional abuse, adult attachment, and depression to several aspects of romantic relationship quality, including overall dyadic adjustment and psychological aggression by the respondent or by the partner (i.e., victimization of the respondent).

Due to definitional problems in the literature, two instruments were used to assess early emotional maltreatment. The Childhood Trauma Questionnaire (CTQ; Bernstein & Fink, 1998) measures different forms of child abuse, including physical, sexual, and emotional abuse. However, as mentioned previously, it is often difficult to determine where "normal" becomes "abusive" on the continuum of parental treatment, and treatment by different caregivers is likely to vary. Consequently, to better capture the broad range of possible parenting behaviors by both mothers and fathers, the Parental Bonding Instrument (PBI; Parker, Tupling, & Brown, 1979) was also included. The PBI is a widely used measure of parental bonding assessing the dimensions of warmth/rejection and independence/control. Emotional maltreatment was conceptualized to fall on the low end of the PBI Care scale, which would reflect excessive coldness and rejection, but on the high end of the PBI Control scale, which would reflect intrusive overcontrol and denial of autonomy (Parker, 2008).

The first hypothesis predicted that a history of childhood emotional abuse would be significantly associated with insecure adult attachment style. The next set of analyses tested three multivariate models shown in Figure 1. Each regression model controlled for physical and sexual abuse to ensure that the unique effects of emotional abuse were assessed, then sequentially added the independent variables (emotional maltreatment, attachment style, depression) to predict a different outcome (dyadic adjustment, psychological aggression, psychological victimization). The order of entry was determined by the expected developmental sequence; that is, emotional maltreatment occurs in childhood, adult attachment style develops in adolescence, and depression can emerge in adulthood partly due to insecure attachment strategies and subsequently increase the risk for poor relational outcomes. The hypothesized models predicted that after other forms of early abuse are controlled for, the combination of childhood emotional maltreatment, adult attachment styles, and symptoms of depression would predict a significant amount of variance in the functioning of romantic relationships. Moreover, each set of predictors was expected to add unique variance to the total variance accounted for in each model.

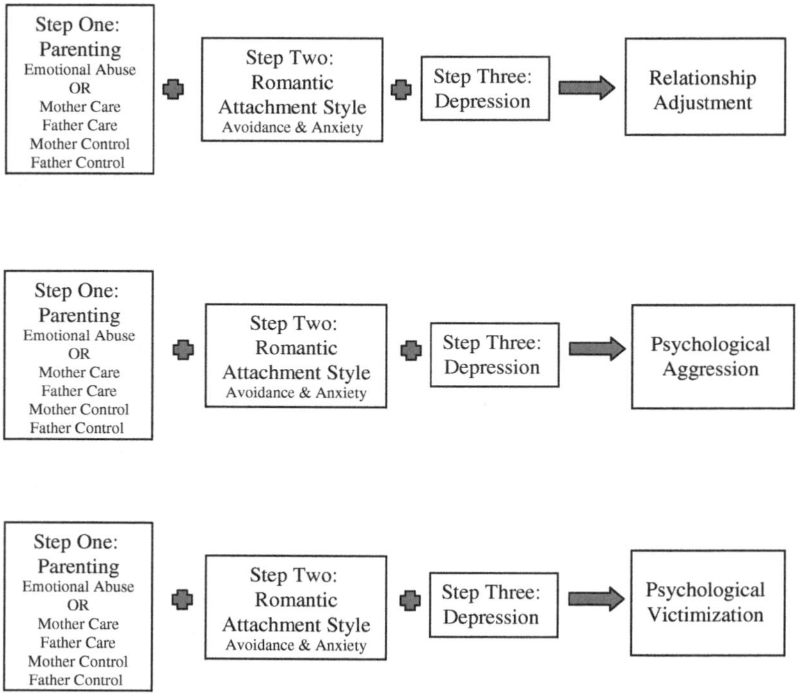

FIGURE 1 Hierarchical regression models for relationship adjustment, psychological aggression, and psychological victimization.

METHOD

Participants

This study is part of a larger project examining romantic attachment relationships of college students and their dating partners of 5 or more months at the time of assessment (range = 5–211 months; *M* = 25 months, median = 18 months, mode = 8 months). All procedures were reviewed and approved by the university's institutional review board. For the purposes of this study, only the college students' responses were considered (*N* = 285) to explore dyadic adjustment as well as psychological aggression and victimization, which were not assessed for partners. After reading and agreeing to the informed consent describing the risks and limits of confidentiality, students completed an online survey in exchange for research credit in psychology courses. Women made up 77% of the sample with a mean age of 21.9 years (*SD* = 3.70), and men made up the remaining 23% of the sample with a mean age of 21.4 years (*SD* = 4.25). The ethnic and racial composition of the sample was 68.5% European American, 10.8% African American, 9.8% Hispanic, 5.6% Asian or Pacific Islander, and 3.4% of participants indicating multiracial or other ethnic or racial background. In terms of annual family income level, 15% of the participants reported below $15,000, 8.8% reported between $15,000 and $30,000, 15% reported between $30,000 and $45,000, 14% reported between $45,000 and $60,000, 12% reported between $60,000 and $75,000, and 35% reported over $75,000. The majority of participants (64%) indicated that their parents were still married, with 30% reporting parental divorce before they were 16 years of age and 6% reporting a divorce after they were 16.

Measures

The Background Information Questionnaire was developed for this study to provide basic demographic information such as age, race, family income level, and so on. The questionnaire also requested information on the length of the current romantic relationships and family background variables, such as parental divorce, number of siblings, and deaths in the family.

The PBI (Parker et al., 1979) is a 25-item retrospective self-report measure assessing the respondent's recollections of their parents' attitudes and behaviors prior to age 16. Two parenting dimensions (Care and Control/Overprotection) are assessed separately for mother and father. Twelve items are included in the Care scale (e.g., "Was affectionate to me"), which represents a continuum of parental style from coldness and rejection (low scores) to affection and emotional warmth (high scores). The Control/Overprotection scale consists of 13 items (e.g., "Tried to control everything I did") representing a continuum ranging from psychological autonomy (low scores) to psychological control and intrusion (high scores). Respondents answer statements about their parents on a scale ranging from very unlike, moderately unlike, moderately like, to very like. The test–retest reliability of the PBI scales ranges from r = .63 to .76, and both scales demonstrate high construct validity in correlations with other measures of parental behavior (i.e., r = .69–.85; Parker, 1983). Cronbach alphas for the current sample were .96 for father Care, .96 for mother Care, .85 for father Control/Overprotection, and .87 for mother Control/Overprotection.

The CTQ (Bernstein & Fink, 1998) is a 28-item retrospective self-report questionnaire designed to assess childhood or adolescent abuse and neglect when the respondent was growing up. The CTQ produces five subscales: physical abuse (e.g., "I was punished with a belt, a board, a cord, or some other hard object"), sexual abuse (e.g., "Someone molested me"), emotional abuse (e.g., "I thought that my parents wished I had never been born"), emotional neglect (e.g., reverse-scored "My family was a source of strength and support"), and physical neglect (e.g., "I didn't have enough to eat"). There is also a three-item minimization-denial subscale to assess for extreme response bias, and attempts to deny experiences of childhood abuse. A 5-point frequency of occurrence scale is used on all items, ranging from 1 (*never true*) to 5 (*very often true*). The test–retest reliability coefficients range from r = .79 to .86. The CTQ reliability coefficients for the current sample were .79 for physical abuse, .94 for sexual abuse, .89 for emotional abuse, .91 for emotional neglect, and .79 for physical neglect.

The Experiences in Close Relationships Scale (ECR; Brennan et al., 1998) is the latest benchmark self-report measuring adult romantic attachment style. To create the ECR, the authors combined existing self-report measures and then used factor analysis to narrow 482 items to 36 representative items with high construct validity. Each item is rated on a 7-point Likert scale ranging from 1 (*not at all like me*) to 7 (*very much like me*). The two higher order scales of Avoidance (e.g., "I get uncomfortable when a romantic partner wants to be very close") and Anxiety (e.g., "I worry about being abandoned") are almost independent (i.e., $r = .11$) and demonstrated coefficient alphas above .90. Item-total correlations ranged from $r = .50$ to .73. Crowell, Fraley, and Shaver (1999) reported that the two scales demonstrate internal consistency and test–retest reliability, and have high construct, predictive, and discriminant validity. For the sample in this study, the Cronbach alphas were .94 for attachment avoidance and .92 for attachment anxiety.

The Hopkins Symptom Checklist (HSCL; Derogatis, Lipman, & Covi, 1973) is a 58-item self-report instrument assessing the extent to which psychological symptoms have been experienced within the last 7 days. Each item is rated on a 5-point scale, ranging from 0 (*not at all*) to 4 (*extremely*). Higher scores indicate the presence of more symptoms, whereas lower scores indicate fewer symptoms. Five subscales can be created, but based on consistent findings establishing robust associations between depression and romantic relationship quality, this study used only the Depression subscale (e.g., "feeling lonely," "feeling no interest in things"), which demonstrated good internal consistency in the current sample ($\alpha = .83$). Derogatis et al. (1973) also reported strong evidence of factorial invariance, construct validity, and test–retest reliability ($r = .81$).

The Dyadic Adjustment Scale (DAS; Spanier, 1976) is one of the most widely used and well-researched measures of relationship quality. Respondents are asked to rate most items on a 6-point scale. Items include questions regarding the extent of agreement or disagreement with partner on various issues (e.g., finances, demonstrations of affection, recreation), frequency of events or behaviors (e.g., confiding to partner, laugh together, quarreling), and expectations for the future of the relationship. In addition, the degree of happiness or agreement in the relationship is rated on a 6-point scale and there are two yes–no items regarding disagreements about "being too tired for sex" and "not showing love." Although the 32-item DAS yields four subscales, only the Total Adjustment subscale was used in this study. According to the author, research supports the DAS Total Adjustment subscale's concurrent and predictive validity and test–retest reliability ($r = .96$). A meta-analytic review of 91 studies ($N = 25{,}035$) found strong internal consistency for the Total Adjustment subscale ($\alpha = .91$); the Cronbach alpha for the current sample was .88.

The revised Conflict Tactics Scale (CTS2; Straus, Hamby, Boney-McCoy, & Sugarman, 1996) is a 39-item self-report assessing interpersonal problem-resolution behaviors in romantic relationships. The questions are asked in terms of both the respondent's and his or her partner's behavior and are rated on an 8-point frequency scale. The instrument produces five subscales (i.e., Psychological Aggression, Negotiation, Physical Assault, Sexual Coercion, Physical Injury), which demonstrate good reliability (α = .74–.89) and construct validity among college students across various cultures (Straus, 2004). Test–retest reliability (r = .60–.76) has also been established for the Psychological Aggression, Physical Assault, Injury, and Negotiation subscales (Vega & O'Leary, 2007). For the purpose of this study, only the Psychological Aggression scales for self and partner were used (e.g., "I insulted or swore at my partner" followed by "My partner did this to me"), demonstrating alphas of .78 and .79, respectively. Psychological Aggression-Self represents the respondent's self-reported perpetration of psychological aggression toward a partner and Psychological Aggression-Partner represents the respondent's perception of psychological aggression perpetrated by the partner toward the respondent (i.e., victimization).

RESULTS

Means, standard deviations, and intercorrelations for all major variables of interest are presented in Table 1. Prior to conducting the primary analyses, preliminary analyses were conducted to determine the need to control for background variables in the primary analyses. With few exceptions, background variables (i.e., age, ethnicity, family income, parental divorce) were not significantly related to the dependent variables. However, age and duration of current romantic relationship were significantly and negatively correlated with DAS Total Adjustment, $r = -.138$ ($p = .02$) and $r = -.146$ ($p = .014$), respectively. In addition, gender was significantly related to CTS2 Psychological Aggression scales for self, $F(1, 284) = 6.36$, $p = .012$, and partner, $F(1, 284) = 4.05$, $p = .045$, with women reporting that they perpetrated and received higher levels of psychological aggression in their current romantic relationships than men.

All predictor variables were centered before proceeding with the primary analyses. In the first set of analyses, simultaneous regressions tested the direct associations between childhood maltreatment, operationalized by either the five CTQ or four PBI scales, and the two adult attachment styles. The next set of analyses used hierarchical regression to test the theoretical models depicted in Figure 1. Based on preliminary findings, gender and length of relationship were included as control variables in the first step of each regression, along with childhood physical and sexual abuse. Age was not controlled because of its strong correlation with length of relationship ($r = .45$, $p < .001$).

TABLE 1 Correlations, Means, and Standard Deviations

	1	2	3	4	5	6	7	8	9	10	11	12	13
1. Dyadic Adjustment	1												
2. Psy Aggression-Self	−.082	1											
3. Psy Aggression-Partner	−.053	.819***	1										
4. Physical Abuse	−.170**	−.007	−.024	1									
5. Sexual Abuse	.020	.119*	.115*	.321***	1								
6. Emotional Abuse	−.307***	.045	.005	.641***	.283***	1							
7. Father Control	−.103	.107	.028	.151**	.193***	.327***	1						
8. Father Care	.250***	−.021	−.003	−.277***	−.093	−.520***	−.331***	1					
9. Mother Control	−.154**	.016	.005	.258***	.106	.316***	.457***	−.100	1				
10. Mother Care	.277***	−.034	.019	−.501***	−.259***	−.721***	−.230***	.335***	−.387***	1			
11. Attachment Avoidance	−.407***	−.440	.017	.330***	.213***	.465***	.207***	−.408***	.110	−.419***	1		
12. Attachment Anxiety	−.345***	.160**	.145*	.245***	.101	.440***	.333***	−.298***	.373***	−.267***	.277***	1	
13. Depression	.014	.321***	.234***	.048	.115*	.041	.000	−.045	.075	−.037	.058	.132*	1
M	44.27	11.94	11.66	7.28	6.35	8.96	13.69	24.24	14.50	28.69	1.51	2.85	17.36
SD	7.50	8.93	9.24	3.26	3.50	4.73	7.36	10.40	7.68	8.91	1.13	1.19	5.21

*$p < .05$. **$p < .01$. ***$p < .001$.

The simultaneous regression model using the four PBI scales to predict adult attachment anxiety was significant, $F(5, 280) = 15.97, p < .001, R^2 = .22$. In terms of their unique contributions to the variance in adult attachment anxiety, father and mother control were positive predictors ($\beta = .12, t = 1.9, p = .05, sr^2 = .01$ and $\beta = .27, t = 4.2, p < .001, sr^2 = .05$, respectively), whereas father care was a negative predictor ($\beta = -.21, t = -3.5, p < .001, sr^2 = .03$) and mother care was not a significant unique contributor. Similarly, the simultaneous regression model using PBI variables to predict adult attachment avoidance was significant, $F(5, 280) = 19.94, p < .001, R^2 = .26$, indicating that father and mother care ($\beta = -.28, t = -4.8, p < .001, sr^2 = .06$ and $\beta = -.34, t = -5.8, p < .001, sr^2 = .09$, respectively), but not father and mother control, each significantly and negatively contributed to the variance in attachment avoidance.

The combination of five CTQ scales in the third simultaneous regression significantly predicted adult attachment anxiety, $F(6, 279) = 11.82, p < .001, R^2 = .20$, but Emotional Abuse emerged as the only significant predictor of unique variance in adult attachment anxiety ($\beta = .50, t = 5.1, p < .001, sr^2 = .08$). For adult attachment avoidance, the regression model with all five CTQ scales was significant, $F(6, 279) = 14.80, p < .001, R^2 = .24$. Both Emotional Abuse and Emotional Neglect were significant unique contributors to the variance ($\beta = .26, t = 2.8, p < .01, sr^2 = .02$ and $\beta = .21, t = 2.2, p < .05, sr^2 = .01$, respectively).

Based on theoretical constructs supported by previous research, a series of hierarchical multiple regression analyses were conducted to test the primary hypotheses regarding the contributions of childhood emotional maltreatment, adult attachment styles, and depression to the prediction of romantic relationship functioning as assessed by DAS Total Adjustment, CTS Psychological Aggression by Self, and CTS Psychological Aggression by Partner. The control variables (gender, length of relationship, physical abuse, sexual abuse) were entered in the first step of the regression. The second step of the regressions included either CTQ Emotional Abuse or the four PBI scales (i.e., Father Control, Father Care, Mother Control, Mother Care) to represent childhood emotional maltreatment by parents. The ECR Attachment and Avoidance scales were added in the third step as measures of attachment style, followed by the HSCL Depression scale in the fourth and final step of the equation.

The first set of hierarchical multiple regressions used DAS Total Adjustment as the outcome variable. The full model of the first regression included the four control variables, Emotional Abuse, the two attachment styles, and depression as predictors in four steps. Results of the full model were significant, $F(8, 276) = 15.69, p < .001, R^2 = .31$, and are presented in Table 2. After controlling for gender, relationship length, and other forms of maltreatment, the entry of Emotional Abuse in the second step showed a significant change in effect size, increasing the variance accounted for by

TABLE 2 Multiple Regressions for DAS-Total, CTS Psychological Aggression-Self, and CTS Psychological Aggression-Partner

Criterion	Step/Predictors	*df*	R^2	*F*	Initial β	Final β	R^2 change
DAS Total Adjustment	1. Gender	4, 280	.06	4.21**	.07	.12*	.057**
	Sexual abuse				.07	.13*	
	Physical abuse				–.18*	.08	
	Relationship length				–.13*	–.23***	
	2. Emotional abuse	5, 279	.14	9.38***	–.39***	–.12	.087***
	3. ECR Avoidance	7, 277	.31	17.89***	–.37***	–.37***	.167***
	ECR Anxiety				–.25***	–.26***	
	4. Depression	8, 276	.31	15.69***	.03	.03	.001
DAS Total Adjustment	1. Gender	4, 280	.06	4.21**	.07	.11*	.057**
	Sexual abuse				.07	.12*	
	Physical abuse				–.18**	.07	
	Relationship length				–.13*	–.22***	
	2. Father Control	8, 276	.14	5.76***	.004	.07	.086***
	Father Care				.17**	.02	
	Mother Control				–.06	–.03	
	Mother Care				.22**	.11	
	3. ECR Avoidance	10, 274	.32	12.64***	–.37***	–.37***	.173***
	ECR Anxiety				–.28***	–.28***	
	4. Depression	11, 273	.32	11.55***	.04	.04	.002
CTS Psych Aggression - Self	1. Gender	4, 280	.033	2.41*	.13*	.11*	.033*
	Sexual abuse				.11†	.07	
	Physical abuse				–.04	–.08	
	Relationship length				.005	.05	
	2. Emotional abuse	5, 279	.034	1.98†	–.04	–.03	.001
	3. ECR Avoidance	7, 277	.059	2.48*	.03	.02	.025*
	ECR Anxiety				.17**	.13*	
	4. Depression	8, 276	.141	5.68***	.29***	.29***	.083***
CTS Psych Aggression - Self	1. Gender	4, 280	.03	2.41*	.13*	.10†	.033*
	Sexual abuse				.11	.06	
	Physical abuse				–.04	–.07	
	Relationship length				.005	.06	

	2. Father Control	8, 276	.04	1.39	.08	.10	.005
	Father Care				.002	.06	
	Mother Control				−.04	−.11	
	Mother Care				−.03	−.02	
	3. ECR Avoidance	10, 274	.06	1.85*	.02	.01	.025*
	ECR Anxiety				.18**	.14*	
	4. Depression	11, 273	.15	4.42***	.30***	.30***	.088***
CTS Psych Aggression - Partner	1. Gender	4, 280	.03	2.10†	.10†	.09	.029†
	Sexual abuse				.12†	.09	
	Physical abuse				−.07	−.07	
	Relationship length				.04	.08	
	2. Emotional abuse	5, 279	.03	4.67	.001	−.08	.000
	3. ECR Avoidance	7, 277	.06	2.35*	.02	.01	.027*
	ECR Anxiety				.18**	.16*	
	4. Depression	8, 276	.10	3.71***	.21***	.21***	.041***
CTS Psych Aggression – Partner	1. Gender	4, 280	.03	2.10†	.10†	.09	.029†
	Sexual abuse				.12†	.10	
	Physical abuse				−.07	−.08	
	Relationship length				.04	.09	
	2. Father Control	8, 276	.03	1.09	−.02	−.02	.001
	Father Care				−.02	.03	
	Mother Control				.02	−.04	
	Mother Care				.04	.05	
	3. ECR Avoidance	10, 274	.06	1.73†	.03	.02	.029*
	ECR Anxiety				.19**	.17**	
	4. Depression	11, 273	.10	2.78**	.21***	.21***	.042***

Note: DAS = Dyadic Adjustment Scale; CTS = Conflict Tactics Scale; ECR = Experiences in Close Relationships Scale.
†$p < .10$. *$p < .05$. **$p < .01$. ***$p < .001$.

8%. In the third step, the inclusion of the attachment style variables in the equation produced another highly significant change in effect size, adding 17% to the explained variance. Including the HSCL Depression scores in the fourth step did not significantly improve the model, which accounted for a total of 31% of the variance in DAS Total Adjustment. Results of the full model indicated that higher levels of adult attachment avoidance (sr^2 = .10) and anxiety (sr^2 = .05), longer relationship length (sr^2 = .05), being male (sr^2 = .01), and a history of childhood sexual abuse (sr^2 = .01) were significant predictors of lower DAS Adjustment scores. Despite significantly and negatively contributing to the variance when initially entered in the equation, physical abuse and emotional abuse dropped to nonsignificance in the second and third steps, respectively. Conversely, gender and childhood sexual abuse were nonsignificant in the first step, but increased to significance in the second and third steps, respectively, and remained significant contributors in the full regression model.

The full model of the second hierarchical regression predicting DAS Total Adjustment included the four control variables, PBI mother and father Care and Control, the two attachment styles, and depression as predictors in four steps. Results of the full model were significant, $F(11, 273) = 11.55$, $p < .001$, $R^2 = .32$ (see Table 2). After accounting for the control variables, the addition of the PBI variables in the second step increased the effect size by 8%, representing a significant change in the variance explained. When attachment avoidance and anxiety were entered in the third step, the effect size rose significantly by 18%. However, no significant change was noted when depression was added in the fourth step. Similar to the previous regression, the results of the full hierarchical model indicated that lower DAS Total Adjustment scores were significantly related to higher levels of adult attachment avoidance (sr^2 = .09) and anxiety (sr^2 = .06), longer relationship length (sr^2 = .04), being male (sr^2 = .01), and a history of childhood sexual abuse (sr^2 = .01). Although childhood physical abuse and both mother and father Care were significant predictors when first entered into the equation, these variables dropped to nonsignificance in the second and third steps, respectively. Once again, gender and childhood sexual abuse were nonsignificant in the first and second steps, but increased to significance in the third step after attachment anxiety and avoidance were entered into the equation, and they remained significant contributors in the full regression model.

The second set of hierarchical regressions used CTS Psychological Aggression perpetrated by the respondent as the outcome variable. In the first regression of this set, the predictors were entered in four steps and included the four control variables, Emotional Abuse, the two attachment styles, and depression. The full model for Psychological Aggression-Self was significant, $F(8, 276) = 5.69$, $p < .001$, $R^2 = .14$ (see Table 2). Contrary to predictions, the inclusion of Emotional Abuse in the second step did not significantly increase the 3% of the variance accounted for in the first step by the control variables (specifically gender). However, the addition of the two attachment styles in the third step significantly improved the model, accounting for an additional 2.5% of the variance. The biggest jump in effect size occurred when depression was included in the final step, adding 8% to the variance accounted for in Psychological Aggression-Self. Results of the full hierarchical model indicated that higher depression scores (sr^2 = .08), higher adult attachment anxiety (sr^2 = .01), and being female (sr^2 = .01) were significant predictors of higher Psychological Aggression-Self scores.

The full model of the second hierarchical regression predicting CTS Psychological Aggression-Self included the four control variables, PBI mother and father Care and Control, the two attachment styles, and depression as predictors in four steps. The full regression model was significant, $F(11, 273) = 4.42$, $p < .001$, $R^2 = .15$ (see Table 2), and similar to the previous analysis. Specifically, the addition of the mother and father Care and Control scales in the second step did not significantly increase the effect size, but both the third and fourth step significantly improved the model. Results of the full hierarchical model indicated that higher levels of depressive symptoms and adult attachment anxiety significantly contributed to higher Psychological Aggression-Self scores (sr^2 = .09 and sr^2 = .01, respectively). Although female gender was a significant predictor in the first step of the equation, it dropped to nonsignificance in the third step after the attachment scales were entered.

The third set of hierarchical multiple regressions used the respondents' reports of Psychological Aggression perpetrated on them by their partners (i.e., victimization) as the outcome variable. The full model of the initial regression in this set included the four control variables, Emotional Abuse, the two attachment styles, and depression as predictors in four steps. The full regression model for Psychological Aggression-Partner was significant, $F(8, 276) = 3.71$, $p < .001$, $R^2 = .10$ (see Table 2). The first two steps of the equation were nonsignificant. However, the addition of the two attachment styles in the third step significantly improved the model, accounting for an additional 3% of the variance. The entry of depression in the fourth step significantly increased the variance accounted for by 4%. Only HSCL depression (sr^2 = .04) and ECR attachment anxiety (sr^2 = .02) emerged as significant positive predictors of Psychological Aggression-Partner. The second analysis for Psychological Aggression-Partner replaced Emotional Abuse with the four PBI scales in the second step, but otherwise was the same. The full hierarchical regression model was also significant, $F(11, 273) = 2.78$, $p < .001$, $R^2 = .10$ (see Table 2), with higher levels of depressive symptoms (sr^2 = .04) and adult attachment anxiety (sr^2 = .02) emerging once again as significant predictors of Psychological Aggression-Partner scores.

DISCUSSION

Findings were mixed, with some hypotheses clearly supported by the results, whereas others were not. First, the hypothesis that a history of childhood emotional maltreatment directly predicts insecure adult attachment style was consistently supported. However, when testing the full models predicting romantic relationship outcomes, the contribution of childhood emotional maltreatment by parents varied considerably. Consistent with hypotheses, adult attachment style emerged as an important predictor of relationship adjustment, psychological aggression, and psychological victimization. Finally, although depression was not a significant predictor of overall relationship adjustment, it proved to be the most influential factor in the models for reported psychological aggression by self and partner. Findings are discussed in light of theory and research, beginning with the direct associations found between childhood experiences and adult attachment style, followed by the results for the full hierarchical regression models, and concluding with limitations and recommendations for future research.

Direct Associations: Childhood Emotional Maltreatment and Adult Attachment Style

First the direct relationship of early parenting experiences with adult attachment styles was examined. When the CTQ was used to operationalize childhood maltreatment, results indicated that together the five scales accounted for 20% of the variance in attachment anxiety and 24% of the variance in attachment avoidance. However, only the emotional maltreatment variables accounted for a significant amount of unique variance in the prediction of adult attachment style. Specifically, emotional abuse uniquely predicted high levels of adult attachment anxiety, whereas emotional abuse and emotional neglect uniquely predicted high levels of attachment avoidance. Taken together, these findings are consistent with previous suggestions that emotional maltreatment might be comparatively more harmful with respect to its impact on the adult romantic attachment system (Allen, 2001; McGee & Wolfe, 1991; Riggs, 2010). That is, although all forms of childhood maltreatment can be significantly related to insecure adult attachment outcomes when examined alone, only emotional maltreatment appears to add additional risk when the negative effects of other forms of maltreatment are considered.

To more closely examine the continuum of childhood treatment by both mothers and fathers, the PBI was also used, with low scores on the Care scale conceptualized as excessive coldness or rejection and high scores on the Control scale conceptualized as intrusive overcontrol, both forms of emotional abuse identified in the literature. Like previous retrospective research (Feeney & Noller, 1990; Hazan & Shaver, 1987; Rothbard & Shaver, 1994), adults who reported higher levels of attachment anxiety and avoidance in their romantic relationships generally recalled their parents as being more rejecting, more controlling, or both than did other participants in this sample. Together, the PBI scales predicted more than 20% of the variance in adult attachment anxiety and more than 25% of the variance in adult attachment avoidance. When examining unique variance accounted for by the PBI scales, results indicated that high levels of both mother and father Control were significant predictors of adult attachment anxiety, but not adult attachment avoidance. These findings are consistent with early research and theory (e.g., Ainsworth et al., 1978; Bowlby, 1973), suggesting that inconsistent and intrusive parental behavior engenders ambivalent infant attachment, which is the expected precursor to negative models of self and attachment anxiety in adults. Maternal overcontrol was an especially strong predictor, uniquely accounting for 5% of the variance in attachment anxiety, versus only 1% accounted for by paternal overcontrol. However, memories of greater rejection (low Care) by fathers, but not mothers, also contributed uniquely to attachment anxiety. In contrast, an examination of unique contributions to adult attachment avoidance indicated that low ratings of both mother and father on the Care dimension were significant predictors, which is consistent with previous theory and research (Ainsworth et al., 1978; Main & Hesse, 1990; Main, Kaplan, & Cassidy, 1985) indicating that parental rejection or neglect contributes to avoidant infant attachment, the expected precursor to negative models of others and attachment avoidance in adults.

A final consideration is the relative strength of maternal and paternal abuse and neglect variables on each type of insecure adult attachment. A summary of the relevant squared semipartial correlations (i.e., sr^2) across analyses suggests that maternal variables account for 15% of the unique variance in insecure adult attachment and paternal variables uniquely account for 11%. Additional research is needed to determine if emotional maltreatment by mothers has more of a negative impact on future adult attachment than similar treatment by fathers. This hypothesis is reasonable given that mothers continue to be in the role of primary caregiver more often than fathers, so their impact on the attachment system is greater. Thus, the failure of a mother to respond sensitively and her actions that psychologically injure her child might have more of a negative impact than if that same maltreatment came from the secondary caregiver. An exception in the data was the unique impact of paternal rejection or neglect on anxious adult attachment style. It is possible that maternal overcontrol, but not rejection, is the key ingredient that contributes to the development of attachment anxiety, whereas any kind of aversive treatment by fathers, whether controlling or intrusive or rejecting or neglecting, might increase the risk for anxious adult attachment style. Further research is needed, however, to explain why a lack of paternal warmth and care, but not a lack of maternal warmth and care, was uniquely predictive of anxious adult attachment style.

Contributions of Emotional Maltreatment, Adult Attachment, and Depression to Relational Outcomes

The models hypothesized that childhood emotional maltreatment, adult attachment style, and symptoms of depression would each account for significant additional variance in dyadic adjustment, perpetration of psychological aggression, and psychological victimization. Because the results of the analyses employing the CTQ and the PBI were so similar, they are discussed simultaneously.

Accounting for an additional 9% of the variance, emotional abuse was a significant predictor of dyadic adjustment above and beyond that of the covariates, including the other maltreatment variables. This finding is consistent with previous research demonstrating the unique effects of childhood emotional abuse compared to physical or sexual abuse (Briere & Runtz, 1988, 1990; Gross & Keller, 1992). However, when the adult attachment variables were added in the third step of the DAS model, not only did they predict significant additional variance as expected based on previous theory and research (e.g., Collins & Read, 1990; Senchak & Leonard, 1992), but their inclusion nullified the unique impact of the childhood maltreatment variables entered in the second step. Although no firm conclusions can be drawn based on the specific type of analyses conducted, this pattern in the data suggests that future researchers might wish to test potential meditation effects of adult attachment style on the relationship between childhood emotional maltreatment on adult dyadic functioning. Such a finding is consistent with the idea that emotional maltreatment profoundly affects the adult attachment system, which in turn affects the quality of romantic relationships. Moreover, these findings suggest that when people are able to develop secure romantic attachment styles, they have a better chance of circumventing the negative outcomes stemming from childhood maltreatment and associated insecure parent–child attachment patterns. The additional finding that gender and sexual abuse initially were nonsignificant, but became significant when the adult attachment styles were included, is intriguing but also puzzling. Once again, the analyses prevent specific interpretations, but one tentative explanation suggests that although these two variables do not directly contribute to romantic relationship functioning per se, they might interact with adult attachment style to produce different outcomes. Future research might productively explore the potential mediating and moderating role of romantic attachment style when examining associations between childhood maltreatment and adult relationship functioning.

The hypothesis that depression would further contribute to the DAS model when added in the fourth step was not upheld. Moreover, these two variables were not even significantly correlated. This finding is contrary to previous research demonstrating associations between depression and romantic relationship functioning (Christian et al., 1994; Schmaling & Jacobson, 1990). One possible explanation is that this study used cross-sectional data and tested a unidirectional model, so any mutual influence or interaction between mental health and relationship functioning over time was not measured. It is conceivable that the association between adult relationship dysfunction and depression is bidirectional and strengthens over time, with poor relational functioning contributing to depressive symptoms as much as the reverse and the two interacting to exacerbate both the individual's and the couple's problems. If this is the case, a statistical relationship between depression and romantic relationship functioning might not yet be apparent in this college student sample who, although required to have been in a romantic relationship for 5 months or more to participate, reported a modal relationship length of 8 months. This explanation is consistent with the current finding of a negative association between length of the dating relationship and overall dyadic adjustment (i.e., the longer partners dated, the lower they rated the quality of their romantic relationship).

The last two sets of hierarchical regressions used the same independent variables to test predictive models for psychological aggression perpetrated by the self or the partner. The findings contrasted sharply with the results for the DAS analyses, but the pattern of results for each of the psychological aggression models was similar, with the relative contributions of the first three sets of independent variables (i.e., the covariates, emotional maltreatment, and adult attachment) to the prediction of psychological aggression and psychological victimization almost identical. Most important, despite what previous research and theory would predict (e.g., Berzenski & Yates, in press; Crawford & Wright, 2007; Wekerle & Wolfe, 1998), neither the CTQ scales nor the PBI scales significantly contributed to outcomes. However, attachment anxiety emerged as a unique predictor of both psychological aggression and victimization, lending support to theoretical conjectures that negative models of self are related to abusive behaviors in romantic relationships due to chronic fears of rejection and abandonment that trigger anger, jealousy, and violence (Dutton et al., 1994). In contrast, avoidant attachment style did not contribute uniquely to psychological aggression or victimization, which was surprising given previous findings that attachment avoidance, especially fearful attachment (which combines both attachment anxiety and avoidance) is related to verbal and psychological aggression in couple relationships (Dutton et al., 1994; Wekerle & Wolfe, 1998). Discrepancies between current findings and previous research might be related to sample differences and varying operational definitions of constructs. For example, Wekerle and Wolfe (1998) used a younger population of high school students and found attachment avoidance only relevant to female aggression and victimization. The latter study also operationalized adult attachment style using a less sophisticated measure with weaker psychometric properties (i.e., Hazan & Shaver's [1987] original three-category instrument) and created a total childhood maltreatment score by combining observations of domestic violence with physical and sexual abuse. A final consideration is that college students with the high levels of attachment avoidance might be less likely than their peers to be in long-term relationships, and therefore, underrepresented among the sample reported here.

The total variance accounted for by the combination of all maltreatment and adult attachment predictors in both sets of psychological aggression models was modest (i.e., ~6%), and it was not until symptoms of depression were added in the fourth step that the effect size became noteworthy. The strength of the effect of depression in the two models differed, however, such that the additional variance explained by depression for psychological victimization (i.e., ~4%) was less than half of what was observed in the prediction of psychological aggression (i.e., ~8–9%). Once again, these findings diverge substantially from the results of the DAS analyses. Specifically, although depression did not contribute to overall dyadic adjustment in dating relationships, it did contribute to psychological aggression, especially female perpetration of psychological aggression against a partner. Although the evidence is mixed, current findings are consistent with previous research demonstrating that depressive symptomatology is associated with high levels of total anger and overt expression of hostility (Koh, Kim, & Park, 2002) and an increased probability of severe aggression toward a spouse (Feldbau-Kohn, Heyman, & O'Leary, 1998; Pan, Neidig, & O'Leary, 1994). Bowlby (1973) proposed that attachment models play a critical role in the experience of anger. In the context of secure attachment, anger can be conceptualized as a functional protest reaction to others' negative attachment behavior; however, in the context of insecure attachment models, the angry protest response can be based on distorted perceptions and exaggerated to the degree that it becomes dysfunctional and damaging to adult attachment relationships. Current findings specifically suggest that anxiously attached females who are depressed might tend to express overt anger toward dating partners in a psychologically abusive manner and to experience similar abuse from partners.

Limitations and Recommendations

Like all cross-sectional research, this study is correlational in nature and no causal conclusions can be drawn. This is particularly true for associations between depression and relational outcomes; the direction or mutual interaction of these two variables remains a question for future research. In addition, retrospective reports of childhood emotional maltreatment might have introduced subjective biases related to faulty memories or lack of self-disclosure. In particular, this study did not use any corroborating evidence of childhood emotional maltreatment. Longitudinal studies following maltreated infants with disorganized attachment relationships are ongoing (e.g., Lyons-Ruth, Melnick, Bronfman, Sherry, & Llanas, 2004; Lyons-Ruth, Repacholi, McLeod, & Silva, 1991) and will hopefully continue to be funded to address important questions regarding the impact of emotional abuse on adult functioning and romantic relationships (see Dodge Reyome, in press).

The exclusive use of self-report instruments also creates the potential for biased reporting and inflated findings due to common method variance. Possibly the most parsimonious explanation for the unexpected findings related to psychological aggression is because of this study's reliance on self-report data. Many individuals might not be accurate reporters of the frequency with which they psychologically mistreat their romantic partners. Such inaccuracies could be a result of unconscious psychological defenses, a social desirability bias, a genuine lack of awareness, or some combination of all of these reasons. Another limitation of this study is sample characteristics that constrain generalizability to college students in dating relationships. Future researchers could strengthen a replication of this study by using a diverse community sample with greater variability in age and length of relationship or commitment. Oversampling participants with known histories of childhood maltreatment or psychological aggression in their current romantic relationship and assessing social desirability might also be helpful. Finally, to minimize self-report bias and common method variance, researchers could include alternative assessment methods, such as interviews (e.g., Adult Attachment Interview, structured diagnostic interviews) and reports from both romantic partners regarding their own and their partner's behavior.

Taken as a whole, the findings reported here support a theoretical model linking emotional maltreatment in childhood to insecure romantic attachment in adulthood. In turn, insecure adult attachment style significantly contributed to overall relationship adjustment, psychological aggression, and psychological victimization. In particular, attachment anxiety characterized by negative internal models of self predicted psychological aggression and victimization. Further research is needed to explore the potential mediating or moderating role of adult attachment in explaining the links between childhood emotional abuse and romantic relationship functioning. In addition, although previous research clearly supports links among insecure adult attachment, depression, and poor relationship functioning (e.g., Carnelley et al., 1994; Cole-Detke & Kobak, 1996; Collins & Read, 1990; Shaver, Schachner, & Mikulincer, 2005), in this study, mixed findings regarding the differential predictive power of depression in overall relationship adjustment versus more specific forms of maladjustment (i.e., psychological aggression) suggest that further study is warranted to clarify the role of depression in romantic relationships. Specifically, although adult attachment likely contributes to both mental health and relational adjustment, the directionality of associations between the latter two constructs remains a question for future longitudinal research.

REFERENCES

Ainsworth, M. D. S., Blehar, M. C., Waters, E., & Wall, S. (1978). *Patterns of attachment: A psychological study of the strange situation.* Oxford, UK: Lawrence Erlbaum Associates.

Allen, J. A. (2001). *Traumatic relationships and serious mental disorders.* Chichester, UK: Wiley.

Arias, I., & Pape, K. (1999). Psychological abuse: Implications for adjustment and commitment to leave violent partners. *Violence and Victims, 14*(1), 55–67.

Bartholomew, K., & Horowitz, L. M. (1991). Attachment styles among young adults: A test of four-category model. *Journal of Personality and Social Psychology, 61*, 226–244.

Bemporad, J. R., & Romano, S. J. (1992). Childhood maltreatment and adult depression: A review of research. In D. Cicchetti & S. L. Toth (Eds.), *Rochester Symposium on Developmental Psychopathology: Vol. 4. Developmental perspectives on depression* (pp. 351–375). Rochester, NY: University of Rochester Press.

Bernstein, D. P. (2002). Cognitive therapy of personality disorders in patients with histories of emotional abuse or neglect. *Psychiatric Annals, 32*, 618–628.

Bernstein, D., & Fink, L. (1998). *Childhood Trauma Questionnaire: A retrospective self-report manual.* San Antonio, TX: Psychological Corporation.

Berzenski, S. R., & Yates, T. M. (in press). A developmental process analysis of the contribution of childhood emotional abuse to relationship violence. *Journal of Aggression, Maltreatment and Trauma.*

Blatt, S. J., & Levy, K. N. (2003). Attachment theory, psychoanalysis, personality development and psychopathology. *Psychoanalytic Inquiry, 23*, 102–150.

Bowlby, J. (1969). *Attachment and loss: Vol. 1. Attachment.* New York: Basic Books

Bowlby, J. (1973). *Attachment and loss: Vol. 2. Separation.* New York: Basic Books.

Bowlby, J. (1980). *Attachment and loss: Vol. 3. Loss.* New York: Basic Books.

Brennan, K. A., Clark, C. L., & Shaver, P. R. (1998). Self-report measurement of adult attachment: An integrative overview. In J. A. Simpson & W. S. Rholes (Eds.), *Attachment theory and close relationships* (pp. 46–76). New York: Guilford.

Brennan, K. A., & Shaver, P. R. (1998). Attachment styles and personality disorders: Their connections to each other and to parental divorce, parental death, and perceptions of parental caregiving. *Journal of Personality, 66*, 835–878.

Briere, J., & Runtz, M. (1988). Multivariate correlates of childhood psychological and physical maltreatment among university women. *Child Abuse & Neglect, 12*, 331–341.

Briere, J., & Runtz, M. (1990). Differential adult symptomatology associated with three types of child abuse histories. *Child Abuse & Neglect, 14*, 257–364.

Brown, G. W., & Harris, T. (1978). *Social origins of depression: A study of psychiatric disorders in women.* New York: Free Press.

Carbone, D. J. (2010). Using cognitive therapies to treat unstable attachment patterns in adults with childhood histories of social rejection. *Journal of Aggression, Maltreatment and Trauma, 19*(1), 105–134.

Carlson, E. A., & Sroufe, L. A. (1995). Contributions of attachment theory to developmental psychopathology. In E. Cicchetti & D. J. Cohen (Eds.), *Developmental psychopathology* (Vol. 1, pp. 581–617). New York: Wiley.

Carnelley, K., Peitromonaco, P., & Jaffe, K. (1994). Depression, working models of others, and relationship functioning. *Journal of Personality and Social Psychology, 66*, 127–140.

Caspi, A., & Elder, G. H. (1988). Developmental history, personality, and family relationships: Toward an emergent family system. In R. Hinde & J. Stevenson-Hinde (Eds.), *Relationships within families: Mutual influences* (pp. 218–240). Oxford, UK: Oxford University Press.

Christian, J. L., O'Leary, K. D., & Vivian, D. (1994). Depressive symptomatology in maritally discordant women and men: The role of individual and relationship variables. *Journal of Family Psychology, 8*, 32–42.

Cicchetti, D., & Rizley, R. (1981). Developmental perspectives on the etiology, intergenerational transmission, and sequelae of child maltreatment. *New Directions for Child Development, 111*, 35–55.

Clemmons, J. (2005). *Multiple forms of child maltreatment and abuse-specific characteristics: Relationships to adult adjustment.* Unpublished doctoral dissertation, University of Nebraska, Lincoln, NE.

Cohn, D. A., Cowan, P. A., Cowan, C. P., & Pearson, J. (1992). Mothers' and fathers' working models of childhood attachment relationships, parenting styles, and child behavior. *Development and Psychopathology, 4*, 417–431.

Cole-Detke, H., & Kobak, R. (1996). Attachment processes in eating disorder and depression. *Journal of Consulting and Clinical Psychology, 64*, 282–290.

Collins, N., & Read, S. (1990). Adult attachment relationships, working models, and relationship quality in dating couples. *Journal of Personality and Social Psychology, 58*, 644–683.

Collins, W. A., & Sroufe, L. A. (1999). Capacity for intimate relationships: A developmental construction. In W. Furman, B. B. Brown, & C. Feiring (Eds.), *The development of romantic relationships in adolescence* (pp. 125–147). New York: Cambridge University Press.

Crawford, E., & Wright, M. O. (2007). The impact of childhood psychological maltreatment on interpersonal schemas and subsequent experiences of relationship aggression. *Journal of Emotional Abuse, 7*, 93–116.

Crowell, J. A., Fraley, R. C., & Shaver, P. R. (1999). Measurement of individual differences in adolescent and adult attachment. In J. Cassidy & P. Shaver (Eds.), *Handbook of attachment: Theory, research, and clinical applications* (pp. 434–465). New York: Guilford.

Davis, J. L., Petretic-Jackson, P. A., & Ting, L. (2001). Intimacy dysfunction and trauma symptomatology: Long-term correlates of different types of child abuse. *Journal of Traumatic Stress, 14*, 63–79.

Derogatis, L. R., Lipman, R. S., & Covi, L. (1973). SCL-90: An outpatient psychiatric rating scale-preliminary report. *Psychopharmacology Bulletin, 9*, 13–27.

DeWolff, M. S., & van IJzendoorn, M. (1997). Sensitivity and attachment: A meta-analysis on parental antecedents of infant attachment. *Child Development, 68*, 571–591.

Diehl, M., Elnick, A., Bourbeau, L., & Labouvie-Vief, G. (1998). Adult attachment styles: Their relations to family context and personality. *Journal of Personality and Social Psychology, 74*, 1656–1669.

DiLillo, D. (2001). Interpersonal functioning among women reporting a history of childhood sexual abuse: Empirical findings and methodological issues. *Clinical Psychology Review, 21*, 553–576.

DiLillo, D., Lewis, T., & Di Loreto-Colgan, A. (2007). Child maltreatment history and subsequent romantic relationships: Exploring a psychological route to dyadic difficulties. *Journal of Aggression, Maltreatment and Trauma, 15*, 19–36.

Dodge Reyome, N. (in press). Childhood emotional maltreatment and later intimate relationships: Themes from the empirical literature. *Journal of Aggression, Maltreatment and Trauma*.

Dodge Reyome, N., Ward, K. S., & Witkiewitz, K. (in press). Psychosocial variables as mediators of the relationship between childhood emotional maltreatment, codependency, and self silencing. *Journal of Aggression, Maltreatment and Trauma*.

Dozier, M., Stovall, C., & Albus, K. (1999). Attachment and psychopathology in adulthood. In J. Cassidy & P. Shaver (Eds.), *Handbook of attachment: Theory, research, and clinical applications* (pp. 497–519). New York: Guilford.

Dutton, D. G., Saunders, K., Starzomski, A., & Bartholomew, K. (1994). Intimacy-anger and insecure attachment as precursors of abuse in intimate relationships. *Journal of Applied Social Psychology, 24*, 1367–1386.

Eiden, R. D., Teti, D. M., & Corns, K. M. (1995). Maternal working models of attachment, marital adjustment, and the parent–child relationship. *Child Development, 66*, 1504–1518.

Eng, W., Heimberg, R. G., Hart, T. A., Schneier, F. R., & Liebowitz, M. R. (2001). Attachment in individuals with social anxiety disorder: The relationship among adult attachment styles, social anxiety, and depression. *Emotion, 1*, 365–380.

Feeney, J. A., & Noller, P. (1990). Attachment style as a predictor of adult romantic relationships. *Journal of Personality and Social Psychology, 58*, 281–291.

Feldbau-Kohn, S., Heyman, R. E., & O'Leary, K. (1998). Major depressive disorder and depressive symptomatology as predictors of husband to wife physical aggression. *Violence and Victims, 13*, 347–360.

Florian, V., Mikulincer, M., & Burcholtz, I. (1995). Effects of adult attachment style on the perception and search for social support. *Journal of Psychology, 129*, 665–676.

Follingstad, D. R., Rutledge, L., Berg, B. J., Hause, E. S., & Polek, D. S. (1990). The role of emotional abuse in physically abusive relationships. *Journal of Family Violence, 5*, 107–120.

Foran, H., & O'Leary, K. (2008). Alcohol and intimate partner violence: A meta-analytic review. *Clinical Psychology Review, 28*, 1222–1234.

Garbarino, J., Guttman, E., & Seely, J. W. (1986). *The psychologically battered child: Strategies for identification, assessment, and intervention.* San Francisco: Jossey-Bass.

Garmezy, N. (1987). Stress, competence, and development: Continuities in the study of schizophrenic adults, children vulnerable to psychopathology, and the search for stress-resistant children. *American Journal of Orthopsychiatry, 57*, 159–174.

Gauthier, L., Stollak, G., Messe, L., & Aronoff, J. (1996). Recall of childhood neglect and physical abuse as differential predictors of current psychological functioning. *Child Abuse & Neglect, 21*, 549–559.

Gilbert, L., El-Bassel, N., Schilling, R. F., & Friedman, E. (1997). Childhood abuse as a risk for partner abuse among women in methadone maintenance. *American Journal of Drug and Alcohol Abuse, 23*, 581–595.

Greenberg, M. T. (1999). Attachment and psychopathology in childhood. In J. Cassidy & P. R. Shaver (Eds.), *Handbook of attachment: Theory, research, and clinical applications* (pp. 469–496). New York: Guilford.

Gross, A. B., & Keller, H. R. (1992). Long-term consequences of childhood physical and psychological maltreatment. *Aggressive Behavior, 18*, 171–185.

Hart, S. N., Brassard, M. R., Binggeli, N. J., & Davidson, H. A. (2002). Psychological maltreatment. In J. E. B. Myers, L. Berliner, J. Briere, C. T. Hendrix, C. Jenny, et al. (Eds.), *The APSAC handbook on child maltreatment* (2nd ed., pp. 79–103). Thousand Oaks, CA: Sage.

Hazan, C., & Shaver, P. (1987). Romantic love conceptualized as an attachment process. *Journal of Personality and Social Psychology, 52*, 511–524.

Kaufman, J. (1991). Depressive disorders in maltreated children. *Journal of the American Academy of Child and Adolescent Psychiatry, 30*, 257–265.

Koh, K. B., Kim, C. H., & Park, J. K. (2002). Predominance of anger in depressive disorders compared with anxiety disorders and somatoform disorders. *Journal of Clinical Psychiatry, 63*, 486–492.

Lopez, F., Melendez, M., Sauer, E., Berger, E., & Wyssmann, J. (1998). IWMs, self-reported problems, and help-seeking attitudes among college students. *Journal of Counseling Psychology, 45*, 79–83.

Losel, F., & Bliesener, T. (1994). Some high-risk adolescents do not develop conduct problems: A study of protective factors. *International Journal of Behavior Development, 17*, 753–777.

Lyons-Ruth, K., & Block, D. (1996). The disturbed caregiving system: Relations among childhood trauma, maternal caregiving, and infant affect and attachment. *Infant Mental Health Journal, 17*, 257–275.

Lyons-Ruth, K., Melnick, S., Bronfman, E., Sherry, S., & Llanas, L. (2004). Hostile-helpless relational models and disorganized attachment patterns between parents and their young children: Review of research and implications for clinical work. In L. Atkinson & S. Goldberg (Eds.), *Attachment issues in psychopathology and intervention* (pp. 65–94). Mahwah, NJ: Lawrence Erlbaum Associates, Inc.

Lyons-Ruth, K., Repacholi, B., McLeod, S., & Silva, E. (1991). Disorganized attachment behavior in infancy: Short-term stability, maternal and infant correlates, and risk-related subtypes. *Development and Psychopathology, 3*, 377–396.

Main, M., & Hesse, E. (1990). Parents' unresolved traumatic experiences are related to infant disorganized attachment status: Is frightened and/or frightening parental behavior the linking mechanism? In M. T. Greenberg, D. Cicchetti, & E. M. Cummings (Eds.), *Attachment in the preschool years* (pp. 161–182). Chicago: University of Chicago Press.

Main, M., Kaplan, N., & Cassidy, J. (1985). Security in infancy, childhood and adulthood: A move to the level of representation. In I. Bretherton & E. Waters

(Eds.), *Growing points of attachment theory and research* (pp. 66–104). *Monographs of the Society for Research in Child Development, 50*(1–2, Serial No. 209).

Masten, A. S., Morison, P., Pellegrini, D., & Tellegen, A. (1990). Competence under stress: Risk and protective factors. In J. Rolf, J. Matsen, J. Cicchetti, K. Nuechterlein, & S. Weintraub (Eds.), *Risk and protective factors in the development of psychopathology* (pp. 236–256). New York: Cambridge University Press.

McCloskey, L. A. (2001). The Medea complex among men: The instrumental abuse of children to injure wives. *Violence and Victims, 16*, 1–19.

McGee, R. A., & Wolfe, D. A. (1991). Psychological maltreatment: Toward an operational definition. *Development and Psychopathology, 3*, 3–18.

Messman-Moore, T. L., & Coates, A. A. (2007). The impact of childhood psychological abuse on adult interpersonal conflict: The role of early maladaptive schemas and patterns of interpersonal behavior. *Journal of Emotional Abuse, 7*, 75–92.

Mickelson, K., Kessler, R., & Shaver, P. (1997). Adult attachment in a nationally representative sample. *Journal of Personality and Social Psychology, 73*, 1092–1106.

Mikulincer, M., & Florian, V. (1998). The relationship between adult attachment styles and emotional and cognitive reactions to stressful events. In J. A. Simpson & W. J. Rholes (Eds.), *Attachment theory and close relationships* (pp. 143–165). New York: Guilford.

Morimoto, Y., & Sharma, A. (2004). Long-term outcomes of verbal aggression: The role of protective factors. *Journal of Emotional Abuse, 4*, 71–99.

Navarre, E. L. (1987). Psychological maltreatment: The core component of child abuse. In M. R. Brassard, R. Germain, & S. N. Hart (Eds.), *Psychological maltreatment of children and youth* (pp. 45–56). New York: Pergamon.

Ney, P. G. (1987). Does verbal abuse leave deeper scars: A study of children and parents. *Canadian Journal of Psychiatry, 32*, 371–378.

Ney, P. G., Fung, T., & Wickett, A. R. (1994). The worst combinations of child abuse and neglect. *Child Abuse & Neglect, 18*, 705–714.

Nicholas, K. B., & Bieber, S. L. (1996). Parental abusive versus supportive behaviors and their relation to hostility and aggression in young adults. *Child Abuse & Neglect, 20*, 1195–1211.

Onishi, M., Gjerde, P. F., & Block, J. (2001). Personality implications of romantic attachment patterns in young adults: A multi-method, multi-informant study. *Personality and Social Psychology Bulletin, 27*, 1097–1110.

Paley, B., Cox, M. J., Burchinal, M. R., & Payne, C. C. (1999). Attachment and marital functioning: Comparison of spouses with continuous-secure, earned-secure, dismissing, and preoccupied attachment stances. *Journal of Family Psychology, 13*, 580–597.

Pan, H., Neidig, P., & O'Leary, D. (1994). Predicting mild to severe husband to wife physical aggression. *Journal of Consulting and Clinical Psychology, 62*, 975–981.

Paradis, A., & Boucher, S. (in press). Child maltreatment history and interpersonal problems in adult couple relationships. *Journal of Aggression, Maltreatment and Trauma*.

Parker, G. (1983). *Parental overprotection: A risk factor in psychosocial development*. New York: Grune & Stratton.

Parker, G. (2008). *The Parental Bonding Instrument: An annotated bibliography.* Retrieved October 2, 2008, from http://www.blackdoginstitute.org.au/research/tools/index.cfm#PBI

Parker, G., Tupling, H., & Brown, L. (1979). A parental bonding instrument. *British Journal of Medical Psychology, 52*, 1–10.

Rholes, W. S., & Simpson, J. A. (2004). Ambivalent attachment and depressive symptoms: The role of romantic and parent–child relationships. *Journal of Cognitive Psychotherapy, 18*, 67–78.

Riggs, S. A. (2010). Childhood emotional abuse and the attachment system across the life cycle: What theory and research tell us. *Journal of Aggression, Maltreatment and Trauma, 19*(1), 5–51.

Riggs, S. A., & Jacobvitz, D. (2002). Expectant parents' representations of early attachment relationships: Associations with mental health and family history. *Journal of Consulting and Clinical Psychology, 70*, 195–204.

Riggs, S. A., Jacobvitz, D., & Hazen, N. (2002). Adult attachment and history of psychotherapy in a normative sample. *Psychotherapy, 39*, 344–353.

Rosen, L. N., & Martin, L. (1996). Impact of childhood abuse history on psychological symptoms among male and female soldiers in the U.S. Army. *Child Abuse & Neglect, 20*, 1149–1160.

Rosenstein, D. H., & Horowitz, H. A. (1996). Adolescent attachment and psychopathology. *Journal of Consulting and Clinical Psychology, 64*, 244–253.

Rothbard, J. C., & Shaver, P. R. (1994). Continuity of attachment across the life span. In M. B. Sperling & W. H. Berman (Eds.), *Attachment in adults: Clinical and developmental perspectives* (pp. 31–71). New York: Guilford.

Sackett, L. A., & Saunders, D. G. (1999). The impact of different forms of psychological abuse on battered women. *Violence and Victims, 14*, 105–117.

Scher, C. D., Forde, D. R., McQuaid, J. R., & Stein, M. B. (2004). Prevalence and demographic correlates of childhood maltreatment in an adult community sample. *Child Abuse & Neglect, 28*, 167–180.

Schmaling, K. B., & Jacobson, N. S. (1990). Marital interaction and depression. *Journal of Abnormal Psychology, 99*, 229–236.

Senchak, M., & Leonard, K. E. (1992). Attachment styles and marital adjustment among newlywed couples. *Journal of Social and Personal Relationships, 9*, 51–64.

Shaver, P., Schachner, D., & Mikulincer, M. (2005). Attachment style, excessive reassurance seeking, relationship processes, and depression. *Personality and Social Psychology Bulletin, 31*, 343–359.

Simpson, J. A., & Rholes, W. S. (2002). Fearful-avoidance, disorganization, and multiple working models: Some directions for future theory and research. *Attachment and Human Development, 4*, 223–229.

Simpson, J. A., Rholes, W. S., Orina, M., & Grich, J. (2002). Working models of attachment, support giving, and support seeking in a stressful situation. *Personality and Social Psychology Bulletin, 28*, 598–608.

Simpson, J. A., Rholes, W. S., & Phillips, D. (1996). Conflict in close relationships: An attachment perspective. *Journal of Personality and Social Psychology, 71*, 899–914.

Solomon, C. R., & Serres, F. (1999). Effects of parental verbal aggression on children's self-esteem and school marks. *Child Abuse & Neglect, 23*, 339–351.

Spanier, G. B. (1976). Measuring dyadic adjustment: New scales for assessing the quality of marriage and similar dyads. *Journal of Marriage and the Family, 38*, 15–28.

Straus, M. A., Hamby, S. L, Boney-McCoy, S., & Sugarman, D. B. (1996). The revised Conflict Tactics Scales (CTS2): Development & preliminary psychometric data. *Journal of Family Issues, 17*, 283–316.

Straus, M. A. (2004). Cross-cultural reliability and validity of the Revised Conflict Tactic Scales: A study of university study dating couples in 17 nations. *Cross-Cultural Research: The Journal of Comparative Social Science, 38*(4), 407–432.

Stuewig, J., & McCloskey, L. A. (2005). The relation of child maltreatment to shame and guilt among adolescents: Psychological routes to depression and delinquency. *Child Maltreatment, 10*, 324–336.

Thompson, R. A. (1991). Attachment theory and research. In M. Lewis (Ed.), *Child and adolescent psychiatry: A comprehensive textbook* (pp. 100–108). Baltimore: Williams & Wilkins.

Tutty, L. M. (1999). Considering emotional abuse in the link between spouse and child abuse: A review and exploratory study. *Journal of Emotional Abuse, 1*(4), 53–79.

U.S. Department of Health and Human Services. (2007). *Definitions of child abuse and neglect: State statutes series.* Retrieved October 6, 2008, from http://www.childwelfare.gov/systemwide/laws_policies/statutes/define.cfm

Vega, E. M., & O'Leary, K. D. (2007). Test–retest reliability of the Revised Conflict Tactics Scales (CTS2). *Journal of Family Violence, 22*, 703–708.

Wekerle, C., & Wolfe, D. A. (1998). The role of child maltreatment and attachment style in adolescent relationship violence. *Development and Psychopathology, 10*, 571–586.

Whitfield, C. L., Anda, R. F., Dube, S. R., & Felitti, V. J. (2003). Violent childhood experiences and the risk of intimate partner violence in adults: Assessment in a large health maintenance organization. *Journal of Interpersonal Violence, 18*, 166–185.

Williams, N. L., & Riskind, J. H. (2004). Adult romantic attachment and cognitive vulnerabilities to anxiety and depression: Examining the interpersonal basis of vulnerability models. *Journal of Cognitive Psychotherapy, 18*, 7–24.

Wind, T. W., & Silvern, L. (1994). Parenting and family stress as mediators of the long-term effects of child abuse. *Child Abuse & Neglect, 18*, 439–453.

Wright, M. O. (2007). The long-term impact of emotional abuse in childhood: Identifying mediating and moderating processes. *Journal of Emotional Abuse, 7*, 1–8.

Zurbriggen, E. L., Gobin, R., & Freyd, J. J. (in press). Childhood emotional abuse and late adolescent sexual aggression perpetration and victimization. *Journal of Aggression, Maltreatment and Trauma.*

CURRENT INTERVENTION

Using Cognitive Therapies to Treat Unstable Attachment Patterns in Adults With Childhood Histories of Social Rejection

DOMINIC J. CARBONE

State University of New York—Fashion Institute of Technology, New York, New York, USA

This article describes the treatment of 5 adults exhibiting unstable attachment patterns, attributed to their repeated experiences with childhood social rejection from their family and peers. A child's attachment to his or her caregiver often determines the quality of his or her peer relationships, which serve to develop the child's self-beliefs and his or her social environment. This social cognition has been shown to influence one's choice of friends and intimate relationships. Satisfying social affiliations are a key component to achieving positive physical and mental health outcomes throughout life. In the cases described in this article, treatment was focused on changing social cognition to a more functional template from which the person could transact satisfying intimate social relationships, thereby yielding more positive outcomes.

This article describes the treatment of a clinical sample of five adults exhibiting unstable attachment patterns, attributed to their repeated experiences with childhood social rejection from their family of origin and peer network. This first section briefly reviews the empirical literature concerning the relationship among early childhood attachment status, childhood peer attachments, and adult intimate attachments. The concept of *social cognition,* or one's beliefs about oneself and his or her social environment, are introduced as a mediating factor between these relationships. This concept is further elaborated by the clinical treatment literature and referred to as *anchoring cognitions*. A treatment model is discussed that focuses on changing the acquired set of negative anchoring cognitions about the self and social world, derived in childhood, as a result of childhood emotional maltreatment in the form of social rejection from the family of origin and peer group. More specifically, the treatment model proposes that it is possible to restructure negative anchoring cognitions in adulthood using a psychotherapeutic relationship and three modalities of cognitive therapy, to provide a corrective attachment experience. Five cases, treated with this model, are discussed. The article concludes with a discussion of the treatment model and directions for further study.

EARLY ATTACHMENT STATUS AND SOCIAL COGNITION

In the classic theoretical literature on infant–caregiver attachment, both Erikson (1963) and Bowlby (1988) posited that a secure and trusting attachment to the primary caregiver would fortify the developing child with a positive attitude toward the self and the social world (see Riggs, 2010; Riggs & Kaminski, 2010). The quality of infant–caregiver attachment has been well documented and categorized in the empirical literature as *secure* and *insecure* by Ainsworth (1989). Insecure attachments are further characterized into two subtypes: *anxious-ambivalent* and *avoidant*. A final category of attachment, *unresolved/disorganized,* is the result of a parenting pattern characterized as irrational and inconsistent (Main, 1996). The quality of attachment begins to shape the child's view of himself or herself and his or her social world, referred to as social cognition. Social cognition helps us to understand our social world and set expectations for all subsequent social interactions, especially for significant others. It is expected that one with a securely attached orientation from childhood would develop a positive social cognition, thereby entering into relationships in adulthood with an expectation that one's needs would be met and that he or she would be willing to meet the needs of the significant other. Conversely, insecurely attached children would develop a negative social cognition and not expect others to respect their emotional needs and they would be reticent to risk meeting the needs of a significant other.

EARLY ATTACHMENT STATUS AND CHILDHOOD PEER RELATIONSHIPS

Early childhood attachment status has been shown to effect peer relations in childhood, which in turn provide the child with opportunities to test social cognitive schemas about the self and the social world (Taussig & Culhane,

2010). Sroufe (1989) found that securely attached children tend to be more self-confident, have more friends, and have better social skills than their insecurely attached counterparts (Riggs, 2010). Positive social relationships in childhood have been posited as necessary for the child to gain experience in learning about others' points of view (Piaget, 1965) and contribute to the child's sense of security and connectedness (Berndt, 1982), thereby fostering the development of a healthy self-concept (Harter, 1999). Children deemed to be popular by their peers have been found to exhibit a healthier self-concept and higher levels of self-efficacy (Harter, 1999). Some of the features that make children popular have been found to be a willingness to work well with others, the experience of enjoyment when being with others, and intelligence (Burkowski & Hoza, 1989). Physical attractiveness has also been associated with popularity among peers (Langlois & Stephan, 1981).

Whereas positive social experiences with peers can provide the child with a host of desired competencies needed for intimate adult social functioning, negative social experiences can have equally powerful effects. Rejected children develop a social cognition that is wrought with hostility (Bierman, 1986) and withdrawal (Parkhurst & Asher, 1992). Children who have experienced peer neglect and social ostracism exhibit lower levels of peer interaction and become barely visible to their peer group (Newcomb, Bukowski, & Pattee, 1993). Coupled with an insecure attachment pattern at home, the child is left without the social support necessary to buffer them from the social stress encountered outside of the home. They launch into adulthood with a negative social cognitive scheme, which they will use in selecting significant others into their social network.

CHILDHOOD EMOTIONAL ABUSE, PEER ATTACHMENT, AND SOCIAL COGNITION

The experience of childhood emotional abuse plays an important role in the quality of the child–caregiver attachment and childhood peer attachments (see Riggs, 2010; Riggs & Kaminski, 2010; Taussig & Culhane, 2010). This type of maltreatment is especially problematic when derived from both the caregiver and peer attachment systems. Of particular interest in this clinical sample was the concept of *total social rejection,* or the chronic neglect received from caregivers coupled with rejection received from the peer group. This combination has been found to be predictive of an inclination for the child to generate negative and hostile social cognitive schema (Crick & Dodge, 1994), whereas nonrejected children tend to maintain more prosocial cognitive schema (Nelson & Crick, 1999). With repeated emotional abuse and peer rejection, the child is left to employ his or her cognitive schema by using defensive social strategies that become recalcitrant (Crick & Dodge, 1996; Hodges & Perry, 1999) and carried forward into adulthood.

EARLY ATTACHMENT STATUS, EMOTIONAL ABUSE, AND LATER INTIMATE RELATIONSHIPS

The quality of the attachment to the primary caregiver has been shown to pave the way for later psychosocial functioning in intimate adult relationships (Ainsworth, 1989; Riggs, 2010; Riggs & Kaminski, 2010; Sroufe, 1989). Steinberg and Avenevoli (2000) identified two functions that the parent–child relationship context performs in the development of later adult intimate relationships. First, the parent–child context (secure vs. insecure attachment) works to establish a particular pattern of behavior, cognition, and affect. The context simultaneously functions to maintain the established pattern by providing the circumstances that allow the specific patterns to be repeated and reinforced as anchoring social cognitive schema. Simpson (1990) found that different relationship experiences were associated with three attachment patterns. Secure individuals experienced more positive and less negative emotion in relationships than those who were insecure. Avoidant individuals were less interdependent and less committed to their partners than secure individuals. Anxious-ambivalent adults were more likely to report that their relationships lacked trust.

In adulthood, people tend to seek attachments with individuals who are physical and mental representations of past attachment figures (Mikulincer & Shaver, 2003). The tendency to affiliate with individuals perceived to be similar to the maltreating caregiver and rejecting peer group has been widely documented (Baumeister & Leary, 1995). However, this same study found evidence of attachment-seeking behavior for persons perceived to be highly unlike one's past source of rejection, especially if a high probability of acceptance is appraised. If the attachment is appraised as supportive, it is maintained, whereas if it is appraised as threatening, a hyperactivation of the attachment system occurs. Hyperactivation exists when efforts to connect with a desired person are at first thwarted and then intensified to such an extent that the attachment-seeker's psychological functioning becomes severely compromised. This is referred to in the clinical literature as a romantic obsession (Carnes, 1992; Tennov, 1999). Whereas some adults with childhood histories of emotional abuse and peer rejection seek to re-create and reenact these dynamics in adulthood, some elect to withdraw, resulting in a decrease of proximity-seeking behaviors (Maner, DeWall, Baumeister, & Schaller, 2007), resulting in a self-inflicted state of social isolation.

ATTACHMENTS, INTIMACY, AND PSYCHOLOGICAL WELL-BEING

One's social cognitive orientation is typically reinforced by repeatedly choosing similar partners. Senchak and Leonard (1992) found that husbands and wives tended to pair on the basis of similarity in attachment security (see Riggs, 2010). Couples in which both partners were securely attached evidenced better overall marital adjustment than couples in which one or both partners were insecurely attached. Insecurely attached adults were found to partner with other insecurely attached adults and these couples evidenced poor marital adjustment. These findings, along with attachment theory and social cognitive theory, predict that individuals are likely to select partners who confirm their anchoring social cognitions.

Partner choice, in turn, affects the quality of the relationship. It has been found that the attachment status of one partner influences the satisfaction of the other partner and thereby the overall satisfaction of the couple (Collins & Read, 1990; Simpson, 1990). Bartholomew put forth a model that brings together attachment theory and social cognitive theory, and applies these to partner choice and relationship dynamics. Bartholomew and Horowitz (1991) proposed a conceptual framework of five categories of adult attachment (see Riggs, 2010; Riggs & Kaminski, 2010). *Secure* individuals maintain positive beliefs about themselves and others, thereby enabling them to form interdependent relationships with others. *Preoccupied* individuals maintain negative beliefs about themselves and positive beliefs about others, thereby yielding an emotionally demanding and anxious relationship pattern with others. *Avoidant* individuals can be either dismissing or fearful. The *dismissing* subtype holds a positive view of the self and a negative view of others, thereby denying their need for a significant other. *Fearful* subtypes maintain a negative view of the self and others, thereby desiring a relationship with a significant other but seeing it as impossibility, resulting in withdrawal.

The quality of one's relationship exerts an effect on one's mental health status. High-quality partnerships, characterized by low conflict and high satisfaction, have been shown to yield positive physical and psychological outcomes for both partners (Horowitz & White, 1998; Ross, 1995). Just being partnered, irrespective of quality, seems to yield positive effects for the individual. Partnered people report higher levels of happiness than unmarried people (Waite & Joyner, 2001). They have lower rates of mental illness, drug and alcohol abuse, and physical illness than their unmarried counterparts. They report higher levels of sexual and emotional satisfaction (Waite & Joyner, 2001), and tend to live longer (Friedman et al., 1995).

COGNITIVE THERAPIES AND ATTACHMENT DISTURBANCES

It follows from this literature review that adults who are in poor quality relationships are replicating relationship patterns rooted in negative anchoring cognitions about the self. They might struggle to cope with their relationships using maladaptive coping strategies rooted in negative social cognition.

The effects of early attachment are not immutable and it is believed that they can be modified later in childhood (see Riggs, 2010; Sroufe, 1989). If the quality of care that the child receives remains irregular, both theoretical and empirical explanations predict that the original, insecure position will be strengthened. This article argues that cognitive psychotherapy, directed at changing the anchoring cognitions, can play this role later in life to correct insecure attachments. By modifying the social cognition, one can reduce opportunities for negative patterns to be repeated and weaken the chance that the anchoring cognitions will persist over time. Cognitive therapies, such as cognitive behavioral therapy (CBT) and rational emotive behavior therapy (REBT; Bishop, 2001; Ellis, 2005), have been shown to be effective treatments for changing negative beliefs about the self, thereby yielding a more adaptive set of behaviors and emotions about the self and the social world (Clark & Ehlers, 2004; Riskind, 2004).

The analysis of anchoring cognitions becomes the focus of treatment of negative social cognition and the resulting mental health outcomes such as anxiety, depression, and associated physical illnesses. The technique of examining and restructuring social cognition is the cornerstone of CBT and REBT. CBT is a technique based on the assumption that negative cognitions give rise to negative affective states. In an attempt to cope with the negative affective states, the person enacts a set of coping behaviors, some of which might be ineffective in reducing the negative affect. Some of these coping behaviors might also be self-destructive, causing further negative affect along with reinforcing the existing negative cognitions. CBT aims to help the person explore the negative thoughts and understand the effects of negative thinking on affect and behavior. It is through this therapeutic exploration that the person develops insights about himself or herself that are less negative, thereby reducing negative affect. New coping behaviors are suggested, assigned as homework, practiced, and then evaluated in subsequent treatment sessions when modifications are made when clinically indicated. The success of the treatment is evaluated weekly by examining the self-reports of the client regarding his or her new positive cognitions, more positive affect, and more functional coping behavior.

REBT, like CBT, is based on the theoretical assumptions regarding the relationships among affect, cognition, and behavior. In REBT, the therapist aggressively challenges the client to examine the rationality of his or her cognitions by scrutinizing the evidence one has for holding onto irrational beliefs about the self. Homework, designed to test the irrational belief, is often assigned to the client who is resistant to adopting alternative, more rational, and positive beliefs about himself or herself. The goal of REBT is to have the client become a "scientist," moving about the world testing his or her social cognition by performing experiments regarding the rationality of his or her beliefs. Over time this becomes a portable skill, allowing the client to work through the crippling negative cognitions that might arise between treatment sessions. In conflict-ridden intimate relationships, irrational cognitions are often derived from assumptions that partners make as a result of poor communication patterns. The therapist encourages communication between partners, so that they can test their assumptions and develop more rational and accurate thoughts about each other's behaviors. As thoughts become more rational, intimate relationships become easier to negotiate, less conflict ridden, and tend to last longer.

With CBT and REBT as tools in helping the client to change negative social cognition to positive, the therapist can begin to help the client transact more satisfying intimate relationships. In some instances where the client is having difficulty in changing his or her social cognition, eye movement desensitization and reprocessing (EMDR), a highly specialized form of cognitive therapy, has been shown to be effective in positively changing social cognition (Shapiro, 2001). EMDR is a focused attention technique designed to help people reinterpret their beliefs regarding past traumatic events. The technique requires a trained therapist who is certified to use EMDR, equipment for alternating sensory stimulation, and a consenting client. The treatment requires that the client invent a visual representation of the disturbing event, as well as a "safe space" to escape to should he or she become emotionally overwhelmed during the treatment. An associated negative cognition is assigned to the visual image and rated numerically on a Likert scale in terms of subjective units of discomfort (SUDs). A corresponding positive cognition is developed by the client to reflect what he or she would like to believe about the disturbing visual image. The client assigns this positive cognition a numerical level of veracity known as the validity of the cognition (VoC). The SUD and VoC are numerical values used to indicate to the therapist the level of reprocessing that has taken place and are part of the determination of the overall treatment outcome.

While imagining the disturbing event, the client receives bilateral sensory stimulation in one of three possible alternating forms: (a) eye movements, (b) tactile stimulation, or (c) auditory stimulation. For this clinical sample, auditory stimulation was used due to its simplicity of use. It is believed that this bilateral sensory stimulation causes the brain to reprocess the cognitive interpretation of the event while having the person experience the associated negative emotions. With the help of the therapist, the client is guided through an exploration of the thoughts associated with the event as these shift from negative to positive whereby the SUDs become lower in value as the VoC value increases. When the client reports a significant reduction in the amount of distress associated with the memory (SUD of 1 or 0), the treatment is deemed successful and the event is considered reprocessed. Successful outcomes are validated further by reported decreases in self-destructive coping behaviors and negative emotional states with accompanying increases in prosocial behaviors and satisfying attachments. The veracity of these self-reported outcomes is assessed over the course of several sessions with particular attention paid to the client's iconic (general) versus episodic (specific) accounts of posttreatment attachments. The amount of discrepancy between the subjects' iconic versus episodic accounts is taken as an indicator of veracity whereby few discrepancies (iconic vs. episodic) indicate high veracity, and frequent discrepancies indicate low veracity and therefore the need for further treatment for the attachment disturbance.

The EMDR phase of treatment can take place over several sessions and frequently other related memories surface that require additional reprocessing. EMDR has also been shown to dramatically decrease the symptoms associated with many psychological disorders (Shapiro, 2001). Because there is no prior research in this area, the application of these techniques to the treatment of attachment disorders in adulthood to create functional and satisfying intimate relationships was of particular interest in this study.

CLINICAL CASE PRESENTATIONS

The following clinical case presentations illustrate the connections among early childhood attachment, social cognition, social rejection, adult attachment seeking, and psychological disorders, offering a treatment model that was successful in changing existing social cognitive schema. Changing the social cognitive schema from negative to positive yielded an increase in positive emotional states, prosocial behaviors, and a reduction in psychological symptoms.

The clinical sample was derived from a larger sample of clients who referred themselves for treatment to a private practice in New York City for a variety of problems involving intimate relationships. The methodology was reviewed by an ad hoc research committee and was exempt from institutional review board review under exemption 45 CFR 46.101(b)(4) and from all 45 CFR part 46 requirements. The treatment approach involved the following components: (a) an exploration of the reason for referral, (b) a review of past and current symptoms, (c) an assessment of emotional abuse history, (d) a review of past and present coping strategies, (e) the establishment of existing anchoring social cognitive schema, (f) the use of cognitive restructuring techniques designed to change these schema (i.e., CBT, REBT and EMDR), and (g) an evaluation of the treatment outcomes.

What follows is a discussion of five cases from a clinical sample designed to illustrate the relationship among early childhood attachment status, childhood peer relations, and adult intimate relationships (Table 1). The author conducted the treatment in all cases. The first case, Patty, illustrates how past social cognitive schemas get reenacted as partner choices in adulthood in an attempt to reconcile attachment hunger from childhood. The second case, Sam, illustrates the effects of social rejection, as a result of

TABLE 1 Pretreatment–Posttreatment Comparison of Anchoring Cognitions and Attachments

Case name	Pretreatment anchoring cognition(s)	Pretreatment attachments	Posttreatment anchoring cognitions	Posttreatment attachments
Dara	"Men always abandon you and cannot be trusted to tell the truth."	Unavailable men No female friends Romantic obsessions Unresolved and disorganized	"I can trust myself to be there for me?"	Unresolved
Sam	"Sex with men is dirty and bad."	Compulsive sex Sexual masochist Superficial attachments Prostitutions Avoidant and fearful	"I like me, so what?" "I am safe from my parents."	Platonic friends Romantic dates Secure attachments
Patty	"Women are crazy and cannot be trusted." "I can control another." "Men are hostile and abandoning."	Unavailable men Fostering dependencies Compulsive sex Superficial attachments No female friends Unresolved and disorganized	"I cannot control another."	Platonic friends Male and female friends No casual sex Secure attachments
Mary	"Men demand sex in exchange for intimacy." "Women are less demanding and safer."	Compulsive sex with men Superficial attachments Reactive attraction to women Unresolved and disorganized	"I am more than just my body."	Platonic friends with men and women Secure attachments
Randy	"Only physically perfect men are worthy of love." "Relationships with men are not real and must be hidden."	Body dysmorphia Cyber relationships Anxious and ambivalent Preoccupied	"I only need one person to be attracted to me to find true love." "Relations with men can be real."	Romantic relationships Friendships Secure attachments

gender nonconformity, on the formation of social cognition and his retreat from the social world. The third case, Randy, illustrates a man's desperate search for social connections in adulthood, after a childhood wrought with rejection from both peers and family. The fourth case, Mary, illustrates how violations in child–caretaker sexual boundaries can lead to long-standing mistrusting social cognition and conflict-ridden intimate adult relationships. Lastly, the case of Dara illustrates how parental rejection and early loss affect later attachment patterns in adulthood.

Patty: Reenacting Past Social Cognition

Reason for referral

Patty was a White, married, German immigrant who began treatment when she was 38 years old. She presented as an anxious, tall, attractive blond with a slight German accent. She immigrated to the United States 10 years prior to take a job in the biotechnology industry. She was referred for individual psychotherapy from couples therapy, where she had been in treatment for the past year. It was discovered in that treatment that she had a "complicated" childhood history that appeared to be affecting her relationship.

Review of past and current symptoms

Patty had a long-standing history of anxiety, which she feared meant she suffered from bipolar illness, similar to her mother. Her anxiety became worse when she was in intimate relationships and was intolerable at times. It was the heightened anxiety she experienced in her relationship at the time that motivated her to seek couples therapy.

Relationship and emotional abuse history

Prior to adulthood Patty had little experience with intimate relationships outside of her family of origin. A review of her early childhood revealed that before Patty was born, her mother was diagnosed with bipolar illness and her father left shortly thereafter, leaving her mother's brother to assist in raising her. She described her mother as "unstable and crazy," and her uncle as "stern and physically abusive." He often used corporal punishment and psychological threats to withhold love to gain behavioral compliance, especially in regard to gender role compliance. She described herself as a "tomboy" and as the object of ridicule from both her family and peers. As a tomboy, the other girls at school would tease her and referred to her by unflattering nicknames. All of her friends were boys throughout grammar school, but after her arrival in high school the story changed. Patty felt that she was never thought of in a sexual way by boys and was abandoned by her male friends in favor of "the real girls." She linked these experiences to her present situation, where this social template was reenacted. Numerous short-term sexual relationships with various men became an attempt to defeat this social cognition.

Patty had no history of relationships with female friends and a long-standing history of dating older men for short periods of time. She met these men while traveling for business. These relationships would always start with casual sex and then turn into a long-distance dating situation. All of these relationships ended due to the man's romantic obsessive behavior, such as harassing phone calls, threats of physical violence, and accusations of her infidelity.

At the time she started treatment, Patty was married to Paul, 10 years her junior. She described him as a "pretty boy" and "irresponsible." They had been married for just over one year, after knowing each other for six months prior. Unlike her numerous other short-term relationships, she initiated the courtship and their engagement. This surprised her, as she never imagined herself as "the marrying kind." Shortly after meeting, Paul moved from his parents' home into the house that Patty owned. Paul had no source of steady income and was unable to afford a place of his own. Shortly after they married, their sex life came to a sudden halt. They decided to address this by opening up their relationship to other sexual partners. They had sexual encounters with other people individually, but never together or with a third. She continued to support her husband financially, while secretly dating other men outside of their open marriage agreement. This was accompanied by an exacerbation of her anxiety. When Paul discovered that her outside sexual encounters became more serious emotional affairs, he confronted her and they decided to enter couples therapy to explore trust issues in their relationship.

Coping strategies

Patty has a long-standing history of coping with her anxiety by having multiple sexual partners. She described sex as a "silver bullet" that made her feel better when she was feeling bored, anxious, tired, lonely, or depressed. She felt connected to men during sex, even when nothing else came of the encounter.

Anchoring social cognitive schema and EMDR

In her individual treatment, we began exploring Patty's existing cognitive schema for relationships with friends and romantic figures. For Patty, her social cognition for women was that they were "crazy and not to be trusted." Men were "abandoning and hostile." EMDR treatment was used to change this anchoring cognition. Patty was asked to develop two separate visual images representative of her disturbing relationship with her mother and with men. These images would also be subtitled with the respective negative cognition. She described an image of her mother being carried away in a straightjacket by the police in the middle of a cold night while she stood watching in her pajamas. The other image was of her uncle and some schoolboys standing around her in a circle, yelling at her because she was dressed "like a boy." Over the course of six treatment sessions, Patty was asked to recall each image and corresponding negative anchoring cognition while she listened to recorded music containing imbedded bilateral stimulation sounds. She was instructed to report any thoughts that came into her mind regarding the image. The therapist sought clarifications when she became vague in her descriptions. Her responses were recorded and a shift occurred in Patty's interpretation of these two events from negative to positive.

During the treatment, Patty reprocessed her thoughts about men that were formed in early childhood and carried forth to adulthood. She realized that in her present relationship she was defending against both cognitive schemas. By marrying a powerless and dependent younger man, she could ensure that he would not abandon or abuse her. Having never had female friends, her "pretty boy" husband was the closest that she came to a female friend, cast in the schema of her "crazy" mother. Prior to the EMDR treatment, Patty believed that she could control his potential "craziness" by having all of the power in the relationship. The treatment yielded the new anchoring cognition: "I cannot control another adult, I can only protect myself." However, after the shift in anchoring cognition, this mother–child formatted relationship with her husband became unsavory to her. She applied the restructured cognition to make a major positive change in her life, as we will see in the next phase of her treatment.

Cognitive restructuring with CBT/REBT

The CBT/REBT phase of treatment progressed by exploring Patty's social cognitive schema. She began viewing her marriage as a mother–child dyad and decided to end it. She allowed Paul to continue to live with her, feeling sorry for him and not wanting to put him out on the street. She continued to infantilize him by holding no expectation that he was able to financially support himself and find another living situation. One year after their decision to separate, Paul came home and announced that he had met another woman and was moving in with her. Patty felt abandoned for a moment then began dating frantically shortly thereafter.

Patty's next relationship was with Bill, a married coworker. She had known Bill for three years and he had petitioned her for sex repeatedly over that period of time. Patty had refused each time because he was known as "the office stud" and boasted having had sexual relations with more than 20 women at work, unknown to his wife. By repeatedly refusing Bill, Patty felt superior to the other women in the office who gave into his advances. In reaction to Paul's departure, Patty decided to accept Bill's pleas to have sex in exchange for dating. Patty wanted to show the other women in the office that she was as attractive as they were, again attempting to defeat a previous aspect of her social cognition. She continued this relationship despite his emerging possessive and abusive nature, similar to that of her uncle. She also described him as erratic and irrational, similar to her mother.

Attachment outcome

During the 12 months of treatment, Patty was able to come to an understanding of the origins of her social cognitive schema. She found it difficult to enact the behavioral changes designed to change the cognitive schema because the physical and social reinforcement garnered from the sexual encounters was very powerful. Over time she ended the relationship with Bill and declared a moratorium on dating. She began focusing on developing platonic relationships with men and women. She reported a decrease in casual sexual activity and anxiety symptoms.

Sam: Social Ridicule and Ostracism in Response to Gender Variant Behaviors

This case that represents an example of how social cognition develops in response to forceful gender norm compliance strategies enacted by both parents and peers.

Reason for referral

Sam came to treatment as a result of intolerable anxiety that had worsened over the past year. Sam was a 35-year-old gay White male who had never been in an intimate relationship outside of his family of origin.

Review of past and current symptoms

Sam presented with symptoms of social anxiety and depression. For as long as he could remember, he desired a close intimate relationship with someone. He found himself spending huge amounts of leisure time engaged in tearful lamentation about his situation. In the few social situations in which he found himself, he would experience intense anxiety and then retreat into his own thoughts or find some way to leave the situation.

Relationship and emotional abuse history

Sam reported years of peer ridicule from age 3 to 23. He attributed the source of ridicule to his behavior and appearance. As a boy he was not interested in the type of play activities characteristic of most boys. Rather than sports, he preferred to play with arts and crafts. Through his interactions with peers, he came to understand that he behaved differently than other boys, as he was often teased for looking "girly." His parents offered him little comfort, as they were preoccupied with work and consuming large amounts of alcohol. When they did attend to his situation with peers, they merely reinforced the themes found in the peer ridicule.

As Sam's sexuality emerged, he found himself in the company of an adult neighbor whom he found physically attractive because of the man's masculinity and dissimilarity to Sam's understanding of himself. Sam was 13 and the neighbor was in his early 20s. Sam had no interest in playing with his male peers, but enjoyed spending time with this neighbor. They started having sex and Sam remembers liking it and feeling gratitude for the opportunity to explore his emerging sexuality with this older man. The sexual activity began spontaneously and was limited to mutual masturbation. They would eat meals together, watch TV, and play games. For the first time in his life Sam felt attended to and cared for by another person. In his perception, his parents did not seem to mind because they were preoccupied with work or alcohol. As this relationship continued and as Sam entered high school, he reported that he began to act more effeminately and his parents scolded him for this. He said:

> They did not give a shit about anything else in my life except for the way I acted. It was never, "Did you do your homework or how are the kids in school?" Just "Carry your books like a man and stop acting like a girl."

At the age of 15, Sam started feeling attraction to his peers and told a schoolmate that he wanted to kiss him, thinking that this would be their special secret. His schoolmate responded by punching Sam and told the teacher. The teacher ruled the punch justified and Sam believed he learned that day that his attraction to men was shameful and wrong. He learned that it was not "normal" to want to kiss men or have feelings toward them. The school called his home and he was punished and beaten by his parents and they figured out that something was going on with him and the neighbor. The entire family quickly moved across town. Sam never saw his neighbor again but has spent most of his adult life wondering about this man. Subsequently Sam's interactions with men were limited to sexual relations in exchange for money.

Coping strategies

Sam found himself coping with his social anxiety by attempting to have complete control over his social encounters. In the role of an escort, he could modulate the intimacy to his liking. Because most of his clients were married and "in the closet" he was assured that he had the upper hand as they came to depend on him as their sole source of pleasure. He had many recidivist clients who he came to know well and he considered them "like family." In this format he could continue to reenact his secret shameful life.

Anchoring social cognitive schema and EMDR

When Sam entered treatment his social cognition reflected that he was a shameful person because of his sexual attractions. Sex with men was "dirty and bad" and therefore only done in secret so that he would not get caught and have to move away. Sam also believed that he could completely control social situations with men by using sex and "the closet" to guard against abandonment. EMDR treatment was used to reprocess this anchoring cognition. Sam was asked to develop a visual image representative of his belief that "sex with men is dirty and bad." Sam described an image of himself as a child eating at the dinner table with his parents in complete silence. He felt alone, upset, and disturbed by this image. Over the course of four treatment sessions, Sam was asked to recall this image and the corresponding negative anchoring cognition while he listened to the bilateral stimulation sounds. During the treatment sessions his thoughts evolved from extreme shame toward himself to anger toward his parents, then to an appreciation of their limitations. He reprocessed their harshness toward him as their naive way of trying to protect him from scorn and ridicule outside of the home. He forgave his parents during the treatment and later wrote them about this matter.

After this treatment, Sam's thoughts about himself changed to reflect a less shameful understanding of his attractions. He concluded with a new anchoring cognition that stated: "I like men and given my history, I'm thankful for being able to find pleasure with any other person." He found comfort and a sense of mental health as a survivor who could connect with others, despite an emotionally abusive childhood. Sam also began to accept that he was now safe from his parents and did not have to control social situations and guard against abandonment.

Cognitive restructuring with CBT/REBT

The next phase of treatment was directed at further changing his anchoring cognitions regarding men, relationships, sexuality, and nurturing. After exploring the origins of his social cognition, he was assigned behaviors that would change his peer group participation. He became part of a peer support group and experienced the nurturing of other men in a nonsexual format. He changed the venues for transacting social relationships and developed a peer support network that worked to change his beliefs about himself and other gay men. With psychoeducational sessions, he came to understand his same-sex attraction as part of the wide spectrum of human sexual responses.

Attachment outcome

In total, Sam's treatment lasted eight months. With a newly formed social cognitive schema, Sam was able to transact healthier romantic and platonic relationships. He was able to meet other men for friendship in a variety of venues that were not mediated by alcohol, drugs, or sex. He expanded his social network to include women and heterosexual men. Dating took on a romantic tone rather than a coercive, sexual struggle.

Randy: Escaping Intimacy by Having a Cyber-Relationship

Reason for referral

Randy, a 33-year-old gay White male, referred himself for treatment because he desperately wanted to be in a relationship and could not seem to make one work. Randy suffered from body dysmorphic disorder (BDD) and social anxiety with a history of suicidal ideation, but he had no history of attempts. At the start of treatment, Randy wanted to feel better about his looks, specifically focusing on the width of his nose. Randy felt frequently rejected by his childhood peers because of his looks. This helped to formulate a distorted cognitive schema regarding his physical appearance.

Review of past and current symptoms

Randy reported a high degree of discomfort in social settings that was expressed in the form of panic attacks. Although he reported a long-standing history of anxiety in all social situations, it was not until recently that he experienced full-blown panic attacks. Over time, he felt defeated by his inability to control his anxiety and withdrew from all social situations. During adolescence, Randy attempted to manage his anxiety by focusing in on his body. He became fixated on the width of his nose, spending hours looking in the mirror and imagining how cosmetic surgery on his nose would greatly improve his attractiveness and social life. His fixation on his nose was then generalized to his entire physical appearance, which he felt was too skinny. He attempted to correct this situation by joining a gym, working out, and using protein supplements to "bulk up." Randy became consumed with guilt if he missed a session at the gym and working out became a centrally organizing activity of his day.

Coping strategies

Randy coped with his symptoms by retreating into his work, his workouts at the gym, and a fantasy social realm, which involved the cyberworld. Supplements containing large amounts of ephedrine and caffeine were used to elevate his mood.

RELATIONSHIP AND EMOTIONAL ABUSE HISTORY

Randy was born an identical twin and grew up in a small, rural farming community in upstate New York. His father rejected him at an early age in favor of his heterosexual twin brother because Randy was "different." Randy loved to draw rather than play sports or work on the family farm. He experienced his mother as a passive nonentity who was always working on the farm. As his sexuality emerged during the early teen years, Randy had several secret sexual relationships with schoolmates. Most of these relationships ended when the other boys began dating girls in the later teen years. Because Randy showed no interest in dating girls, he became the target of ridicule by these same boys who had previously had sexual relations with him.

After high school, Randy retreated into his work and studied architecture at a local college. After graduating, he moved to New York City to escape a lifelong reputation in his small town as a "fag." He attempted to have intimate relationships, but these always seemed to start with sex and end after a few dates. Many of these men became part of his social network. He attributed his single status to being physically unattractive, although never having explicitly been told this by anyone. Social situations were wrought with anxiety for Randy, given the social cognition that he maintained.

Fed up with his inability to control his social anxiety, Randy began pursuing men online and met Todd, who was nothing more than a "fuzzy picture." Randy fell in love instantly because he could make out from this fuzzy picture that Todd had a "gorgeous" body. Todd claimed to be a fashion model living in western Canada. Randy quickly began referring to Todd as his "boyfriend" and friends, family, and coworkers warned him to be cautious about this online relationship.

As they began speaking to each other several times during the day, Randy relied exclusively on Todd for affiliation and support. He distanced himself from his social network because of their suspicious inquiries regarding Todd. His own suspicions grew, as a result of questions carefully raised in his therapy and he attempted to garner a clearer photograph of Todd, who made excuses for not complying with this simple request. Despite the ambiguity of the situation, they began talking about planning a trip together to meet in person. Several plans were made over the course of 6 months, but each time the date of the union grew closer, Todd would suddenly cancel the trip for various reasons that, at first, seemed acceptable to Randy. The phone relationship continued, as did the e-mails. Randy started to grow impatient and hungry for a live meeting with his "boyfriend." He decided to assert himself and buy a ticket to Vancouver to visit Todd. Todd replied that it was not a good time for Randy to visit because he was recently diagnosed with leukemia and would be starting a round of aggressive chemotherapy. Randy was devastated and feared losing Todd to this disease. His peers explored the veracity of this chain of events at length and Randy reacted by further dissociating from reality to defend his position.

The phone calls and e-mails continued. Randy insisted on going to Vancouver to be with Todd during the treatment to meet and to celebrate their one-year anniversary. On the day that Randy was set to leave for Vancouver, he received an e-mail from someone claiming to be Todd's brother. The e-mail stated that Todd died suddenly as a result of the chemotherapy treatment for his leukemia. Randy replied and insisted on taking the trip and going to the funeral to see his lover's body, but a subsequent e-mail indicated that Todd was to be cremated and a viewing would be reserved for family members only. Randy was devastated and went into a deep depression. His functioning at work and at home was compromised. Once again, his peers explored the veracity of this chain of events at length and he maintained his position that all the events were true.

Anchoring social cognitive schema and EMDR

Randy's social cognitive schema reflected the belief that "relationships with men are not real or possible and they must be hidden." This case clearly illustrates the level of cognitive distortion that someone can enact to cope with his or her attachment hunger originating in childhood. Randy was already capable of gross distortions in body image, and this was an extension of that level of distorted thinking. It became clear during the assessment phase of Randy's treatment that the social rejection and peer ridicule that he experienced played a powerful role in the development of his beliefs about himself and his social world. He appeared ill equipped to cope with the social realities of competition and rejection, so he retreated into a fantasy world whereby he could modulate the amount of intimacy so as not to compete and risk rejection.

During the restructuring phase of the treatment, EMDR was used to process Randy's anchoring cognitions about himself and his social world, which were reflected in the statement: "I must be attractive to everyone to be loved by them and protected from harm." Randy was asked to develop a visual image representative of this belief and he described an image of himself as an adult looking in a mirror while kids from his past looked on at him in horror. In the mirror he saw his father's face with elements of his mother's face that he deemed unflattering. Over the course of four treatment sessions, Randy was asked to recall this image and corresponding negative anchoring cognition while he listened to the bilateral stimulation sounds.

The treatment yielded a change in social cognition about his body that did not require that he be attractive to everyone. He arrived at the more rational position that he offered more to the relationship equation than just a sexual contribution, sought through having a "perfect" face and body. The new anchoring cognition became: "Only one person has to find me attractive for me to find true love." This statement released him from feeling like he had to be physically attractive to everyone to guard against gaining attention and therefore ridicule.

Cognitive restructuring with CBT/REBT

Randy's continued treatment revolved around working through grief issues and changing his social cognition so that he could believe that relationships are possible in real time with real people. He was assigned homework that placed him in stressful social contexts where he was sure he would encounter attractive men. While recognizing his tendency to think of himself as unattractive and unworthy of such men, he was instructed to act as if he were one of the attractive men he sought. He practiced in sessions the social skills associated with self-confidence and rehearsed some conversation points. After repeatedly doing this in social settings, the results were reviewed in treatment. He had collected enough evidence to refute his original cognition about himself and began believing that he was socially competent and attractive. His cognitive schema regarding his body image was restructured to yield an acceptance of himself as worthy of love irrespective of the appearance of certain parts of his body.

Attachment outcome

Randy's treatment lasted a total of 13 months. As a result of this new schema, he became less fearful of social situations when he no longer conceptualized social interactions as litmus tests of his worthiness as a person. Randy connected with a peer network that was primarily focused on commonalities in activity interests rather than physical appearances. He began to develop a social cognition that was prosocial, which served to reduce his anxiety, depression, and BDD symptoms.

Mary: A History of Mistrust in Relationships as a Result of Childhood Sexual Abuse

Reason for referral

Mary was a 24-year-old Hispanic woman who began treatment for depression after having had seven therapy relationships in her recent past, each ending after a perceived breach of trust. She identified the source of her depression as the recent end of a 3-year relationship with an older woman who suddenly left. This was Mary's only long-term, intimate relationship to date.

Review of past and current symptoms

Mary had a long-standing history of depression, suicidal ideation, anxiety, and posttraumatic stress disorder. At the time she began this episode of treatment, she reported a baseline of generalized anxiety and recurrent night terrors depicting episodes from the sexual abuse she experienced as a child. These symptoms became worse over the course of her most recent relationship.

Relationship and emotional abuse history

An exploration of her past revealed that Mary was sexually abused when she was 4 years old, for 3 years, by a 50-year-old man who was a family friend. During the abuse, she experienced a high degree of shame and withdrew from her peers and family while telling no one. As a result of this withdrawal, she became the target of peer ridicule in school for reasons that she could not clearly identify. Many years after the abuse ended and the perpetrator died, Mary disclosed her abuse history to her parents at the age of 17. Her parents responded by forcing her to go to therapy and as a result of this therapy, Mary gained an understanding of her emerging bisexuality. When she disclosed this to her parents they terminated her therapy relationship and sent her to another therapist whom they believed would "cure" her of these feelings. Her parents ended this therapeutic relationship after the therapist deemed Mary's bisexual feelings a normal part of development.

While in high school, Mary never dated or showed interest in romantic relationships. After high school she had several short-term relationships with older men. All of these relationships ended when she refused to have sexual relations with them. At the age of 21, she began her first relationship with a woman, Marjorie.

Shortly after their relationship began, Marjorie proposed involving other women in their sexual relationship as a solution to her boredom. Mary objected to an open relationship but she went along with it to save the relationship, which ultimately caused its demise. Mary stated that her biggest fear was being abandoned by her partner. During the process of negotiating three-way sexual encounters, some of her partner's flirtations with the prospective third frightened Mary and brought up fears of abandonment. She began to withdraw sexually from the partnership. Her partner ended the relationship and left.

Coping strategies

Mary moved back in with her parents as a result of the end of her relationship with Marjorie. Shortly after moving in with them again, Mary began going online to meet men for sex. She acquired numerous offers but did not actually going through with meeting any of them because she feared catching a sexually transmitted disease. She felt compelled to have straight sex to please her parents and recover from her breakup. Possible pregnancy was not a concern that she considered until it was mentioned in therapy. As a result of this compulsive sexual behavior, she began suffering from flashbacks of the childhood abuse. She used marijuana every night to help her sleep, and she drank alcohol on the weekends to get drunk and forget her situation.

Anchoring social cognitive schema and EMDR

As a result of her trauma history, Mary came to understand that "intimacy with men is gained through sex," even if it is nonconsensual on her part. Women were considered "a safer sexual refuge from men," but they were capable of sudden abandonment. Both sexes can be harshly critical and rejecting at any time, so she prepared herself for this inevitable course by avoiding intimacy by engaging in casual sexual relations with men. EMDR was used to help Mary restructure her social cognitive scheme derived from her childhood sexual abuse and parental criticism. Mary was asked to develop a visual image representative of her belief that "men demand sex in exchange for intimacy." Mary described an image of herself as a child, undressing in her basement in front of the man who sexually abused her. Her parents and some other children populated the windows opening into the basement from above. The children were laughing at her, as they did in her real-life history. Her parents manifested indifference in their faces. Over the course of five treatment sessions, Mary was asked to recall this image and corresponding negative anchoring cognition while she listened to the bilateral stimulation sounds. During the treatment sessions the image changed so that she became the director of the action in the scene. Her thoughts shifted from self-shame to anger and blame toward her parents. She empathized with the children who were looking on because she believed that they were using humor to help them cope with seeing something that they did not understand. She was able to come to an understanding of the image that was significantly less disturbing than in the past, although she had some residual anger toward her parents that required further reprocessing.

Mary was able to restructure her thoughts to reflect a more secure interpretation of her social world and the people in it. EMDR treatment yielded a new anchoring cognition for Mary that stated: "I am more than just my body." With this new anchoring cognition the next phase of treatment could take place.

Cognitive restructuring with CBT/REBT

During the next phase of treatment, it became essential that Mary experience a positive, nonsexual relationship, first with the therapist and then with others outside of the treatment setting. Psychoeducation was used to explore and normalize her bisexual attractions, a counterpoint to the information she received from her parents. Her homework outside of the treatment setting was to connect with a new social network that was not mediated by sex or drugs, but rather by activities that she enjoyed. She agreed to review petitions for sex in treatment before acting on these overtures, to provide her with a portable cognitive skill designed to deduce the appropriateness of the situation to her in the course of treatment.

Attachment outcome

Mary left 8 months of treatment with a better understanding of her attractiveness and how it can cause others to respond to her in both positive and exploitative ways. In this last stage of treatment, Mary developed realistic strategies for seeking healthy attachments and protecting herself from threats to her attachment system. She joined a variety of activity groups where she met people of various ages for intimate relations that were centered around common activities, mutual support, and mentorship.

Dara: Satisfying Attachment Hunger From Childhood

Reason for referral

Dara entered treatment at the age of 34 while in the midst of a relationship with Ben, a married coworker. She entered treatment because she was experiencing severe bouts of shortness of breath and heart palpitations that had been diagnosed by her medical doctor as panic attacks. All medical causes for her symptoms were ruled out and she was referred for psychotherapy treatment for an anxiety disorder.

Review of past and current symptoms

After an in-depth review of Dara's symptoms, it was discovered that these panic attacks were experienced previously in childhood in response to the impending death of her father. These attacks reemerged recently during her boyfriend's departures from their weekends together.

Relationship and emotional abuse history

After a relatively uneventful early childhood, at the age of 4, Dara learned that her father was very sick. Over the course of the next five years, she watched her father become progressively more disabled, as he was suffering from many forms of cancer. She watched her mother care for her father as he went from ambulatory and alert to bedridden and intermittently conscious.

Dara experienced her father distancing himself from her during the last two years of his life. Her mother was overwhelmed with caring for both her husband and Dara, so Dara was sent to live with her maternal grandmother. Her mother then became a source of rage and was seen as an obstacle between Dara and her father. Dara was told that she would return to the home when her father recovered from his illness. While he was dying, Dara was not allowed to visit her father. She escaped further into a fantasy world whereby she imagined her father as a healthy man and attentive to her exclusively. She looked forward to the day when he would recover. When her father finally died, Dara felt betrayed when told and further outraged when she was forbidden to attend the wake or funeral. She was told that she was too young to attend these ceremonies, which resulted in her feeling more anger and estrangement. She was left to wonder what she did wrong to make her father sick and get sent away.

Dara spent the rest of her childhood and adolescence depressed and withdrawn. Her peers rejected her at school because of her social withdrawal into a fantasy world where her father was alive and well. Her mother was preoccupied and bereft, rendering her unable to comfort Dara. She was confused as to what to do with Dara and became focused on dwindling finances and remarriage possibilities.

Dara's adulthood relationships were characterized by dating unavailable men. Dara's relationship with Ben started out as a friendship that she initiated when he began working at her law firm. She was in the process of ending a three-year relationship with a man she described as "inadequate." Dara and Ben frequently admitted to each other that there was "a lot of chemistry" between them and if they were both to become single in the future they believed that they would have a great relationship. After a year of friendship, they both confessed their love for each other during a romantic dinner and began what Dara believed would be a smooth transition into an intimate relationship.

For the majority of their three-year relationship, Ben had been married and would return to his married life during the week, reserving his weekends for Dara. Prior to starting treatment and three years into the relationship, Dara confronted him about leaving his wife to be with her exclusively. He asked Dara for extra time to handle the situation with his wife while continuing their relationship on the weekends. Over the course of many months, Dara fluctuated from discussing his wife directly with him to saying nothing about it and escaping into a fantasy world in which they were both committed only to each other. It was established in treatment that it was after these fantasy weekends, when Ben returned to his wife, that Dara had her panic attacks.

Coping strategies

A review of Dara's coping history indicated that she had a childhood history of retreating into a fantasy world and staying there for long periods of time, longer than is normal for a child. This type of escape coping began at the age of 4 when she learned that her father was very sick.

Anchoring social cognitive schema and EMDR

Dara's cognitive schema reflected a belief that she was not lovable and was someone who men distanced themselves from without an apparent reason. She felt inadequate to be the sole object of desire so she affiliated with men who were not available to her exclusively. She believed that men would always leave intimate situations and cannot be trusted to say the truth, as they maintain secrets from women in relationships. Dara was asked to develop a visual image representative of her belief that "men always abandon you and cannot be trusted to tell the truth." Dara described a scene where she was being taken out of her home by her mother and walked past her father's empty hospital bed that was set up in the living room. Seeing this image she felt alone, betrayed, and confused. Over the course of four treatment sessions, Dara was asked to recall this image and corresponding negative anchoring cognition while she listened to the bilateral stimulation sounds. Dara was able to reinterpret the family secrecy as a misguided protective device. She came to understand that her parents tried not to overwhelm her with information about her father's illness and she agreed that she probably was too immature to have understood what she was capable of understanding as an adult. A more forgiving interpretation was adopted regarding this anchoring event in her life. EMDR treatment was successful in restructuring her anchoring cognitions and yielded the new belief: "I am not the sole cause of my unsuccessful relationships." With this new belief, Dara was ready to continue with the next phase of treatment.

Cognitive restructuring with CBT/REBT

During the CBT/REBT phase of the treatment, Dara came to understand that her previous history predisposed her to pick men who would eventually disappoint her and serve to validate her existing cognitive schema. By identifying the early warning signs of someone who has a low probability of meeting her attachment hunger, she would be equipped to make better choices in subsequent relationships. In making these changes to her cognitive schema, Dara became aware of how profoundly unfulfilling her present relationship was for her. This resulted in an increase in depressive symptoms, hopelessness, and helplessness. She began fixating on the thought: "Why can't I just have him to myself?" This was considered a symptom substitution, whereby an anchoring cognition is changed only temporarily to a more functional version and then replaced outside of treatment by a similarly dysfunctional cognition to the original anchoring belief.

ATTACHMENT OUTCOME

Dara ended four months of treatment abruptly after a week without a session due to a national holiday. This unavoidable interruption in treatment was attributed as the cause of the symptom substitution. Dara stated that she knew what she needed to do to feel better but lacked the desire to follow through on the course of action. The treatment ended at this point. Although the techniques were effective in changing social cognition, the interruption in treatment caused Dara to experience an abandonment reaction, whereby the therapist was cast in the role of the disappointing father figure. Treatment was incomplete for this case.

DISCUSSION

The previous clinical case presentations illustrate the relationships among early childhood attachment status, childhood peer attachments, and adult intimate relationships, all of which have been thoroughly documented in the clinical, theoretical, and empirical literature regarding adult relationships. These relationships are mediated through the development and employment of cognitive schema. Attachment disturbances in childhood carry forward into adulthood by way of anchoring cognitive schema that are negative, resulting in negative emotional states, self-destructive coping behaviors, and negative social behaviors. The treatment phase of each case focused on changing existing cognitive schema about the self and the social world, from negative to positive, using three cognitive behavioral modalities: CBT, REBT, and EMDR. Changes in anchoring cognitive schema from negative to positive resulted in positive psychological outcomes, including more satisfying attachments and social intimacy.

The cases that were reviewed illustrate theoretical formulations reflecting the idea that a trusting attachment to the primary caregiver serves to assist the child in developing a positive attitude toward the self and the social world (Bowlby, 1988; Erikson, 1963; Riggs, 2010). All five of the individuals in the cases reviewed reported insecure attachments to their primary caregiver systems in early childhood. The effects of a poor quality attachment system resulted in a crystallized set of beliefs about themselves and the social world that were reflected in their pretreatment anchoring cognitions (see Table 1). These anchoring cognitions were frequently negative appraisals of people along gender lines. For example, both Dara and Patty held anchoring cognitions about men as primarily unreliable and hostile. Sam believed that his sexual attraction to men rendered him "bad and dirty," and Patty felt women were "crazy" and not to be trusted. These social templates were carried forward into childhood, adolescence, and adulthood, guiding attractions and expectations for peers and partners alike. The therapeutic treatments were effective in changing these anchoring cognitions and allowing the clients to make behavioral changes consistent with the posttreatment cognitive schema.

All of the cases presented in this article reported chronic parental emotional abuse, which then determined their social cognitions. Sam and Randy were ridiculed by their early attachment systems for their gender nonconformity. Mary was a victim of emotional neglect from her caretakers, thereby paving the way for her childhood sexual abuse. One or more caretakers abandoned both Patty and Dara, for reasons that were not clear to them as children. This further illustrates findings in the empirical literature regarding the experience of childhood emotional abuse on social cognition. Their maltreatment was especially problematic because it was experienced from both their caregivers and their peer group.

Characteristic of all cases in this clinical sample was the concept of total social rejection, which is the chronic neglect from caregivers coupled with rejection from the peer group. This combination has been found to be predictive of an inclination for the child to generate negative and hostile social cognitive schema (Crick & Dodge, 1994). This was evident in all five cases; in childhood and adolescence they ventured out from their family of origin and entered their peer networks with an understanding of the social world as being a hostile and rejecting place. Sam, Patty, and Randy experienced peer ridicule in response to gender nonconformity. Mary carried around a secret about a loss of innocence and a mistrust of the opposite sex. Dara's depression made her appear strange to the other children and therefore a target of ridicule and ostracism. The empirical literature informs us that with repeated emotional abuse and peer rejection, the child is left to employ his or her cognitive schema by using defensive social strategies that become recalcitrant (Crick & Dodge, 1996; Hodges & Perry, 1999). These coping strategies are rooted in anchoring cognitions that are difficult to change as they serve to reinforce one's existing social cognition. After experiencing repeatedly reinforced social cognitions in childhood and adolescence, the adult must now transact social relationships and establish attachments with these beliefs rooted in early social experiences with the caregivers and peers. When their social cognition failed them, in that they could not find satisfaction in their intimate social relationships, they experienced feelings of defeat and helplessness (see Riggs & Kaminski, 2010). This often resulted in depression and anxiety, which led the individuals in this sample to seek professional help.

Studies on adult attachment systems have found that adults tend to seek attachments with persons who are physical and mental representations of past attachment figures (Mikulincer & Shaver, 2003). There is a tendency to affiliate with persons perceived to be similar to the maltreating caregiver and rejecting peer group (Baumeister & Leary, 1995). This was seen in all five cases. Randy sought out men who he perceived as perfect, the very same type he feared would reject him, as they had in the past. Mary had compulsive sexual encounters with men to avoid intimacy and by default enacted reactive attachments to women in nonsexual relationship formats. Patty and Dara had relationships with unavailable men and became romantically obsessed with possessing them, in spite of their detachment. Sam had superficial attachments as a prostitute who reenacted versions of his adolescent relationship with his neighbor.

Baumeister and Leary (1995) also found that people have an affinity for persons perceived to be highly unlike one's past source of rejection, especially if a high probability of social acceptance is appraised. This was not evidenced in any of the cases except in their connection to the therapist and later posttreatment attachments. After successful treatment when an attachment was appraised as potentially supportive, it was pursued and maintained. Prior to treatment, if an attachment figure was appraised as threatening or rejecting, hyperactivation of the attachment system occurred or what is referred to in the clinical literature as a romantic obsessive behavior (Carnes, 1992; Tennov, 1999); Dara and Randy evidenced this. As they felt their attachment to threatening figures slipping away from them, they activated an obsessive attachment-seeking orientation toward the love object. After treatment, if an attachment figure were appraised as potentially threatening or rejecting, the client would dismiss this person as a potential attachment figure.

Adult attachment research has demonstrated that whereas some adults with childhood histories of emotional abuse and peer rejection seek to repair their insecure attachment status by re-creating and reenacting these dynamics in adulthood, some elect to withdraw, resulting in a decrease in proximity-seeking behaviors (Maner et al., 2007; Riggs, 2010). This was the case with Sam, who gave up on having a supportive intimate relationship with another man in place of counterdependent casual sexual relationships with clients as a prostitute. This served as a protective device against the psychological pain suffered during previous attempts at attaching to male love objects, similar to his teenage sexual exploration with his neighbor. He carried this avoidant cognitive schema for nearly 20 years before receiving treatment to change his beliefs to a social cognition that resulted in more prosocial attachment-seeking behaviors.

Sroufe (1989) believed that the effects of early attachment might be modified later in childhood. None of the cases in this clinical sample had experiences with peers, teachers, or mentors that served to modify or correct their negative social cognition. Sam attempted to have a seemingly corrective adolescent experience with his neighbor, but the secondary trauma that ensued after he was made to feel ashamed of his behavior served to undo any corrective effects that this relationship might have had on his social cognition. This article argues that psychotherapy, directed at changing the anchoring cognitions, can play this role later in life to correct insecure attachments. By modifying the social cognition in four of the five cases, the therapist was able to reduce opportunities for negative patterns to be repeated and weaken the chance that the anchoring cognitions would persist over time as evidenced by the posttreatment attachments for each case (see Table 1).

The application of CBT, REBT, and EMDR to the treatment of attachment disturbances in adults with childhood histories of social rejection from peers and caregivers should be studied further. A larger sample size of clients and therapists from geographically, ethnically, and culturally diverse populations should be studied in an empirical format. The measurement of all variables previously discussed (i.e., attachment status, treatment outcomes, etc.) should be empirically validated as well. A more rigorous consideration of the relationship between emotional abuse and later intimate attachments could yield important findings for prevention and intervention efforts with at-risk populations.

REFERENCES

Ainsworth, M. D. S. (1989). Attachments beyond infancy. *American Psychologist, 44*, 709–716.

Bartholomew, K., & Horowitz, L. (1991). Attachment styles among young adults: A test of the four category model. *Journal of Personality and Social Psychology, 61*, 226–244.

Baumeister, R. F., & Leary, M. R. (1995). The need to belong: Desire for interpersonal attachments as a fundamental human motivation. *Psychological Bulletin, 117*, 497–529.

Berndt, T. J. (1982). The features and effects of friendship in early adolescence. *Child Development, 53*, 1447–1460.

Bierman, K. (1986). Process of change during social skills training with preadolescents and its relation to treatment outcomes. *Child Development, 55*, 151–162.

Bishop, F. M. (2001). *Managing addictions*. North Bergen, NJ: Aronson.

Bowlby, J. (1988). *A secure base: Parent–child attachment and healthy human development*. New York: Basic Books.

Burkowski, W. M., & Hoza, B. (1989). Popularity and friendship: Issues in theory, measurement, and outcome. In T. J. Berndt & G. Ladd (Eds.), *Peer relations in child development* (pp. 15–45). New York: Wiley.

Carnes, P. (1992). *Don't call it love: Recovery from sexual addiction*. New York: Bantam.

Clark, D. M., & Ehlers, A. (2004). Posttraumatic stress disorder: From cognitive theory to therapy. In R. L. Leahy (Ed.), *Contemporary cognitive therapy: Theory, research and practice* (pp. 141–161). New York: Guilford.

Collins, N. L., & Read S. J. (1990). Adult attachment, working models, and relationship quality in dating couples. *Journal of Personality and Social Psychology, 58*, 644–663.

Crick, N. R., & Dodge, K. A. (1994). A review and reformulation of social information-processing mechanisms in children's social adjustment. *Psychological Bulletin, 115*, 74–101.

Crick, N. R., & Dodge, K. A. (1996). Social informational-processing mechanisms in reactive and proactive aggression. *Child Development, 67*, 993–1002.

Ellis, A. (2005). *Rational emotive behavior therapy: A therapist's guide* (2nd ed.). Atascadero, CA: Impact.

Erikson, E. (1963). *Childhood and society* (2nd ed.). New York: Norton.

Friedman, H. S., Tucker, J. S., Schwartz, J. E., Tomlinson-Keasey, C., Martin, L. R., Wingard, D. L., et al. (1995). Psychosocial and behavioral predictors of longevity: The aging and death of the "Termites." *American Psychologist, 50*, 69–78.

Harter, S. (1999). *The construction of the self: A developmental perspective*. New York: Guilford.

Hodges, E. V. E., & Perry, D. G. (1999). Personal and interpersonal antecedents and consequences of victimization by peers. *Journal of Personality and Social Psychology, 76*, 677–685.

Horowitz, A. B., & White, H. R. (1998). The relationship of cohabitation and mental health: A study of a young adult cohort. *Journal of Marriage and the Family, 60*, 505–514.

Langlois, J. H., & Stephan, C. W. (1981). Beauty and the beast: The role of physical attraction in peer relationships and social behavior. In S. S. Brehm, S. M. Kassin, & S. X. Gibbans (Eds.), *Developmental social psychology: Theory and research* (pp.152–168). New York: Oxford University Press.

Main, M. (1996). Overview of the field of attachment. *Journal of Consulting and Clinical Psychology, 64*, 237–243.

Maner, J. K., DeWall, C. N., Baumeister, R. F., & Schaller, M. (2007). Does social exclusion motivate interpersonal reconnection? Resolving the porcupine problem. *Journal of Personality and Social Psychology, 92*, 42–55.

Mikulincer, M., & Shaver, P. R. (2003). The attachment behavioral system in adulthood: Activation, psychodynamics, and interpersonal processes. In M. P. Zanna (Ed.), *Advances in experimental social psychology* (Vol. 35, pp. 52–153). New York: Academic.

Nelson, D. A., & Crick, N. R. (1999). Rose-colored glasses: Examining the social information-processing of prosocial young adolescents. *The Journal of Early Adolescence, 19*, 17–38.

Newcomb, A. F., Bukowski, W. M., & Pattee, L. (1993). Children's peer relations: A meta-analytic review of popular, rejected, neglected, and average sociometric status. *Psychological Bulletin, 113*, 99–128.

Parkhurst, J. T., & Asher, S. R. (1992). Peer rejection in middle school: Subgroup differences in behavior, loneliness, and interpersonal concerns. *Developmental Psychology, 28*, 231–241.

Piaget, J. (1965). *The moral judgment of the child*. New York: Free Press.

Riggs, S. A. (2010). Childhood emotional abuse and the attachment system across the life cycle: What theory and research tell us. *Journal of Aggression, Maltreatment and Trauma, 19*(1), 5–51.

Riggs, S. A., & Kaminski, P. (2010). Childhood emotional abuse, adult attachment, and depression as predictors of relational adjustment and psychological aggression. *Journal of Aggression, Maltreatment and Trauma, 19*(1), 75–104.

Riskind, J. H. (2004). Cognitive theory and research. In R. L. Leahy (Ed.), *Contemporary cognitive therapy: Theory, research and practice* (pp. 62–86). New York: Guilford.

Ross, C. E. (1995). Reconceptualizing marital status as a continuum of social attachment. *Journal of Marriage and the Family, 57*, 129–140.

Senchak, M., & Leonard, K. E. (1992). Attachment styles and marital adjustment among newlywed couples. *Journal of Personality and Social Psychology, 9*, 51–64.

Shapiro, F. (2001). *Eye movement desensitization and reprocessing: Basic principles, protocols, and procedures* (2nd ed.). New York: Guilford.

Simpson, J. A. (1990). Influence of attachment styles on romantic relationships. *Journal of Personality and Social Psychology, 59*, 971–980.

Sroufe, L. A. (1989). Pathways to adaptation and maladaptation: Psychopathology as developmental deviation: The roots of maladaption and competence. In D. Cicchetti (Ed.), *Rochester Symposium on Developmental Psychopathology: Vol. 1. The emergence of discipline* (pp. 13–40). Hillsdale, NJ: Lawrence Erlbaum Associates.

Steinberg, L., & Avenevoli, S. (2000). The role of context in the development of psychopathology: A conceptual framework and some speculative propositions. *Child Development, 71*, 66–74.

Taussig, H. N., & Culhane, S. E. (2010). Emotional maltreatment and psychosocial functioning in preadolescent youth placed in out-of-home care. *Journal of Aggression, Maltreatment and Trauma, 19*(1), 52–74.

Tennov, D. (1999). *Love and limerance: The experience of being loved* (2nd ed.). New York: Scarborough House.

Waite, L. J., & Joyner, K. (2001). Emotional satisfaction and physical pleasure in sexual unions: Time horizon, sexual behavior, and sexual exclusivity. *Journal of Marriage and the Family, 63*, 247–264.

INTRODUCTION TO PART 2

NANCY DODGE REYOME
State University of New York College at Potsdam, Potsdam, New York, USA

This is the second part of a special double issue focusing on the effects that childhood emotional maltreatment has on intimate relationships. It explores the relational difficulties often encountered by emotional abuse survivors. The empirically based articles in this issue look at the association between childhood emotional maltreatment and the relational difficulties of self-sacrifice, codependency, intimate partner violence, and sexual aggression. This introduction provides a brief summary of each article in this special issue.

This issue of the *Journal of Aggression, Maltreatment and Trauma* is the second issue of two special issues concerned with the influence of childhood emotional maltreatment on the formation and maintenance of intimate relationships in adolescence and adulthood. This issue focuses on the association between childhood emotional maltreatment and relational difficulties in adolescence and adulthood. For some time, researchers and clinicians have understood that childhood emotional maltreatment is a serious form of child maltreatment and perhaps the most developmentally deleterious form of maltreatment (Ney, Fung, & Wickett, 1994; Spertus, Yehuda, Wong, Halligan, & Seremetis, 2003). Yet research on the long-term relational consequences of childhood emotional maltreatment has lagged behind research on other forms of child maltreatment such as sexual and physical abuse (Egeland, 2009). This issue contains five articles that investigate many of the relational difficulties associated with a history of childhood emotional maltreatment. The first article looks at psychosocial mediators of the relationship between a history of emotional maltreatment and codependency in adulthood. The second article looks at the association between child maltreatment history and interpersonal problems in couple relationships. The third and fourth articles focus on the connection between childhood emotional maltreatment and relationship violence. The final article reviews the research literature on the effect of childhood emotional maltreatment on relationship functioning and makes suggestions for further research on this very important topic.

In the first article, Paradis and Boucher explore the relationship between child maltreatment history and relationship problems in adult couple relationships. They discovered that victims of childhood maltreatment reported more interpersonal problems than nonmaltreated individuals. They also found that male abuse victims experienced more interpersonal problems than female abuse victims. Further, emotional neglect in males was associated with being distant and nonassertive in close relationships, whereas emotional neglect in females was associated with distance, a lack of assertiveness, and self-sacrifice in close relationships. Finally, females with emotional abuse histories were more likely to report being distant and domineering in couple relationships.

In the second article, Dodge Reyome, Ward, and Witkiewitz consider the role of depression, self-esteem, self-differentiation, and self-concealment as potential mediators of the relationship between a history of emotional maltreatment and codependency as well as the relationship between emotional maltreatment and self-silencing in a sample of upper division nursing students. Prior to their study, both codependency and self-silencing had been previously linked with childhood emotional abuse in the research literature. In their study, they found a moderate relationship between emotional and psychological forms of child maltreatment and both codependency and self-silencing. Also, they discovered depression, self-esteem, self-concealment, and self-differentiation are each partial mediators of the relationship between childhood emotional maltreatment and codependency as well as childhood emotional maltreatment and self-silencing.

Using a developmental process framework, Berzenski and Yates report on the relationship between childhood emotional maltreatment and relationship violence perpetration and victimization in a large, ethnically diverse sample of college students. They found relationship violence perpetration and relationship violence victimization were positively associated with a childhood history of emotional maltreatment. In fact, Berzenski and Yates discovered that of the forms of childhood maltreatment and violence exposure measured in their study, a history of emotional abuse was the strongest predictor of intimate violence. Finally, adding to the significance of this study, these researchers found that emotion regulation (especially impulsivity) serves as a mediator of the relationship between childhood emotional abuse and relationship violence.

In the most comprehensive and focused study to date on the topic, Zurbriggen, Gobin, and Freyd look at the relationship between childhood emotional trauma and sexual aggression perpetration and victimization in a college sample. They compared childhood emotional abuse, childhood sexual abuse, and childhood physical abuse as predictors of sexual violence perpetration and sexual violence victimization. For the entire sample, a history of childhood emotional abuse was significantly related to being both a victim of sexual violence and a perpetrator of sexual violence. When controlling for other forms of child maltreatment, they found childhood emotional abuse significantly predicted perpetration of sexual violence among women and sexual victimization among men.

In the final article, Dodge Reyome provides an overview of the extant literature dealing with the long-term relational consequences of childhood emotional maltreatment. This overview brings together many of the topics addressed in the articles in this issue, including relationship quality and satisfaction, codependency, and relationship violence. While shedding light on some of the main findings to date, she also points out the limitations of the current research literature and makes suggestions for further research investigations to move forward our understanding of the long-term consequences of this often overlooked form of childhood trauma.

The awareness of the harmful consequences of childhood emotional victimization has grown over the last three decades. This issue of the *Journal of Aggression, Maltreatment and Trauma* contains empirically based articles that extend our understanding of these consequences for interpersonal well-being and the health of intimate relationships of emotional abuse survivors. By moving forward our understanding of how childhood emotional abuse influences relational functioning and well-being, professionals in the field can use this new knowledge to provide more effective support and interventions for those individuals with childhood histories of emotional and psychological victimization.

REFERENCES

Egeland, B. (2009). Taking stock: Childhood emotional maltreatment and developmental psychopathology. *Child Abuse and Neglect*, *33*, 22–26.

Ney, P., Fung, T., & Wickett, A. (1994). The worst combinations of child abuse and neglect. *Child Abuse and Neglect*, *18*, 705–714.

Spertus, I., Yehuda, R., Wong, C., Halligan, S., & Seremetis, S. (2003). Childhood emotional abuse and neglect as predictors of psychological and physical symptoms in women presenting to a primary care practice. *Child Abuse and Neglect*, *27*, 1247–1258.

RESEARCH ON INTERPERSONAL PROBLEMS AND CODEPENDENCY

Child Maltreatment History and Interpersonal Problems in Adult Couple Relationships

ALISON PARADIS and SOPHIE BOUCHER
Université du Québec à Montréal, Montréal, Canada

This study examines the relationship between interpersonal problems in adult couple relationships and childhood maltreatment in a sample of 1,728 university students who completed an online questionnaire. Victims of maltreatment reported higher levels of couple interpersonal problems. Also, the experience of childhood maltreatment is more strongly associated with couple interpersonal difficulties for males than for females. For females, emotional neglect is more consistently related to couple interpersonal problems, including problems with being nonassertive, distant, and self-sacrificing. For males, physical abuse is significantly associated with the likelihood of being domineering, distant, and self-sacrificing. The issue of how the different forms of maltreatment might contribute differently to couple interpersonal problems for males and females is addressed and discussed.

The research reported in this article was supported by a grant from the Fonds de Recherche sur la société et la culture (FQRSC) and by a grant from the Centre de recherche interdisciplinaire sur les problèmes conjugaux et les agressions sexuelles (CRIPCAS).

Both attachment theory (Bowlby, 1969/1982) and complex trauma theory (Herman, 1992) support the idea that childhood abuse and neglect can have a powerful impact on how individuals construct their lives and their relationships (see Riggs, 2010). Childhood maltreatment often involves those most needed by the victims. For instance, in cases of physical or sexual abuse, the parent can evoke intense fear, helplessness, and horror, and simultaneously be the person from whom the child seeks protection. These experiences can irrevocably shape the way victims define the world and themselves, and can impact their interpersonal relationships as adults. A deeper understanding of the difficulties arising within couple relationships in victims of childhood maltreatment is even more important because an intimate relationship can provide adult survivors an ideal context in which to heal (Herman, 1992; Walsh, 1996; Whiffen, Judd, & Aube, 1999). Despite the theoretical interests, only recently have researchers begun to systematically examine the relationship between childhood abuse and neglect and subsequent interpersonal difficulties in adulthood (see Dodge Reyome, 2010).

ASSOCIATION BETWEEN CHILDHOOD MALTREATMENT AND COUPLE RELATIONSHIPS

To date, sexual abuse has received more attention in the literature than any of the other forms of childhood maltreatment. Many have suggested that one of the most pervasive consequences of childhood sexual abuse is the development of erroneous relational models that lead to difficulties in interpersonal relationships in adulthood (Cole & Putnam, 1992; Davis & Petretic-Jackson, 2000; Finkelhor & Browne, 1985). Victims of childhood sexual abuse report a wide variety of difficulties in their ability to establish and maintain stable and satisfying intimate relationships. Findings have shown an association between a history of sexual abuse and lower satisfaction in intimate relationships (DiLillo & Long, 1999; Hunter, 1991), higher symptoms of sexual dysfunctions (Hunter, 1991; Mullen, Martin, Anderson, Romans, & Herbison, 1994), lower level of trust in their partners, and poorer communication between spouses (DiLillo & Long, 1999). In addition, victims of sexual abuse are more likely than nonvictims to report higher levels of partner violence (Banyard, Arnold, & Smith, 2000; DiLillo, Giuffre, Tremblay, & Peterson, 2001), as well as separation and divorce (Colman & Widom, 2004; Mullen et al., 1994). Emerging research has only started to demonstrate a similar pattern of association between other types of childhood maltreatment and adult intimate relationships. Childhood physical abuse (Ornduff, Kelsey, & O'Leary, 2001; Wolfe, Wekerle, Reitzel-Jaffe, & Lefebvre, 1998) and psychological maltreatment (Crawford & O'Dougherty-Wright, 2007) are shown to be associated with both victimization and perpetration of adult intimate partner aggression (see Berzenski & Yates, 2010; Dodge Reyome, 2010; Zurbriggen, Gobin, & Freyd, 2010). An association between childhood physical abuse and a greater fear of intimacy has also been reported (Repic, 2007). In addition, studies have shown that victims of psychological maltreatment are more likely to report marital dissatisfaction (Perry, DiLillo, & Peugh, 2007).

Despite the cumulative evidence of the impact of childhood abuse on later interpersonal functioning, few studies have compared the association of different forms of maltreatment with specific relational difficulties. Those that have indicate that the various forms of abuse and neglect lead to similar interpersonal outcomes (Davis, Petretic-Jackson, & Ting, 2001; Wind & Silvern, 1992). However, findings are limited to interpersonal outcomes such as divorce or marital dissatisfaction (Colman & Widom, 2004; Davis et al., 2001; DiLillo, Lewis, & Di Loreto-Colgan, 2007). Briere and Runtz (1990) found that a history of childhood sexual abuse is associated with dysfunctions in the domain of sexuality, physical abuse is related to aggressive behaviors, and psychological maltreatment is associated with dysfunctions in the domain of self-esteem. Thus, it is possible that specific associations could also be found between the different types of maltreatment experiences and specific domains of problems within the couple relationship (e.g., coldness, dominance). These problems could eventually lead to the same interpersonal outcomes (e.g., separation and divorce).

A further limitation of the current research on childhood maltreatment is that the majority of studies have been conducted with female victims (see Dodge Reyome, 2010, for a brief discussion of this limitation of maltreatment research). The few studies that have looked at male victims often show mixed results. Whereas some report similar difficulties in couple functioning for both male and female victims (Finkelhor, Hotaling, Lewis, & Smith, 1990; Repic, 2007), others have found different associations for male victims (Colman & Widom, 2004; DiLillo et al., 2007). Thus, research is needed to clarify if and how males and females with histories of childhood maltreatment differ in their ability to maintain healthy intimate relationships.

THE INTERPERSONAL MODEL

Interpersonal theories (e.g., Horney, 1945; Leary, 1957; Sullivan, 1953) can help explain the impact of maltreatment on the quality of adult couple relationships. They offer a valuable organizational framework for understanding patterns of maladaptive intimate relationships. One current interpretation of the interpersonal theory (Horowitz et al., 2006; Kiesler, 1996), based particularly on Sullivan's (1953) early theoretical concepts, assumes that everything people do in interaction with one another reflects an effort to avoid anxiety and to achieve and maintain self-esteem. These two motives can be

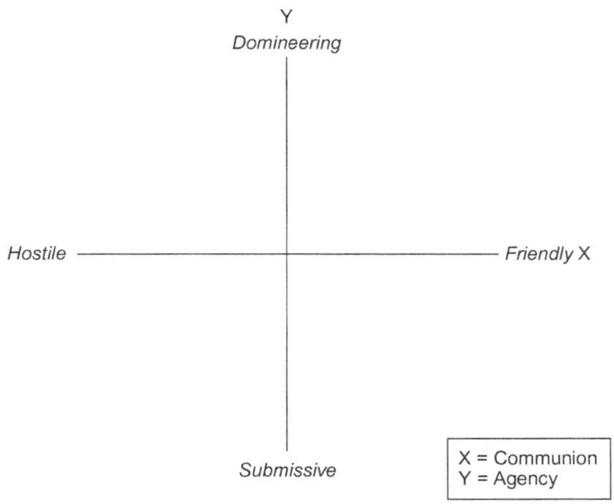

FIGURE 1 The two-dimensional interpersonal space.

organized along two axes that form a circumplex structure, a dimension of affiliation or *communion* that ranges from hostile to friendly behaviors (horizontal axis) and a dimension of dominance or *agency* that ranges from submissive to domineering behaviors (vertical axis; see Figure 1). According to Horowitz et al. (2006), dimensions of communion and agency can be used to organize behaviors, traits, and intentions. They reflect two principal evolutionary challenges: (a) connecting with other people to form a protective community (communion), and (b) achieving a sense of one's own competence and control (agency). Horowitz et al. (2006), referring to Blatt (1990), suggested that personality develops following these two developmental dimensions. Ideally, the first should lead to the conviction that one is loved and can safely enter intimate and lasting relationships with others, whereas the second should contribute to a stable, realistic, independent, and competent self-image. However, when for some reason the development of one or both dimensions is disturbed during childhood, interpersonal difficulties arise (Horowitz et al., 2006).

Specific interpersonal problems that exemplify a range of maladaptive behaviors derived from current interpersonal theory have been identified (Horowitz, Rosenberg, Baer, Ureno, & Villasenor, 1988). Problems related to communion range from being overly cold and distant to being excessively self-sacrificing. Problems related to agency range from being domineering and controlling to being nonassertive when interacting or attempting to interact with others. According to Alden, Wiggins, and Pincus (1990), the two-dimensional interpersonal space can be divided into eight equal octants, each representing a domain of interpersonal problem (see Figure 2). For example, being "overly accommodating" corresponds to being friendly

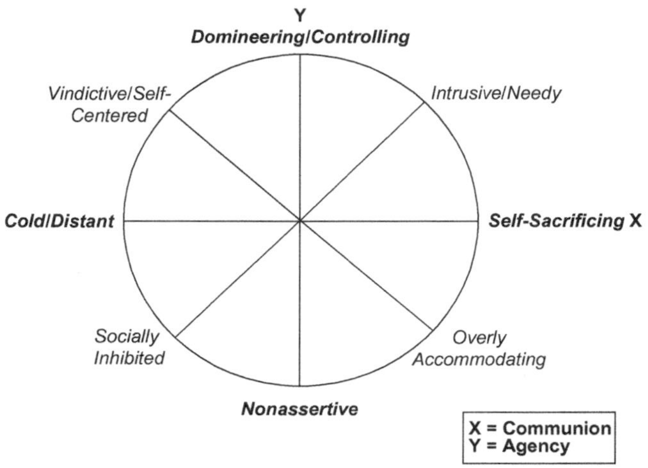

FIGURE 2 Circumplex model of interpersonal problems (Alden et al., 1990).

(positive communion) and submissive (negative agency). This way of describing interpersonal behavior has often been used in the literature. However, few studies on couple relationships have referred to the circumplex model. This can be explained by the fact that the instrument most commonly used to measure interpersonal problems related to agency and communion has been developed to measure a person's most salient interpersonal problems in a global way, not specific to a relationship in particular. Indeed, while completing the Inventory of Interpersonal Problems (IIP–64; Horowitz, Alden, Wiggins, & Pincus, 2000), respondents think of relationships with friends, a spouse, or coworkers. Because the levels of communion and agency can differ according to the type of relationship (e.g., interaction with a friend vs. with a romantic partner), some believe that it is important to take into account the context in which the interaction takes place when assessing the two dimensions (Suh, Moskowitz, Fournier, & Zuroff, 2004).

The circumplex model of interpersonal problems seems to be particularly suited to the study of maltreatment because it can help conceptualize the differing patterns of outcomes seen in the victim's couple relationship. It can be hypothesized that an experience of childhood abuse and neglect will disturb one or both developmental dimensions (communion and agency) and greatly impact the way a person views the world and himself or herself. For instance, a victim of childhood maltreatment might not feel safe or protected when connecting to other people because early experiences have shown them that the people from whom they sought protection cannot be trusted or are not a source of comfort (communion). As a result, these individuals might report difficulty in making long-term commitments and an inability to express affection toward their partner or feel love for their partner in adulthood. According to the circumplex model, they will likely interact with their partner in a cold and distant manner. On the other hand, early experiences of abuse and neglect might also underscore a person's own sense of incompetence and lack of control (agency). Thus, it is possible that once in adulthood, these victims will have difficulties making their needs known and have problems being assertive toward their partner (being nonassertive).

GOALS OF THIS STUDY

The purpose of this study was to assess the problems in adult couple relationships in a sample of males and females who disclosed being victims of abuse, neglect, or both during childhood and compare them to a nonvictimized comparison group. The first aim was to expand on the findings from earlier studies that are often limited to one type of abuse. Therefore, this study examined the relationship among a range of maltreatment experiences (physical abuse, emotional abuse, physical neglect, emotional neglect, and sexual abuse) and interpersonal problems. It is postulated that the victims of childhood abuse and neglect will show more interpersonal problems in their couple relationships than nonvictims. The second aim of this study was to use interpersonal theories as a framework for understanding patterns of maladaptive intimate relationships of victims of childhood maltreatment. As mentioned earlier, it is proposed that the various forms of maltreatment will relate differently to the dimensions of agency and communion in couple relationships. Four domains of interpersonal problems were examined: domineering/controlling, cold/distant, nonassertive, and self-sacrificing. Finally, the third aim of this study was to examine if males and females with histories of childhood maltreatment differ in the types of interpersonal problems they report.

METHODS

Participants

Participants were male and female French-Canadian university students who signed up for this study through an online program. Among the 2,885 respondents, 177 were excluded because they did not meet the inclusion criteria (having been in at least one committed heterosexual relationship for more than a month) and 980 were excluded because of incomplete questionnaires or incongruent responses. The final sample consisted of 1,728 students (320 males and 1,408 females) for whom complete data were available. Participants ranged in age from 18 to 65 years (*M* age for males = 27.3, *SD* = 8.0; *M* age for females = 24.9, *SD* = 6.2). The sample consisted primarily of undergraduates (78%) and most described their ethnic or racial background as Caucasian (92.6%). Although only 7.4% of participants reported being married, another 38.4% mentioned living with their partner without being married. Three quarters of the respondents reported that the duration of the relationship was of 6 months or more (75.4%).

Procedure

Initially, e-mail invitations were sent out to all university students. The e-mail explained the purpose of the study, that participation was voluntary and confidential, and it contained the Web site address (Uniform Resource Locator) to access the Web-based questionnaire. An e-mail address and telephone number were provided for participants to contact if they had any questions about the study or the Web survey. In addition to the e-mail invitations, recruitment was carried out by advertisement placed in a number of university buildings and classrooms. As an incentive to complete the survey, participants were offered a chance to win one cash prize of $200 that was awarded by a drawing. Students who were interested in participating were first directed, via the Internet, to a consent form on which it was indicated that they would be asked to answer personal questions about their couple relationship and their childhood experiences. Upon consent, each respondent completed the online battery of questionnaires. The measures used in this study were part of this battery. With the use of a password, it was possible for participants to take breaks while completing the survey. This study received the approval of the university's institutional review ethics board.

Measures

Intrafamilial childhood sexual abuse

Different aspects of childhood sexual abuse were measured with the Instrument to Measure Sexual Aggression in Childhood—Short Form (ASE; Cyr & Frappier, 2005). This instrument is based on the Incest History Questionnaire (Courtois, 1988) and on the History of Victimization Form (Wolfe, Gentile, & Bourdeau, 1987). It contains 10 specific questions about respondents' sexual abuse histories in the first 18 years of life. A history of sexual abuse is assessed with the following question: "As a child (before the age of 18) did someone ever do something inappropriate sexually with you? By inappropriate, we mean that someone exposed themselves or asked you to expose intimate parts of your body, kissed or fondled you in a sexual manner, or did any other sexual activities, while you did not want to participate. Therefore, those situations have happened against your will; you were subjected to them or you were forced to participate in them." Specific questions about respondents' sexual abuse histories are then asked, including the approximate number of aggressions, the nature of the sexual(s) aggression(s), the age at which they were first victimized, and the nature of their relationship with the perpetrator(s). In this study, only experiences of sexual abuse perpetrated by a member of the victim's family were considered in the analyses (e.g., parents, siblings, grandparents, cousins). In addition, only experiences that included at least one physical contact (i.e., fondling of genitals or breast, attempted or completed penetration) were classified as sexual abuse.

Childhood physical and emotional abuse and neglect

The other forms of childhood abuse and neglect were assessed using the Childhood Trauma Questionnaire–Short Form (CTQ–SF; Bernstein et al., 2003; translated into French by Paquette, Laporte, Bigras, & Zoccolillo, 2004). The CTQ–SF is a self-administered inventory that was developed to measure the severity of different types of childhood trauma. Four subscales were used in this study, including emotional abuse (five items), emotional neglect (four items), physical abuse (five items), and physical neglect (five items). Participants indicate whether they experienced certain events while growing up on a 5-point Likert scale ranging from 1 (*never true*) to 5 (*very often true*), producing four clinical subscales with scores of 5 to 25. Cutoff scores can be applied to identify individuals with histories of abuse and neglect. As recommended by Paquette et al. (2004), the CTQ cutoff scores were defined as scores of 16 or greater for emotional abuse and neglect, 14 or greater for physical neglect, and 11 or greater for physical abuse. The psychometric properties of the CTQ–SF have been well documented and appear to be adequate (Bernstein et al., 2003; Paquette et al., 2004). Reliability coefficients of the four selected subscales are satisfactory and similar to those documented in other studies (e.g., Bernstein et al., 2003; Paquette et al., 2004) with subscale alpha scores of .60 for physical neglect, .82 for physical abuse, .84 for emotional abuse, and .88 for emotional neglect.

Couple interpersonal problems

Interpersonal difficulties in intimate relationships were measured with the Inventory of Interpersonal Problems in Couple Relationships (IIP–Couple; Paradis & Boucher, 2007). The IIP–Couple is a self-report instrument, developed by the authors of this study, adapted from the IIP-64, which measures overall interpersonal problems (IIP–64; Horowitz et al., 2000). The 64 items of the IIP–64 were reworded to apply to "my partner." For instance, the item "It is hard for me to trust other people" became "It is hard for me to trust my partner." The instrument was then translated into French Canadian using the back-translation method (Brislin, 1970; Vallerand, 1989).

The IIP–Couple is designed to assess different domains of interpersonal difficulties that individuals might have while interacting or attempting to interact with their partner. It contains 39 items preceded by the phrase "It is hard for me to . . ." and 25 items describing interpersonal behavior people might do too much when interacting with their partner (e.g., "I fight with my partner too much"). Participants answer on a 5-point Likert scale ranging from 0 (*not at all*) to 4 (*extremely*). The 64 items produce eight subscales with scores of 0 to 32. It is also possible to obtain a total score on the IIP–Couple by calculating the sum of the eight subscale scores. This study reported the results of the four subscales corresponding to the extremities of the two main axes of the interpersonal circumplex: cold/distant (e.g., "It is hard for me to feel close to my partner"), self-sacrificing (e.g., "I try to please my partner too much"), domineering/controlling (e.g., "I am too aggressive toward my partner"), and nonassertive (e.g., "It is hard for me to tell my partner to stop bothering me"). The results of a principal components analysis on the subjects' ipsatized scores (i.e., every item's deviation from the individual's overall mean) suggest that the items provide a close representation of the two-dimensional interpersonal circumplex with its two main components of agency and communion (Paradis & Boucher, 2008). In addition, analyses indicate that the IIP–Couple has the same underlying circumplex structure as for the IIP–64 shown by Alden et al. (1990). The psychometric properties of the IIP–Couple were shown to be similar to that of the original instrument with the internal consistency of each dimension ranging from .79 to .83.

RESULTS

The descriptive statistics of the variables of interest for the 1,728 participants are presented by gender in Table 1. Because the distributions of the scores for the IIP–Couple were positively skewed, square-root and log transformations were applied to normalize the distributions (Tabachnick & Fidell, 2007). There are 64 (20.0%) males and 336 (23.9%) females who indicated having experienced at least one type of childhood maltreatment. Of the total sample, 7.5% of males and 8.8% of females indicated that they had been victims of more than one type of childhood maltreatment. To examine the differences between males and females on the prevalence rates for the different types of childhood trauma and on the subscale scores of the IIP–Couple, chi-square analyses and *t* tests were conducted. Given the number of *t*-test comparisons, Bonferroni corrections were applied ($p < .01$). Significant results indicate that males were more likely to report physical abuse, $\chi^2 = 4.56$, $p < .05$ (df = 1, N = 1728), and females were more likely to report an experience of child sexual abuse, $\chi^2 = 11.55$, $p < .001$ (df = 1, N = 1728). In terms of interpersonal problems, males were also more likely to report being distant

TABLE 1 Means, Standard Deviations, and Prevalence of Childhood Maltreatment and Interpersonal Problems in Couple Relationships by Gender

	Males[a]		Females[b]		
	M (*SD*)	Prevalence (clinical scores)	*M* (*SD*)	Prevalence (clinical scores)	*p*[c]
Type of trauma experience in childhood					
Physical abuse (CTQ)	6.3 (3.1)	25 (7.8%)	5.9 (2.5)	68 (4.8%)	.033
Emotional abuse (CTQ)	7.5 (3.8)	17 (5.3%)	8.2 (4.3)	111 (7.9%)	*ns*
Physical neglect (CTQ)	6.9 (2.7)	7 (2.2%)	6.5 (2.5)	18 (1.3%)	*ns*
Emotional neglect (CTQ)	10.1 (4.7)	47 (14.7%)	10.1 (4.7)	211 (15.0%)	*ns*
Sexual abuse (ASE)		10 (3.1%)		123 (8.7%)	.000
Interpersonal problems in couple relationships (IIP–Couple)					
Domineering	6.7 (5.3)		6.4 (5.2)		*ns*
Distant	5.0 (5.7)		3.7 (4.6)		.001
Nonassertive	9.6 (6.2)		8.0 (6.0)		.000
Self-sacrificing	9.9 (6.1)		7.9 (5.7)		.000
Total score (sum of subscales 1 to 8)	57.6 (34.2)		48.3 (30.3)		.000

Note: CTQ = Childhood Trauma Questionnaire; ASE = Instrument to Measure Sexual Aggression in Childhood—Short Form; IIP–Couple = Inventory of Interpersonal Problems in Couple Relationships.
[a]*n* = 320. [b]*n* 1,408. [c]Differences between males and females on prevalence of trauma experiences in childhood (χ^2) and mean scores of couple interpersonal problems (*t* tests).

toward their partner ($t = 3.35$, $p < .001$), nonassertive ($t = 4.76$, $p < .001$), and self-sacrificing ($t = 5.92$, $p < .001$). They also revealed higher overall rates of couple interpersonal problems than females ($t = 4.81$, $p < .001$). However, both males and females reported similar levels of domineering behaviors while interacting with their partner ($t = 1.137$, *ns*).

To examine the relationship between a range of maltreatment experiences (physical abuse, emotional abuse, physical neglect, emotional neglect, and sexual abuse) and interpersonal problems, separate two-way analyses of variance (Gender × Victimization) were performed to compare the total score on the IIP–Couple for each type of trauma experienced in childhood (victims vs. nonvictims). The means and standard deviations of interpersonal problems in couple relationship for each type of maltreatment are presented by gender in Table 2. Results reveal that victims of childhood physical abuse, $F(1, 1724) = 44.66$, $p < .001$; emotional abuse, $F(1, 1724) = 19.32$, $p < .001$; physical neglect, $F(1, 1724) = 11.71$, $p < .001$; and emotional neglect, $F(1, 1724) = 27.16$, $p < .001$, report significantly more interpersonal problems than nonvictims of childhood maltreatment. Results also show significant main effects of gender on the total number of couple interpersonal problems reported, with males presenting more interpersonal difficulties than females in the analyses involving physical abuse, $F(1, 1724) = 24.19$, $p < .001$; emotional abuse, $F(1, 1724) = 12.18$, $p < .001$; physical neglect, $F(1, 1724) = 14.09$, $p < .001$; and emotional neglect, $F(1, 1724) = 20.16$,

TABLE 2 Mean Total Scores and Standard Deviations of Interpersonal Problems in Couple Relationships by Gender and Maltreatment History

Type of trauma experience in childhood	Males[a]		Females[b]	
	Nonvictims	Victims	Nonvictims	Victims
Physical abuse (CTQ)	54.0 (29.8)	98.8 (52.0)	47.5 (29.7)	63.7 (39.9)
Emotional abuse (CTQ)	56.1 (33.0)	83.2 (44.9)	47.3 (29.5)	60.3 (33.5)
Physical neglect (CTQ)	56.4 (32.6)	108.3 (61.6)	48.2 (30.1)	56.0 (40.9)
Emotional neglect (CTQ)	54.6 (32.3)	74.3 (39.8)	46.5 (28.7)	68.1 (36.5)
Sexual abuse (ASE)	56.1 (32.2)	50.6 (27.5)	47.0 (29.5)	56.5 (32.0)

Note: CTQ = Childhood Trauma Questionnaire; ASE = Instrument to Measure Sexual Aggression in Childhood—Short Form. Inventory of Interpersonal Problems in Couple Relationships means and standard deviations are presented before transformation.
[a]n = 320. [b]n 1,408.

$p < .001$. In addition, significant interaction effects were found between the severity of physical abuse and gender, $F(1, 1724) = 9.06$, $p < .01$, and between the severity of physical neglect and gender, $F(1, 1724) = 6.47$, $p < .05$. This indicates that males and females were affected differently by physical abuse and neglect. Specifically, physical abuse and physical neglect seem to have a significantly greater impact on interpersonal problems in males than in females. Surprisingly, no significant main effects or interactions of trauma or of gender were found for childhood sexual abuse, indicating that males or females with a history of childhood sexual abuse do not report more interpersonal problems.

Stepwise regressions were used to explore whether the various forms of maltreatment would relate differently to the different dimensions of couple interpersonal problems along the dimensions of agency and communion. Table 3 summarizes the results of these analyses for both males and females. In each model, the five different types of childhood trauma experiences served as the predictor variables (continuous) of the four domains of interpersonal problems. Given the size of the sample, the inclusion criterion was limited to a significance level of .01. Results indicated that different forms of maltreatment contribute differently to problems related to dimensions of agency and communion. For both males and females, emotional neglect was most strongly associated with couple interpersonal problems in the submissive southern hemisphere of the circumplex (being nonassertive). On the other hand, physical abuse for males and emotional abuse for females contributed more to couple interpersonal problems in the northern hemisphere (being domineering). Childhood physical neglect as well as an experience of childhood sexual abuse did not add to the prediction of couple interpersonal problems in either males or females. Finally, in regards to the third aim of this study, it appears that males and females with histories of childhood maltreatment differ in terms of the types of interpersonal

TABLE 3 Summary of Stepwise Regressions of Interpersonal Problems in Couple Relationships on Child Maltreatment Experiences

Outcome variables	Males[a]				Females[b]			
	Predictors	ß	t	R^2 adjusted (model)	Predictors	ß	t	R^2 adjusted (model)
Domineering	Physical abuse	.304	5.68**	.089	Emotional abuse	.181	6.90**	.032
Distant	Physical abuse	.173	2.90*	.077	Emotional neglect	.133	3.65**	.051
	Emotional neglect	.167	2.80*		Emotional abuse	.115	3.14*	
Nonassertive	Emotional neglect	.200	3.64**	.037	Emotional neglect	.117	4.40**	.013
Self-sacrificing	Physical abuse	.252	4.65**	.061	Emotional neglect	.125	4.73**	.015

Note: All models summarized in Table 3 were significant, $p < .001$.
[a] $n = 320$. [b] n 1,408.
* $p < .01$. ** $p < .001$.

problems they report. Indeed, results of the stepwise regressions indicate that experiences of child maltreatment contributed more strongly to the prediction of couple interpersonal difficulties in males than in females. For males, physical abuse significantly predicted the likelihood of being domineering, distant, and self-sacrificing. In addition, for males, emotional neglect significantly predicted the likelihood of being distant and nonassertive. For females, emotional neglect significantly predicted the likelihood of being overly distant, nonassertive, and self-sacrificing, whereas emotional abuse significantly predicted the likelihood of being domineering and distant.

DISCUSSION

This study explored the relationship between childhood experiences of abuse and neglect and problems in adult couple relationships in a sample of male and female university students. The aims of the study were to: (a) examine the relationship among a range of maltreatment experiences (sexual, physical, and emotional abuse, and neglect) and couple interpersonal problems, (b) determine if the various forms of maltreatment are related differently to the dimensions of agency and communion in couple relationships, and (c) examine if males and females with histories of childhood maltreatment differed in terms of the different types of couple interpersonal problems they report. Of the individuals in the current sample, 22% reported having experienced at least one childhood trauma, and 8.2% reported having experienced two or more types of such traumas. The proportion of respondents reporting different maltreatment types is consistent with those of previous findings drawn from university samples (Higgins & McCabe, 2001). As shown in previous studies, females reported a higher prevalence of sexual abuse (Finkelhor et al., 1990; Putnam, 2003), whereas males reported more physical abuse in childhood (Edwards, Holden, Felitti, & Anda, 2003; Thompson, Kingree, & Desai, 2004).

Results indicate that male and female victims of childhood physical and emotional abuse and neglect show overall more interpersonal difficulties in their couple relationships than nonvictims (see Dodge Reyome, 2010). These findings are therefore unique in demonstrating empirically that specific childhood maltreatment experiences have a pervasive influence on couple functioning in adulthood. However, no such associations were found when looking at victims of childhood sexual abuse. These results are unexpected given that most studies have reported positive relations between a history of sexual abuse and difficulties in intimate relationship (e.g., Colman & Widom, 2004; DiLillo & Long, 1999; Hunter, 1991; Mullen et al., 1994). There are several potential explanations for these results. First, sexual abuse in childhood was assessed by a single item requiring an answer of "yes" or "no." It is possible that measuring the experience of sexual abuse with the use of a 5-point Likert scale could have provided more accurate and sensitive information by providing a range on which to assess the severity of the trauma. However, this explanation is unlikely given that all previous studies mentioned earlier also measured a history of sexual abuse using a single "yes" or "no" item. Consequently, the differences in the results between other studies and those reported here appear to be more likely due to sample characteristics. For instance, in the Colman and Widom (2004) study, the sample consisted of substantiated cases of sexual abuse drawn from the records of county juvenile and criminal courts. These might represent more severe cases then the ones found in this study. In addition, even if the inclusion criteria in this study were limited to victims of intrafamilial sexual abuse, most of the intrafamilial abuse reported by the victims was perpetrated by a member of their extended family (e.g., cousins, grandparents) rather than by an immediate family member (e.g., parents, siblings). Thus, it is possible that, in this sample, the duration of sexual abuse experience was less chronic than the other types of childhood maltreatment, and therefore perceived by the victim as less severe. Finally, it could be possible that the victims of sexual abuse from this sample possess certain characteristics that make them more resilient, such as coping skills or a higher threshold for trauma-related stress. Subsequently, these characteristics weakened their vulnerability to couple interpersonal difficulties. Further research on the effects of sexual abuse on couple interpersonal functioning should take into account the severity of the abuse and explore other potential contributing factors, such as coping skills.

With respect to the second aim of this study, emotional neglect was most strongly associated with couple interpersonal problems in the submissive southern hemisphere of the circumplex for both males and females. This might show that if one's feelings and needs have been neglected as a child, one might avoid communicating his or her wishes and needs to his or her partner in adulthood. In contrast, physical abuse for males and emotional abuse for females contributed more to couple interpersonal problems in the northern hemisphere (e.g., domineering behaviors). Thus, if as a child someone is subjected to emotional or physical acts of aggression, he or she might feel threatened by others and feel a need to control and manipulate his or her partner to protect his or her sense of worth and self-respect (see Dodge Reyome, Ward, & Witkiewitz, 2010, for a discussion of childhood emotional abuse and codependency). This finding is of particular interest because there is evidence that interpersonal problems located in the northern hemisphere of the circumplex (domineering, vindictive, intrusive) are important mediating factors of the association between violence in the family of origin and violence in intimate relationships in adulthood (Murphy & Blumenthal, 2000). In contrast, childhood sexual abuse and physical neglect did not contribute to the prediction of any of the four specific domains of interpersonal problems for either males or females. As discussed earlier, it is difficult to assume whether the absence of results for sexual abuse reflects differences in sample characteristics or if it is explained by the potential contribution of coping factors not measured in this study. The lack of significant results in the case of physical neglect might be due to the lower prevalence rates of this type of trauma in the current sample. Indeed, physical neglect, considered a more chronic form of maltreatment often associated with poverty (English, 1998), was less common in this sample. It is therefore possible that different associations would have emerged with a more diverse sample. This is consistent with the fact that significant differences were found for victims of physical neglect when examining overall couple interpersonal difficulties, but not when the four specific domains of problems were examined.

Finally, regarding the third aim of this study, results were examined for males and females separately, assessing how males and females differ in the way they experience interpersonal problems while interacting with their partner. Contrary to previous research that failed to show gender differences when looking at interpersonal problems (Bullitt & Farber, 2002; Löffler-Stastka, Ponocny-Seliger, Fischer-Kern, & Leithner, 2005), the results of this study revealed that regardless of maltreatment histories, males tended to report more couple interpersonal problems than females. It is possible that previous studies did not find any significant sex differences because they examined interpersonal difficulties in general, rather than difficulties specific to intimate relationships, as measured in this study. For instance, it is possible that males and females show similar patterns of interpersonal problems when interacting with their friends and coworkers but males report more problems when interacting with their partner. In addition, results stemming from this study show that a history of maltreatment contributes more to couple interpersonal problems in males than in females. These results are in contrast to previous studies that have failed to confirm any gender differences (Finkelhor et al., 1990; Repic, 2007). Furthermore, the results reported here are in stark contrast to those of previous studies that have suggested that female victims of childhood abuse and neglect are more vulnerable to relationship dysfunction than males (Colman & Widom, 2004; DiLillo et al., 2007). It is possible that although males experience more interpersonal problems when interacting with their partner, these difficulties are not perceived when studies limit their investigation to particular outcomes such as divorce or marital dissatisfaction. Lastly, results revealed slightly different patterns of couple interpersonal problems for males and females. Whereas for males, physical abuse seemed more consistently associated with couple interpersonal difficulties, emotional neglect was the best predictor of interpersonal problems in females. At this juncture, it is unclear what processes are responsible for the sex differences. Future research should seek to clarify how and why different types of child maltreatment relate differently to the dimensions of agency and communion for males and females.

Future Directions

Given that victims of abuse and neglect from lower socioeconomic backgrounds might experience more severe forms of maltreatment, and that the sample used in this study was composed mainly of Caucasian French-Canadian university students (92.6%), these results should be generalized with caution. Indeed, it is possible that the patterns of association between childhood traumas and couple interpersonal difficulties are different for this group than for other abuse victims. Thus, further research should include clinical samples as well as representative samples of the general population. Second, the correlational design of the study precludes the possibility of exploring causal relationships, leaving other interpretations open to possibility. Future studies should help delineate the causal factors explaining interpersonal problems in couple relationships of victims of abuse and neglect. Also, self-reports were used to measure childhood maltreatment. Self-reports are commonly used in research on this topic. However, they are not equivalent to court-documented cases of childhood abuse and neglect. Similarly, the participants' perception of their interpersonal problems was not validated by direct observation of their behavior. It is possible that concerns about social desirability have impacted the participants' willingness to report current or past negative experiences, such as difficulties in couple relationships and childhood maltreatment. However, all questionnaires comprised behaviorally specific questions and were completed anonymously to encourage an accurate reporting of information.

Finally, a number of researchers have noted that the role of multiple victimization experiences in explaining responses to childhood maltreatment has largely been ignored in the literature (Finkelhor, Ormrod, & Turner, 2007; Higgins, 2004). Unfortunately, the analyses reported in this article did not assess multitype maltreatment and its combined influence on couple interpersonal behaviors. Indeed, despite the large sample of this study, the sample size would decrease when assessing multitype maltreatment (37% of the victims), which would yield statistically insignificant results due to small sample size. Given the overlap between maltreatment types and the possible negative impact of experiencing more than one type of maltreatment (Davis et al., 2001; Higgins & McCabe, 2000; Ney, Fung, & Wickett, 1994), future research should address the contribution of coexisting traumas.

Conclusions

In summary, despite the vast attention paid by previous studies to the adult intimate relationships of victims of childhood sexual abuse, the male and female victims of sexual abuse in this study did not appear to be more vulnerable to couple interpersonal problems than nonvictims. However, physical abuse, emotional abuse, and emotional neglect were strongly associated with couple interpersonal problems, especially for males. Significant differences in terms of couple interpersonal difficulties were also revealed between those with a history of physical neglect and those without such a history. Intervention programs addressing difficulties in couple relationships should thus consider the history of all types of childhood maltreatment in helping couples build healthier relationships. Additionally, being a victim of emotional neglect was associated with couple interpersonal problems in the submissive southern hemisphere of the circumplex, such as having difficulties expressing needs to a partner and having problems being firm and assertive toward a partner. On the contrary, physical abuse for males and emotional abuse for females contributed more to couple interpersonal problems in the northern hemisphere, with problems related to being controlling, manipulating, and aggressive toward and trying to change a partner. In light of these results, it seems that the different forms of childhood maltreatment have a greater influence on the dimension of agency (submissive to domineering behaviors) than on the dimension of communion (from hostile to friendly behaviors). Different associations could surface with a larger and more diverse sample. Nevertheless, these results suggest that therapists should consider the different types of childhood maltreatment and their association with specific issues in intimate relationships (e.g., nonassertiveness or domineering behaviors) that can be targeted during treatment (see Carbone, 2010, for therapeutic intervention with emotional abuse survivors). Finally, it seems that the differential impact of maltreatment for males and females is also an important factor to be addressed in clinical interventions. Future work should continue to shed further light on the contribution of various forms of childhood abuse and neglect to the development of problems in adult intimate relationships.

REFERENCES

Alden, L. E., Wiggins, J. S., & Pincus, A. L. (1990). Construction of circumplex scales for the Inventory of Interpersonal Problems. *Journal of Personality Assessment, 55*(3–4), 521–536.

Banyard, V. L., Arnold, S., & Smith, J. (2000). Childhood sexual abuse and dating experiences of undergraduate women. *Child Maltreatment, 5*(1), 39–48.

Bernstein, D. P., Stein, J. A., Newcomb, M. D., Walker, E., Pogge, D., Ahluvalia, T., et al. (2003). Development and validation of a brief screening version of the Childhood Trauma Questionnaire. *Child Abuse & Neglect, 27*, 169–190.

Berzenski, S. R., & Yates, T. M. (2010). A developmental process analysis of the contribution of childhood emotional abuse to relationship violence. *Journal of Aggression, Maltreatment and Trauma, 19*(2), 180–203.

Blatt, S. J. (1990). Interpersonal relatedness and self-definition: Two personality configuration and their implications for psychopathology and psychotherapy. In J. L. Singer (Ed.), *Repression and dissociation* (pp. 299–335). Chicago: University of Chicago Press.

Bowlby, J. (1982). *Attachment and loss: Vol. 1. Attachment* (2nd ed.). London: Hogarth. (Original work published 1969)

Briere, J., & Runtz, M. (1990). Differential adult symptomatology associated with three types of child abuse histories. *Child Abuse & Neglect, 14*, 357–364.

Brislin, R. W. (1970). Back-translation for cross-cultural research. *Journal of Cross-Cultural Psychology, 1*, 185–216.

Bullitt, C., & Farber, B. A. (2002). Sex differences in the relationship between interpersonal problems and defensive style. *Psychological Reports, 91*, 767–768.

Carbone, D. J. (2010). Using cognitive therapies to treat unstable attachment patterns in adults with childhood histories of social rejection. *Journal of Aggression, Maltreatment and Trauma, 19*(1), 105–134.

Cole, P. M., & Putnam, F. W. (1992). Effect of incest on self and social functioning: A developmental psychopathology perspective. *Journal of Consulting and Clinical Psychology, 60*, 174–184.

Colman, R. A., & Widom, C. S. (2004). Childhood abuse and neglect and adult intimate relationships: A prospective study. *Child Abuse & Neglect, 28*, 1133–1151.

Courtois, C. A. (1988). *Healing the incest wound: Adult survivors in therapy*. New York: Norton.

Crawford, E., & O'Dougherty-Wright, M. (2007). The impact of childhood psychological maltreatment on interpersonal schemas and subsequent experiences of relationship aggression. *Journal of Emotional Abuse, 7*(2), 93–116.

Cyr, M., & Frappier, J.-Y. (2005). *Instrument pour mesurer l'ASE—Version courte* [Instrument to Measure Sexual Aggression in Childhood—Short Form]. Unpublished manuscript, Université de Montréal, Montréal, Canada.

Davis, J. L., & Petretic-Jackson, P. A. (2000). The impact of child sexual abuse on adult interpersonal functioning: A review and synthesis of the empirical literature. *Aggression and Violent Behavior, 5*, 291–328.

Davis, J. L., Petretic-Jackson, P. A., & Ting, L. (2001). Intimacy dysfunction and trauma symptomatology: Long-term correlates of different types of child abuse. *Journal of Traumatic Stress, 14*(1), 63–79.

DiLillo, D., Giuffre, D., Tremblay, G. C., & Peterson, L. (2001). A closer look at the nature of intimate partner violence reported by women with a history of childhood sexual abuse. *Journal of Interpersonal Violence, 16*, 116–132.

DiLillo, D., Lewis, T., & Di Loreto-Colgan, A. (2007). Child maltreatment history and subsequent romantic relationships: Exploring a psychological route to dyadic difficulties. *Journal of Aggression, Maltreatment & Trauma, 15*, 19–36.

DiLillo, D., & Long, P. J. (1999). Perceptions of couple functioning among female survivors of child sexual abuse. *Journal of Child Sexual Abuse, 7*, 59–76.

Dodge Reyome, N. (2010). Childhood emotional maltreatment and later intimate relationships: Themes from the empirical literature *Journal of Aggression, Maltreatment and Trauma, 19*(2), 224–242.

Dodge Reyome, N., Ward, K. S., & Witkiewitz, K. (2010). Psychosocial variables as mediators of the relationship between childhood emotional maltreatment, codependency, and self silencing. *Journal of Aggression, Maltreatment and Trauma, 19*(2), 159–179.

Edwards, V. J., Holden, G. W., Felitti, V. J., & Anda, R. F. (2003). Relationship between multiple forms of childhood maltreatment and adult mental health in community respondents: Results from the adverse childhood experiences study. *American Journal of Psychiatry, 160*, 1453–1460.

English, D. J. (1998). The extent and consequences of child maltreatment. *Future of Children, 8*(1), 39–53.

Finkelhor, D., & Browne, A. (1985). The traumatic impact of child sexual abuse: A conceptualization. *American Journal of Orthopsychiatry, 55*, 530–541.

Finkelhor, D., Hotaling, G., Lewis, I. A., & Smith, C. (1990). Sexual abuse in a national survey of adult men and women: Prevalence, characteristics, and risk factors. *Child Abuse & Neglect, 14*, 19–28.

Finkelhor, D., Ormrod, R. K., & Turner, H. A. (2007). Poly-victimization: A neglected component in child victimization. *Child Abuse & Neglect, 31*, 7–26.

Herman, J. L. (1992). *Trauma and recovery: The aftermath of violence—From domestic violence to political terror.* New York: HarperCollins.

Higgins, D. (2004). Differentiating between child maltreatment experiences. *Family Matters, 69*, 50–55.

Higgins, D. J., & McCabe, M. P. (2000). Multi-type maltreatment and the long-term adjustment of adults. *Child Abuse Review, 9*, 6–18.

Higgins, D. J., & McCabe, M. P. (2001). Multiple forms of child abuse and neglect: Adult retrospective reports. *Aggression and Violent Behavior, 6*, 547–578.

Horney, K. (1945). *Our inner conflicts.* New York: Norton.

Horowitz, L. M., Alden, L. E., Wiggins, J. S., & Pincus, A. L. (2000). *Inventory of Interpersonal Problems (IIP–32/IIP–64).* San Antonio, TX: Psychological Corporation.

Horowitz, L. M., Rosenberg, S. E., Baer, B. A., Ureno, G., & Villasenor, V. S. (1988). Inventory of Interpersonal Problems: Psychometric properties and clinical applications. *Journal of Consulting and Clinical Psychology, 56*, 885–892.

Horowitz, L. M., Wilson, K. R., Turan, B., Zolotsev, P., Constantino, M. J., & Henderson, L. (2006). How interpersonal motives clarify the meaning of interpersonal behavior: A revised circumplex model. *Personality and Social Psychology Review, 10*(1), 67–86.

Hunter, J. A. (1991). A comparison of the psychosocial maladjustment of adult males and females sexually molested as children. *Journal of Interpersonal Violence, 6*, 205–217.

Kiesler, D. J. (1996). *Contemporary interpersonal theory and research: Personality, psychopathology and psychotherapy.* New York: Wiley.

Leary, T. F. (1957). *Interpersonal diagnosis of personality.* New York: Ronald Press.

Löffler-Stastka, H., Ponocny-Seliger, E., Fischer-Kern, M., & Leithner, K. (2005). Utilization of psychotherapy in patients with personality disorder: The impact of gender, character traits, affect regulation, and quality of object-relations. *Psychology and Psychotherapy: Theory, Research and Practice, 78*, 531–548.

Mullen, P. E., Martin, J. L., Anderson, J. C., Romans, S. E., & Herbison, G. P. (1994). The effect of child sexual abuse on social, interpersonal and sexual function in adult life. *British Journal of Psychiatry, 165*, 35–47.

Murphy, C. M., & Blumenthal, D. R. (2000). The mediating influence of interpersonal problems on the intergenerational transmission of relationship aggression. *Personal Relationships, 7*, 203–218.

Ney, P. G., Fung, T., & Wickett, A. R. (1994). The worst combinations of child abuse and neglect. *Child Abuse & Neglect, 18*, 705–714.

Orndluff, S. R., Kelsey, R. M., & O'Leary, K. D. (2001). Childhood physical abuse, personality, and adult relationship violence: A model of vulnerability to victimization. *American Journal of Orthopsychiatry, 71*, 322–331.

Paquette, D., Laporte, L., Bigras, M., & Zoccolillo, M. (2004). Validation de la version française du CTQ et prévalence de l'histoire de maltraitance [Validation of the French version of the CTQ and prevalence of history of maltreatment]. *Santé mentale au Québec, 29*(1), 201–220.

Paradis, A., & Boucher, S. (2007). Inventaire des problèmes interpersonnels dans les relations de couple (IIP-Couple) [Inventory of interpersonal problems in couple relationships (IIP-Couple)]. Unpublished document, Département de sexologie, Université du Québec à Montréal, Montréal, Canada.

Paradis, A., & Boucher, S. (2008). La structure circomplexe de l'Inventaire des problèmes interpersonnels dans les relations de couple (IIP-Couple) [Circumplex structure of the inventory of interpersonal problems in couple relationships (IIP-Couple)]. Unpublished raw data, Université du Québec à Montréal, Montréal, Canada.

Perry, A. R., DiLillo, D., & Peugh, J. (2007). Childhood psychological maltreatment and quality of marriage: The mediating role of psychological distress. *Journal of Emotional Abuse, 7*, 117–142.

Putnam, F. W. (2003). Ten-year research update review: Child sexual abuse. *Journal of the American Academy of Child and Adolescent Psychiatry, 42*, 269–278.

Repic, T. (2007). Fear of intimacy among married and divorced persons in association with physical abuse in childhood. *Journal of Divorce & Remarriage, 46*(3), 49–62.

Riggs, S. A. (2010). Childhood emotional abuse and the attachment system across the life cycle: What theory and research tell us. *Journal of Aggression, Maltreatment and Trauma, 19*(*1*), 5–51.

Suh, E. J., Moskowitz, D. S., Fournier, M. A., & Zuroff, D. C. (2004). Gender and relationships: Influences on agentic and communal behaviors. *Personal Relationships, 11*, 41–59.

Sullivan, H. S. (1953). *The interpersonal theory of psychiatry*. New York: Norton.

Tabachnick, B. G., & Fidell, L. S. (2007). *Using multivariate statistics* (5th ed.). Boston: Pearson Education.

Thompson, M. P., Kingree, J. B., & Desai, S. (2004). Gender differences in long-term health consequences of physical abuse of children: Data from a nationally representative survey. *American Journal of Public Health, 94*, 599–604.

Vallerand, R. J. (1989). Vers une méthodologie de validation trans-culturelle de questionnaires psychologiques: Implications pour la recherche en langue française [Towards a methodology for the transcultural validation of psychological questionnaires: Implications for French language research]. *Canadian Psychology. 30*, 662–680.

Walsh, F. (1996). The concept of family resilience: Crisis and challenge. *Family Process, 35*, 261–281.

Whiffen, V. E., Judd, M. E., & Aube, J. A. (1999). Intimate relationships moderate the association between childhood sexual abuse and depression. *Journal of Interpersonal Violence, 14*, 940–954.

Wind, T. W., & Silvern, L. (1992). Type and extent of child abuse as predictors of adult functioning. *Journal of Family Violence, 7*, 261–281.

Wolfe, D., Wekerle, C., Reitzel-Jaffe, D., & Lefebvre, L. (1998). Factors associated with abusive relationships among maltreated and nonmaltreated youth. *Development and Psychopathology, 10*, 61–85.

Wolfe, V. V., Gentile, C., & Bourdeau, P. (1987). *History of Victimization form.* Unpublished assessment instrument, London Health Science Centre, London, Canada.

Zurbriggen, E. L., Gobin, R., & Freyd, J. J. (2010). Childhood emotional abuse and late adolescent sexual aggression perpetration and victimization. *Journal of Aggression, Maltreatment and Trauma, 19*(2), 204–223.

Psychosocial Variables as Mediators of the Relationship Between Childhood History of Emotional Maltreatment, Codependency, and Self-Silencing

NANCY DODGE REYOME
State University of New York at Potsdam, Potsdam, New York, USA

KAREN S. WARD
Middle Tennessee State University, Murfreesboro, Tennessee, USA

KATIE WITKIEWITZ
University of Washington, Seattle, Washington, USA

This study investigated the role of psychosocial variables as mediators of the relationship between a childhood history of emotional maltreatment and codependency and a childhood history of emotional maltreatment and self-silencing in a sample of upper division female nursing students. Depression, self-esteem, self-differentiation, and self-concealment were considered as possible mediators of the relationship. Multiple regression analyses revealed that each psychosocial variable partially mediated the relationship between a history of emotional maltreatmentand codependency, and emotional maltreatment and self-silencing.

Recent research has linked a history of childhood abuse and neglect with difficulty in the formation and maintenance of intimate relationships in

An earlier version of this article was presented as a poster in July 2007 at the International Family Violence Research Conference in Portsmouth, NH.

adulthood (Berlin & Dodge, 2004; Colman & Widom, 2004; Dodge Reyome, 2010; Paradis & Boucher, 2010; Riggs, 2010; Riggs & Kaminiski, 2010). Codependency is one type of interpersonal difficulty that has been linked with a history of child maltreatment, especially emotional maltreatment (Carson & Baker, 1994; Cullen & Carr, 1999; Dodge Reyome, 2010; Dodge Reyome & Ward, 2007). At the same time, the emerging psychological construct of self-silencing, which is similar to codependency, has also been linked to a history of emotional trauma (Ali et al., 2000). This study sought to replicate earlier research demonstrating a link among a history of childhood emotional maltreatment, codependency, and self-silencing while looking at possible psychosocial mediators of those relationships.

Childhood emotional abuse is a serious form of maltreatment that involves one or more of the following actions: ignoring and overlooking a child's needs, rejecting and refusing to respond to a child's needs, isolating and confining a child, exploiting or corrupting a child, verbally assaulting a child, terrorizing and threatening a child, and neglecting a child (Garbarino, Eckenrode, & Bolger, 1997; Hart & Brassard, 1987; McGee & Wolfe, 1991). Repeated exposure to psychologically and emotionally abusive actions is considered to be especially deleterious to the growing child's psychological, social, and emotional well-being. It cuts across all forms of child abuse and neglect and is the most harmful form of childhood victimization (Hart & Brassard, 1987; McGee & Wolfe, 1991). Garbarino et al. (1997) asserted that psychological maltreatment destroys a growing child's sense of competence and interferes with the development of intrapersonal and interpersonal skills. Recently, investigators have found that a childhood history of emotional and psychological maltreatment is positively associated with difficulties in intimate relationships in adolescence and adulthood (Berzenski & Yates, 2010; Crawford & Wright, 2007; Dodge Reyome; 2010; Dodge Reyome & Ward, 2007; Messman-Moore & Coates, 2007; Paradis & Boucher, 2010; Perry, DiLillo, & Peugh, 2007; Riggs, 2010; Riggs & Kaminski, 2010; Spertus, Yehuda, Wong, Halligan, & Seremetis, 2003; Zurbriggen, Gobin, & Freyd, 2010).

Codependency is a way of approaching intimate relationships that is characterized by a focus on the needs of others, self-sacrifice, and dysfunctional coping behaviors (Beattie, 1987; Dear, Roberts, & Lange, 2005; Mellody, Miller, & Miller, 1989; Scaturo, Hayes, Sagula, & Walter, 2000). It is said that in this unhealthy and self-defeating approach to human relationships, codependents focus on controlling the other person while overlooking their own needs. Preservation of the relationship, no matter how detrimental and unhealthy, is valued over and above either individual's well-being. Almost all explanations for the origins of codependency trace the development of this unhealthy approach to relationships back to a history of early family dysfunction (Dear et al., 2005). The most widely considered form of family dysfunction cited by theorists and practitioners has been substance abuse.

However, recent empirical investigations examining the link between family-of-origin substance abuse and codependency in adulthood have found little or no relationship (Carson & Baker, 1994; Cullen & Carr, 1999; Gotham & Sher, 1995; Irwin, 1995). Some researchers have found that mental health issues in the family of origin are more important than actual substance use and abuse for predicting codependency in adulthood (Fuller & Warner, 2000).

Investigations looking at the relationship between a history of child abuse and neglect and codependency have proven to be more fruitful than investigations focusing on family history of substance abuse as the roots of codependency. Several researchers have found at least a moderate relationship between child abuse history and codependency, especially a history of childhood emotional maltreatment (Dodge Reyome, 2010; Dodge Reyome & Ward, 2007). Carson and Baker (1994) found that individuals with histories of emotional abuse tended to score high on a measure of codependency. Cullen and Carr (1999) found that early family relationships devoid of appropriate emotional expression were related to codependency. Researchers have also discovered that individuals who report parenting experiences that are high in control and coercion and low in nurturance also tend to score high on measures of codependency (Crothers & Warren, 1996; Fischer & Crawford, 1992). In the most comprehensive study on the relationship between a history of child maltreatment and codependency to date, Dodge Reyome and Ward (2007) found, of the major forms of child abuse and neglect, that codependency was most strongly correlated with physical abuse and emotional abuse and neglect.

Jack (1991) introduced the notion of self-silencing, a psychological construct that appears to have parallels with codependency. According to Jack, self-silencing involves an approach to intimate relationships where the individual seeks connectedness in a manner that does not allow for self-expression and leads to caretaking and self-sacrifice. Further, Jack hypothesized that this manner of viewing and being in intimate relationships is associated with depression in women. According to Jack, women are typically socialized to think about and approach human relationships this way. However, instead of leading to healthy human relationships, self-silencing leads to a loss of self and a lack of true connection with others. At present, only one study has looked at the association of childhood history of emotional abuse and self-silencing in adulthood. Ali et al. (2000) looked at history of emotional abuse, self-blame, self-silencing, and depression in a sample of women with irritable bowel syndrome. Ali and colleagues found a rather robust positive relationship between history of emotional abuse and self-silencing among this sample of women.

In this study, four psychosocial variables were investigated as mediators of the relationship among childhood emotional abuse, codependency, and self-silencing: depression, self-esteem, self-concealment, and self-differentiation.

Two of these variables, depression and self-esteem, were chosen based on already empirically established relationships with emotional abuse, codependency, and self-silencing. The other two variables, self-concealment and self-differentiation, were chosen based on the likelihood of establishing such relationships. Childhood history of emotional maltreatment has been linked with a variety of internalizing problems, externalizing problems, and self-system impairments including low self-esteem and negative self-beliefs (Kim & Cicchetti, 2006; Schneider, Rosa, Graham, & Zielinski, 2005; Showers, Zeigler-Hill, & Limke, 2006), depression and self-criticism (Chapman et al., 2004; Sachs-Ericsson, Verona, Joiner, & Preacher, 2006; Schneider et al., 2005; Spertus et al., 2003; Teicher, Samson, Polcari, & McGreenery, 2006; Uhrlass & Gibb, 2007; Webb, Heisler, Call, Chickering, & Colburn, 2007), anxiety (Sachs-Ericsson et al., 2006; Schneider et al., 2005; Spertus et al., 2003; Teicher et al., 2006; Uhrlass & Gibb, 2007), anger (Schneider et al., 2005; Teicher et al., 2006), dissociation (Schneider et al., 2005; Teicher et al., 2006), posttraumatic stress disorder (Schneider et al., 2005; Spertus et al., 2003), eating problems (Kent & Waller, 2000; Witkiewitz & Dodge Reyome, 2000), and substance abuse (Moran, Vuchinich, & Hall, 2004).

Similarly, codependency and self-silencing have been linked with various internalizing problems, externalizing problems, and self-system difficulties. Codependency is directly associated with low self-esteem and self-confidence (Cullen & Carr, 1999; Lindley, Giordano, & Hammer, 1999; Springer, Britt, & Schlenker, 1998; Wells, Glickauf-Hughes, & Jones, 1999), depression (Cullen & Carr, 1999; Fischer, Spann, & Crawford, 1991; Hughes-Hammer, Martsolf, & Zeller, 1998), anxiety (Cullen & Carr, 1999; Fischer et al., 1991; Springer et al., 1998), negative affectivity (Gotham & Sher, 1995), shame-proneness (Wells et al., 1999), self-defeating personality characteristics (Wells, Glickauf-Hughes, & Bruss, 1998; Wells, Hill, Brack, Brack, & Firestone, 2006), borderline and dependent personality characteristics (Hoenigmann-Lion & Whitehead, 2006; Wells et al., 1998), and narcissistic personality disorder and covert narcissism (Irwin, 1995; Wells et al., 2006). Although not as much research has been conducted on the psychological correlates of self-silencing, it has been discovered that self-silencing is related to low self-esteem (Haemmerlie, Montgomery, Williams, & Winborn, 2001), depression (Cramer, Gallant, & Langlois, 2005; Flett, Besser, Hewitt, & Davis, 2007; Haemmerlie et al., 2001; Jack & Dill, 1992; Page, Stevens, & Galvin, 1996; Thompson, 1995), anxiety (Haemmerlie et al., 2001), self-blame and self-criticism (Ali et al., 2000; Besser, Flett, & Davis, 2003), perfectionism (Flett et al., 2007), and neuroticism (Witte, Sherman, & Flynn, 2001).

Unlike depression and self-esteem, neither self-concealment nor self-differentiation has been previously investigated as a correlate of childhood emotional maltreatment, codependency, or self-silencing. Larson and Chastain (1990) pointed out that self-concealment "involves the conscious concealment of personal information (thoughts, feelings, actions, or events) that is highly intimate and negative in valence" (p. 440). Those who engage in self-concealment tend to take negatively charged personal information and hold it inside. They have found that self-concealment is related to the tendency to engage in self-disclosure but that the two constructs are distinct psychological phenomenon. Individuals high in self-concealment tend to be high in physical complaints, shyness, anxiety, and depression, and low in social support and self-esteem (Ichiyama et al., 1993; Larson & Chastain, 1990). Differentiation of the self emerges from Bowen theory (Skowron & Friedlander, 1998). According to Skowron and Friedlander (1998), those who are highly differentiated are able to "balance emotional and intellectual functioning and intimacy and autonomy in relationships" (p. 235). Low levels of self-differentiation have been associated with higher levels of distress and psychological symptoms and poorer psychosocial development (Bartle-Haring, Rosen, & Stith, 2002; Jenkins, Buboltz, Schwartz, & Johnson, 2005; Skowron, Wester, & Azen, 2004).

Difficulties in self-functioning and depression are among the psychological disturbances associated with a history of abuse during childhood (Cicchetti, 1991; Harter, 1998). In particular, victims of childhood emotional abuse are exposed to repeated derogatory activities that negatively influence beliefs about self-worth and competence (Garbarino et al., 1997). These negative beliefs about the self and the surrounding world underlie various psychological problems including depression. According to Cicchetti (1991), the abused child learns that the caregiver is emotionally unresponsive and the self is not lovable. Further, as an abused child grows and develops, it is hypothesized that these negative internal representations about the self and others influence an individual's functioning within close relationships, leading not only to further self-system disturbances, but also to disturbances in interpersonal relationships. Among other things, Cicchetti indicates that young children who have experienced maltreatment struggle with autonomous functioning and engage in "caretaker controlling" relationships with caregivers. Interestingly, self-sacrifice, caretaking, and impaired identity development are all hallmarks of codependent and self-silencing relationships in adulthood. In this research project, it was hypothesized that a history of childhood emotional abuse would be positively associated with codependency and self-silencing in young adulthood and that the relationship between a history of emotional maltreatment and codependency and self-silencing would be mediated by the psychosocial variables of depression, self-esteem, self-differentiation, and self-concealment.

In summary, this investigation focused on replicating previously established relationships between childhood history of emotional abuse and neglect, codependency, and self-silencing. In addition to replicating existing studies that have found childhood emotional maltreatment to be positively related to codependency and self-silencing in adulthood, this research looked at possible psychosocial mediators of the relationship that have both empirical and theoretical promise. Two of the psychosocial variables considered were depression and self-esteem. Both of these variables are well-established correlates of childhood emotional trauma, codependency, and self-silencing. The investigation of two additional psychosocial variables, self-concealment and self-differentiation, was exploratory in nature.

METHOD

Prior to data collection, the research project in question underwent institutional review board review at both the first author's institution and at the institution where the data were collected. During data collection, all participants read and signed an informed consent document. All individuals were told that their participation in the project was voluntary and that their information would be anonymous and confidential. Also, participants were informed of their right to skip questions on the questionnaire and terminate participation at any time without penalty. No identifying information was collected on the questionnaires and all questionnaires were collected separately from informed consent documents. Finally, all participants were provided with the researchers' names and contact information should they want to discuss the study. Also, information regarding local counseling services was provided to all participants.

Participants

One hundred and forty-one upper division female nursing students participated in the project. Virtually all members of four different nursing classes at a medium-sized public university in the Southeastern United States agreed to participate in the study. Of those students, 141 were female, 10 were male, and 1 individual did not report on gender. This study analyzed data from the 141 female participants. The ages of the participants ranged from 18 to 49 years, with the mean age being 24 years. Slightly over 90% of the participants were Caucasian. The demographic background of this sample of nursing students is similar to most student nurse populations throughout the United States.

Measures

A questionnaire format was utilized in this study. The questionnaire was administered in a group setting to students recruited from upper division nursing courses. The questionnaire administered to each participant contained demographic questions and inventories and scales to measure child abuse history, history of emotional maltreatment, depression, self-esteem, self-differentiation, self-concealment, codependency, and self-silencing.

An earlier version of the Childhood Trauma Questionnaire (CTQ; Bernstein et al., 1994) was utilized in the study to measure a history of childhood abuse. This version contains 34 items designed to measure five forms of child maltreatment: emotional abuse ("People in my family said hurtful or insulting things to me"), emotional neglect ("I felt loved," reverse scored), physical abuse ("People in my family hit me so hard that it left me with bruises or marks"), sexual abuse ("Someone molested me"), and physical neglect ("I didn't have enough to eat"). The participant is instructed to "circle the number that best describes how you feel" on a 5-point scale ranging from 1 (*never true*) to 5 (*very often true*). Based on instructions provided by the author of the scale, total score and subscale scores for this version of the CTQ were computed to approximate the total score and subscale scores on a more recently developed 28-item version of the questionnaire. The CTQ is a widely used self-report measure of childhood abuse and neglect. Bernstein, Ahluvalia, Pogge, and Handelsman (1997) demonstrated that child abuse history, as measured by the CTQ, correlates well with clinician ratings of client history. Also, although the CTQ was originally created using a clinical sample, Scher, Stein, Asmundson, McCreary, and Forde (2001) found that the measure has good internal consistency using a community-based sample. In the Scher et al. study, the alpha coefficients for the entire measure and the five subscales were .91 (entire scale), .94 (sexual abuse), .85 (emotional neglect), .83 (emotional abuse), .69 (physical abuse), and .58 (physical neglect).

The Psychological Maltreatment Inventory (PMI), as designed by Engels and Moisan (1994), is a 25-item inventory intended to assess self-reported childhood history of emotional and psychological abuse as well as neglect. The PMI has three subscales: isolation ("kept you from playing with other children"), hostile rejection ("called you names—dummy, fatso, stupid"), and neglect ("interacted with you only when necessary"). The participants were asked to rate each item on a scale ranging from 0 (*this didn't happen*) to 5 (*extreme negative effect on me*) depending on how much they think they had been negatively affected by the action described in each item. The original PMI did not separately assess maternal and paternal psychological maltreatment. In this study, participants were instructed to provide separate ratings for maternal and paternal psychological maltreatment on each item of the PMI. In the original study of the instrument, Engels and Moisan found Cronbach's alphas of .91, .90, and .85 for emotional neglect, hostile rejection, and isolation, respectively. More recently, Webb et al. (2007) found similar estimates of internal consistency for each of the subscales of the PMI. Witkiewitz and Dodge Reyome (2000) utilized the modified version of the PMI, which they found had good split-half reliability and good internal consistency. Finally, the predictive validity of the measure was demonstrated by Swift and Gayton (1996), who discovered significant positive correlations between scores on the PMI and scores on the Beck Depression Inventory.

The Differentiation of Self Inventory (DSI; Skowran & Friedlander, 1998) was also utilized in the study. The DSI is a 43-item self-report inventory that measures the degree of autonomous functioning within interpersonal relationships. Each item is rated on a scale ranging from 1 (*not at all*) to 6 (*very true of me*) scale based on "how much the statement is generally true of you." The DSI yields a total score and four subscale scores: emotional reactivity ("People have remarked that I am overly emotional"), emotional cut-off ("I have difficulty expressing my feelings to people I care for"), fusion with others ("I feel a need for approval from virtually everyone in my life") and I-position ("I tend remain pretty calm even under stress"). Skowran and Friedlander (1998) reported internal consistency reliabilities for the total scale and the four subscales of the DSI: total DSI (.88), emotional reactivity (.88), I-position (.85), emotional cut-off (.79), and fusion with others (.70). The authors also found evidence of construct validity in that those participants who reported functioning in a more autonomous manner within interpersonal relationships as measured by the DSI and the DSI subscales were less anxious, had fewer psychological symptoms, and reported greater marital satisfaction. Due to strong correlations between the DSI subscales ($r = -.20$–$.67$, $ps < .05$) the total DSI score was used in all analyses.

The research instrument also contained the Depressive Experiences Questionnaire for Adolescents (DEQ–A; Blatt, Schaffer, Bers, & Quinlan, 1992). The DEQ–A is a 66-item inventory designed to measure "experiences associated with depression, but usually not considered symptoms of depression" (p. 82). Participants are instructed to rate each item on a 7-point scale based on how well each statement describes him or her. The DEQ–A yields three factors: dependency, self-criticism, and efficacy. All items in the inventory contribute to each factor. Items on the DEQ–A include the following: "Sometimes I feel very big, and other times I feel very small," "It bothers me that relationships with people change," and "I am a very independent person." Blatt et al. (1992) found sufficient short-term and long-term test–retest reliability with all three factors of the DEQ–A. Also, the dependency and self-criticism factors of the DEQ–A were found to directly correlate with other measures of depression and the efficacy factor was found to be positively correlated with a measure of autonomy.

The Self-Concealment Scale (SCS), as created by Larson and Chastain (1990), is a 10-item scale with items focused on the tendency to hide negative and distressing personal information. Items on the SCS are rated on a 5-point scale ranging from 1 (*strongly disagree*) to 5 (*strongly agree*). Some of the items on the SCS are as follows: "I have an important secret I haven't shared with anyone," "There are lots of things about me that I keep to myself," and "My secrets are too embarrassing to share with others." Using correlation and factor analytic techniques on self-concealment and self-disclosure data from the same sample, Larson and Chastain discovered that self-concealment and self-disclosure are related but different constructs. They found a significant inverse relationship between self-disclosure and self-concealment. They also found that when analyzing the data using a maximum-likelihood factor analysis, items from the SCS had relatively high loadings on one factor, whereas items from the self-disclosure scale had high loadings on the other factor. Larson and Chastain concluded from these analyses that actively concealing significant troubling aspects of the self (self-concealment) is related to the tendency to share important self-information (self-disclosure) but not the same. Also, they discovered that self-concealment is positively related to physical symptoms, depression, and anxiety and negatively related to social support. Cramer and Barry (1999) reported a Cronbach internal consistency estimate of .86 for the SCS.

Global self-esteem was assessed in the study using the Rosenberg Self-Esteem Scale (RSE; Rosenberg, 1965). The RSE is a 10-item measure on which participants are asked to rate statements of global self-worth ("On the whole I am satisfied with myself") on a 4-point scale ranging from 0 *(strongly disagree)* to 3 *(strongly agree)*. The RSE has been widely used as a measure of global self-esteem and has been found to be a reliable and valid measure of self-worth. Internal consistency of the RSE has been reported from a Cronbach's alpha of .77 (Dobson, Goudy, Keith, & Powers, 1979) to .88 (Fleming & Courtney, 1984) and test–retest reliability is similar with findings of .82 (Fleming & Courtney, 1984) and .85 (Silber & Tippet, 1965). Face, convergent, and discriminant validity have all been well documented in numerous studies over a long period of time (Robinson, Shaver, & Wrightsman, 1991).

The Silencing the Self Scale (STSS; Jack, 1991; Jack & Dill, 1992) was included in the study as one measure of functioning within intimate relationships. The STSS is a 31-item measure with four subscales: externalized self-perception ("I tend to judge myself by how I think other people see me"), care as self-sacrifice ("Caring means putting the other person's needs in front of my own"), silencing the self ("I don't speak my feelings in an intimate relationship when I know they will cause disagreement"), and divided self ("I find it is harder to be myself when I am in a close relationship than when I am on my own"). Each item on the STSS is rated on a 5-point scale ranging from 1 *(strongly disagree)* to 5 *(strongly agree)*. Jack and Dill (1992) investigated the psychometric properties of the STSS using three samples of women: undergraduate females, women in a battered women's shelter, and women participating in a pregnancy and health study. Internal consistency coefficients for the total STSS score and the four subscale scores across the three samples of women ranged from .60 to .94. Also, Jack and Dill found high test–retest reliability for total STSS score for all three samples of women. Finally, in all three samples, total STSS score had a significant positive relationship with depression scores and the STSS varied across these three samples of women, with the shelter women reporting the highest average levels of self-silencing. Given the high correlations between the subscales of the STSS (r = .43–.71, ps < .005) we used the total STSS score in all analyses.

Codependency was assessed using the Spann–Fischer Codependency Scale (Fischer et al., 1991). The Spann–Fischer Codependency Scale is a 16-question self-report inventory with items rated on a 6-point scale ranging from 1 (*strongly disagree*) to 6 (*strongly agree*). Items on the Spann–Fischer Codependency Scale include "Sometimes I almost feel bored or empty if I don't have problems to focus on," and "I don't usually let others see the 'real' me." Fischer et al. (1991) reported Cronbach's alphas of .73 to .80. Also, the authors found that those who were in recovery for codependency scored lower on the scale than those who were actively codependent. Finally, they found that certain psychological constructs such as self-esteem, anxiety, depression, and external locus of control, which would be expected to be significantly correlated with codependency, did have significant relationships with the Spann–Fischer Codependency Scale.

RESULTS

The first step in the statistical analysis involved examining the correlations and distributions of all measured variables. As expected the scales of the PMI and CTQ were significantly and highly correlated (see Table 1). Given the high correlation, a composite emotional maltreatment factor was created by standardizing and summing the scores of the total PMI and CTQ emotional abuse scales. The composite emotional maltreatment factor was utilized in a series of regression analyses to test for mediation, as outlined later. In addition, as shown in Table 1, the correlations between the emotional abuse scores (CTQ emotional abuse, CTQ emotional neglect, PMI total, PMI rejection, PMI isolation, and PMI neglect) and the codependency/self-silencing scores were highly significant (Spann–Fischer total score, total STSS).

The first step to testing mediating hypotheses was to examine the direct relationship between the emotional maltreatment composite and both the codependency score and scores on the subscales of the STSS scale. As outlined in the first section of Table 2, the emotional maltreatment composite significantly predicted codependency scores and the STSS total scores ($p < .05$). After establishing significant direct relationships between the emotional maltreatment factor and both the codependency score and total scores on the STSS, several regression models were run to test for mediation using the product of coefficients method and the Sobel test (Sobel, 1982). Asymmetric confidence intervals of the mediated effects were calculated using PRODCLIN (MacKinnon, Fritz, Williams, & Lockwood, 2007). The product of coefficients method for testing mediation was used to measure the significance

TABLE 1 Pearson Correlations between Subscales of the CTQ, PMI revised, the Spann–Fischer Codependency Scale, and the STSS

	1	2	3	4	5	6	7	8	9	10	11	12	13	14
1. CTQ Emotional Abuse	1.00													
2. CTQ Emotional Neglect	.72**	1.00												
3. PMI Neglect	.70**	.76**	1.00											
4. PMI Reject	.84**	.65**	.73**	1.00										
5. PMI Isolate	.64**	.47**	.55**	.61**	1.00									
6. PMI Total Score	.82**	.76**	.95**	.89**	.71**	1.00								
7. Codependency	.26**	.15	.09	.24**	.23**	.18*	1.00							
8. STSS Total	.22*	.17	.07	.23*	.19*	.15	.73**	1.00						
9. DSI Composite	.22*	.16	.08	.20*	.31**	.16	.67**	.63**	1.00					
10. Self-Concealment	.19*	.19*	.27**	.24**	.33**	.30**	.46**	.46**	.51**	1.00				
11. Self-Esteem	–30**	–.23*	–.12	–.31**	–.17	–.21*	–.59**	–.59**	–.62**	–.30**	1.00			
12. DEQ–A Dependency	.05	–.16	–.09	.04	.12	–.02	.57**	.61**	.76**	.36**	–.47**	1.00		
13. DEQ–A Self-Criticism	.39**	.47**	.37**	.38**	.31**	.40**	.50**	.47**	.46**	.42**	–.59**	.06	1.00	
14. DEQ–A Self-Efficacy	.19*	.04	.19*	.12	.24**	.20*	.14	.28**	.29**	.36**	–.07	.32**	.07	1.00
M	2.4	11.9	2.9	2.2	0.8	2.0	40.8	78.0	36.1	22.1	23.8	–0.8	–0.7	–0.1
SD	3.6	3.2	5.7	3.3	1.6	3.1	12.7	15.9	6.2	10.3	4.3	1.0	0.9	0.9

Note: CTQ = Childhood Trauma Questionnaire; PMI = Psychological Maltreatment Inventory; STSS = Silencing the Self Scale; DSI = Differentiation of Self Inventory; DEQ–A = Depressive Experiences Questionnaire for Adolescents.

*$p < .05$ (two-tailed). **$p < .01$ (two-tailed).

of the indirect effect of emotional maltreatment in predicting both codependency and self-silencing via the proposed psychosocial measures. Results from these tests confirmed that the relationship between emotional maltreatment and codependency was mediated by the DEQ–A self-criticism subscale score, the SCS score, scores on the RSE, and the DSI. Similarly, the relationship between emotional maltreatment and the STSS total score was mediated by the self-criticism subscale of the DEQ–A, the SCS, the RSE, and the DSI. The Sobel test statistics and the confidence limits of the indirect effects from all sets of regressions are provided in Table 2.

DISCUSSION

This study was conducted to further investigate the association between childhood emotional maltreatment and the relational difficulties of codependency and self-silencing in later intimate relationships and to look at the role of various psychosocial variables as mediators in these relationships. As has been found in previous studies, childhood histories devoid of emotional support or nurturance have been found to be positively related to codependency and self-silencing (Ali et al., 2000; Carson & Baker, 1994; Crothers & Warren, 1996; Cullen & Carr, 1999; Dodge Reyome, 2010; Dodge Reyome & Ward, 2007; Fischer & Crawford, 1992). Individuals who reported histories of parental emotional abuse and neglect tended to report having intimate relationships that were fraught with caretaking, self-sacrifice, and a focus on the other person's needs. Although the relationship between a history of childhood emotional trauma and codependency as well as self-silencing in later adulthood has not been extensively studied, most studies that have considered emotional forms of child maltreatment have found a significant direct relationship between parental emotional maltreatment and codependency as well as self-silencing in adult relationships.

As expected, tests for mediation revealed that the significant correlation between emotional maltreatment and codependency were partially accounted for by self-esteem, self-concealment, depression, and self-differentiation. Also, the association between a history of emotional maltreatment and self-silencing was partially explained by self-esteem, self-concealment, depression, and aspects of self-differentiation. These findings give us a glimpse into how a childhood history of emotional and psychological abuse might be related to psychosocial development and beliefs and approaches to future relationships. In general, the results from these analyses suggest that socioemotional development through adolescence and into young adulthood can be predicted by histories of emotional abuse and neglect. However, given the cross-sectional nature of these

TABLE 2 Results From Multiple Regression Models

Model	R^2	$F(df)$	B(*SE*)	β	*t* test
#1: Emotional abuse/neglect predicting DVs (c-path)					
DV: Codependency	.05	6.17 (1, 115)	2.93 (1.18)	.23	2.48*
IV: Emotional abuse/neglect factor					
DV: STSS Total score	.05	4.98 (1, 106)*	3.36 (1.51)	.21	2.23*
IV: Emotional abuse/neglect factor					
#2: "Self" mediators predicting DVs (b-path)					
DV: Codependency	.55	47.93 (3, 120)**			
IV1: DEQ Dependency			6.89 (.79)	.56	8.68**
IV2: DEQ Self-Criticism			6.99 (.93)	.46	7.45**
IV3: DEQ Self-Efficacy			−.91 (.92)	−.06	−1.00
DV: STSS Total	.56	46.82 (3, 112)**			
IV1: DEQ Dependency			8.69 (1.04)	.56	8.38**
IV2: DEQ Self-Criticism			7.80 (1.18)	.42	6.63**
IV3: DEQ Self-Efficacy			.98 (1.19)	.06	0.82
DV: Codependency	.21	32.94 (1, 126)**	.55 (.10)	.46	5.74**
IV: Self-Concealment Scale					
DV: STSS Total	.22	32.19 (1, 117)**	.71 (.13)	.46	5.67**
IV: Self-Concealment Scale					
DV: Codependency	.35	59.07 (1, 112)**	−1.75 (.23)	−.59	−7.69**
IV: Rosenberg Self-Esteem					
DV: STSS Total	.35	57.40 (1, 105)**	−2.19 (.29)	−.60	−7.58**
IV: Rosenberg Self-Esteem					
DV: Codependency	.45	89.84 (1, 112)**			
IV: Differentiation of Self Total			8.25 (.87)	.67	9.48**
DV: STSS Total	.39	68.10 (1, 105)**			
IV: Differentiation of Self Total			9.67 (1.17)	.63	8.25**
#3: Emotional abuse/neglect predicting self mediators (a-path)					
DV: DEQ Dependency	.00	.02 (1, 123)	−.01 (.09)	−.01	−0.14
IV: Emotional abuse/neglect factor					
DV: DEQ Self-Criticism	.23	35.93 (1, 123)	.40 (.07)	.48	5.99**
IV: Emotional abuse/neglect factor					
DV: DEQ Efficacy	.03	4.37 (1, 123)	.16 (.08)	.19	2.09*
IV: Emotional abuse/neglect factor					
DV: Self-Concealment	.09	11.87 (1, 124)**	3.17 (.92)	.30	3.45**
IV: Emotional abuse/neglect factor					
DV: Rosenberg Self-Esteem Scale	.08	9.27 (1, 110)*	−1.16 (.38)	−.28	−3.05*
IV: Emotional abuse/neglect factor					
DV: Differentiation of Self Total	.04	5.15 (1, 113)*	.24 (.10)	.21	2.27*
IV: Emotional abuse/neglect factor					

	Sobel test	PRODCLIN lower critical value	PRODCLIN upper critical value
#4: Indirect (mediated) effect			
DV: Codependency	2.95**	−6.083	−3.204
IV: Emotional abuse/neglect factor			
Mediator: Self-Concealment			
DV: STSS Total	2.94**	−6.100	−3.197

(Continued)

TABLE 2 *(Continued)*

	Sobel test	PRODCLIN lower critical value	PRODCLIN upper critical value
IV: Emotional abuse/neglect factor Mediator: Self-Concealment DV: Codependency	4.36**	−6.765	−4.552
IV: Emotional abuse/neglect factor Mediator: Self-Criticism DV: STSS Total	4.11**	−6.659	−4.314
IV: Emotional abuse/neglect factor Mediator: Self-Criticism DV: Codependency	2.83**	−5.378	−3.041
IV: Emotional abuse/neglect factor Mediator: Rosenberg Self-Esteem DV: STSS Total	2.82**	−5.406	−3.037
IV: Emotional abuse/neglect factor Mediator: Rosenberg Self-Esteem DV: Codependency	2.21*	−4.389	−2.402
IV: Emotional abuse/neglect factor Mediator: Differentiation of Self total DV: STSS Total	2.20*	−4.664	−2.406
IV: Emotional abuse/neglect factor Mediator: Differentiation of Self total			

Note: DV = dependent variable; IV = independent variable; STSS = Silencing the Self Scale; DEQ–A = Depressive Experiences Questionnaire for Adolescents.
*$p < .05$ and **$p < .01$.

data, it is impossible to determine whether causal relationships exist between these constructs or whether the significant mediated effects observed in this study are simply the reflection of overlapping variance across correlated constructs. Future research that assesses social, relational, and emotional development over time is necessary to test whether causal mediation is supported.

Additionally, it is likely that other variables exist that have not been investigated to date that would more fully account for the association of emotional abuse in childhood with codependent and self-silencing tendencies in adult relationships. One possible variable is anxiety. Although anxiety has been found to be a correlate of childhood emotional trauma (Sachs-Ericsson et al., 2006; Schneider et al., 2005; Spertus et al., 2003; Teicher et al., 2006; Uhrlass & Gibb, 2007), codependency (Cullen & Carr, 1999; Fischer et al., 1991), and self-silencing (Haemmerlie et al., 2001), it was not considered as a mediator in this study. Future research looking at the mediators of the relationship between a history of childhood emotional trauma and codependency or self-silencing in intimate relationships should investigate other psychosocial variables such as anxiety to see if they are more potent mediators of the relationship.

Counseling Implications

These findings have implications for those involved in counseling. Both diagnosis and treatment might be impacted by employing these preliminary results. Certainly it is appropriate to investigate each of the variables even if the client presents with only one. A careful examination of childhood experiences and current patterns of behavior is likely part of most clinicians' intake processing. Making new connections in relationship to maltreatment, traits of codependency, self-silencing, depression, self-esteem, and anxiety is suggested from this study (see Carbone, 2010, for further exploration of clinical interventions with emotional abuse survivors). Although there is much more to be researched, considering these possibilities is advisable.

Depending on why a client comes into counseling, possible treatment options might include ways to tackle the interconnected problems. For example, a woman complaining of depression who has a history of emotional abuse might notice improved self-esteem when she receives treatment for the depressive episodes. Medication accompanied by some form of talk therapy, although alleviating her depression, will have additional benefits that, in turn, will make her life brighter.

As always, clinicians are advised to explore how their own histories affect interactions with clients. In applying findings from this study, noting the potential pathways from one variable to another is an important exercise in self-awareness. Helping clients through difficult content and potentially painful treatment is much more effective if there are no personal issues to intervene.

Limitations of This Study and Suggestions for Future Research

One major limitation of this study is the nature of the sample. The sample was made up of female college students majoring in nursing. Some researchers have found gender differences in the psychological outcomes associated with child abuse and neglect (Banyard, Williams, & Siegel, 2004; Thompson, Kingree, & Desai, 2004). It is possible that there are gender differences in psychological responses to emotional maltreatment and the relationships uncovered in this study using a female sample would not hold true for a sample with a larger representation of male participants. In addition, those who attend college, especially those who persist into the junior and senior year of college, are not representative of the general population. Also, of this college population, those who major in nursing might be different from those who pursue other college majors (Horn & Holzemer, 1991; Silcox & Cummings, 1999). Future studies considering the effect of childhood emotional abuse on the development of codependency and self-silencing in later intimate relationships in nonclinical populations should utilize a noncollege sample of male and female participants.

Also, the methods by which all of the psychological constructs in this study were measured carry their own limitations. All of these constructs were assessed using self-report retrospective measures. Self-report measures are heavily dependent on memory, honesty, and self-awareness. The accuracy of self-report retrospective measures has been questioned in the abuse and neglect literature (Hardt & Rutter, 2004; Widom & Morris, 1997; Widom & Shepard, 1996). Prospective reports of abuse made by others (case records, agency reports) are favored as more accurate assessments of maltreatment status. Similarly with the constructs of codependency and self-silencing, some individuals might be in denial regarding their codependent and self-silencing tendencies or might not have the self-awareness needed to report accurately about the way they view and participate in intimate relationships. To more fully understand the association between childhood history of emotional maltreatment and codependency and self-silencing in adult relationships, future studies should utilize prospective research designs that incorporate multiple measures of emotional maltreatment, codependency, and self-silencing.

REFERENCES

Ali, A., Toner, B., Stuckless, N., Gallop, R., Diamant, N., Gould, M., et al. (2000). Emotional abuse, self-blame, and self-silencing in women with irritable bowel syndrome. *Psychosomatic Medicine, 62*, 76–82.

Banyard, V., Williams, L., & Siegel, J. (2004). Childhood sexual abuse: A gender perspective on context and consequences. *Child Maltreatment, 9*, 223–238.

Bartle-Haring, S., Rosen, K., & Stith, S. (2002). Emotional reactivity and psychological distress. *Journal of Adolescent Research, 17*, 568–585.

Beattie, M. (1987). *Codependent no more: How to stop controlling others and start caring for yourself.* Center City, MN: Hazeldon Press.

Berlin, L., & Dodge, K. (2004). Relations among relationships. *Child Abuse and Neglect, 28*, 1127–1132.

Bernstein, D., Ahluvalia, T., Pogge, D., & Handelsman, L. (1997). Validity of the Childhood Trauma Questionnaire in an adolescent psychiatric population. *Journal of the American Academy of Child and Adolescent Psychiatry, 36*, 340–346.

Bernstein, D., Fink, L., Handelsman, L., Lovejoy, M., Wenzel, K., Saparento, E., et al. (1994). Initial reliability and validity of a new retrospective measure of child abuse and neglect. *American Journal of Psychiatry, 151*, 1132–1136.

Berzenski, S. R., & Yates, T. M. (2010). A developmental process analysis of the contribution of childhood emotional abuse to relationship violence. *Journal of Aggression, Maltreatment and Trauma, 19*(2), 180–203.

Besser, A., Flett, G., & Davis, R. (2003). Self-criticism, dependency, silencing the self, and loneliness: A test of a meditational model. *Personality and Individual Differences, 35*, 1735–1752.

Blatt, S., Schaffer, C., Bers, S., & Quinlan, D. (1992). Psychometric properties of the Adolescent Depressive Experiences Questionnaire. *Journal of Personality Assessment, 59*, 82–98.

Carbone, D. J. (2010). Using cognitive therapies to treat unstable attachment patterns in adults with childhood histories of social rejection. *Journal of Aggression, Maltreatment and Trauma, 19*(1), 105–134.

Carson, A., & Baker, R. (1994). Psychological correlates of codependency in women. *The International Journal of the Addictions, 29*, 395–407.

Chapman, D., Whitfield, C., Felitti, V., Dube, S., Edwards, V., & Anda, R. (2004). Adverse childhood experiences and the risk of depressive disorders in adulthood. *Journal of Affective Disorders, 82*, 217–225.

Cicchetti, D. (1991). Fractures in the crystal: Developmental psychopathology and the emergence of the self. *Developmental Review, 11*, 271–287.

Colman, R., & Widom, C. (2004). Childhood abuse and neglect and adult intimate relationships: A prospective study. *Child Abuse and Neglect, 28*, 1133–1151.

Cramer, K., & Barry, J. (1999). Psychometric properties and confirmatory factor analysis of the self-concealment scale. *Personality and Individual Differences, 27*, 629–637.

Cramer, K., Gallant, M., & Langlois, M. (2005). Self-silencing and depression in women and men: Comparative structural equation models. *Personality and Individual Differences, 39*, 581–592.

Crawford, E., & Wright, M. (2007). The impact of childhood psychological maltreatment on interpersonal schemas and subsequent experiences of relationship aggression. *Journal of Emotional Abuse, 7*, 93–116.

Crothers, M., & Warren, L. (1996). Parental antecedents of adult codependency. *Journal of Clinical Psychology, 52*, 231–239.

Cullen, J., & Carr, A. (1999). Codependency: An empirical study from a systemic perspective. *Contemporary Family Therapy, 21*, 505–526.

Dear, G., Roberts, C., & Lange, L. (2005). Defining codependency: A thematic analysis of published definitions. In S. Shobov (Ed.), *Advances in psychological research*, (Vol. 34, pp. 189–205). Hauppage, NY: Nova Science.

Dobson, C., Goudy, W., Keith, P., & Powers, E. (1979). Further analysis of Rosenberg's Self-Esteem Scale. *Psychological Reports, 44*, 639–641.

Dodge Reyome, N. (2010). Childhood emotional maltreatment and later intimate relationships: Themes from the empirical literature. *Journal of Aggression, Maltreatment and Trauma, 19*(2), 224–242.

Dodge Reyome, N., & Ward, K. (2007). Self-reported history of childhood maltreatment and codependency in undergraduate nursing students. *Journal of Emotional Abuse, 7*, 37–50.

Engels, M., & Moisan, D. (1994). The Psychological Maltreatment Inventory: Development of a measure of psychological maltreatment in childhood for use in adult clinical settings. *Psychological Reports, 74*, 595–604.

Fischer, J., & Crawford, D. (1992). Codependency and parenting styles. *Journal of Adolescent Research, 7*, 352–363.

Fischer, J., Spann, L., & Crawford, D. (1991). Measuring codependency. *Alcoholism Treatment Quarterly, 8*, 87–100.

Fleming, J., & Courtney, B. (1984). The dimensionality of self-esteem: II. Hierarchical facet model for revised measurement scales. *Journal of Personality and Social Psychology, 46*, 404–421.

Flett, G., Besser, A., Hewitt, P., & Davis, R. (2007). Perfectionism, silencing the self, and depression. *Personality and Individual Differences, 43*, 1211–1222.

Fuller, J., & Warner, R. (2000). Family stressors as predictors of codependency. *Genetic, Social and General Psychology Monographs, 126*, 5–22.

Garbarino, J., Eckenrode, J., & Bolger, K. (1997). The elusive crime of psychological maltreatment. In J. Garbarino & J. Eckenrode (Eds.), *Understanding abusive families* (pp. 101–113). San Francisco: Jossey-Bass.

Gotham, H., & Sher, K. (1995). Do codependent traits involve more than basic dimensions of personality and psychopathology? *Journal of Studies on Alcoholism, 57*, 34–39.

Haemmerlie, F., Montgomery, R., Williams, A., & Winborn, K. (2001). Silencing the self in college settings and adjustment. *Psychological Reports, 88*, 587–594.

Hardt, J., & Rutter, M. (2004). Validity of adult retrospective reports of adverse childhood experiences: Review of the evidence. *Journal of Child Psychology and Psychiatry, 45*, 260–273.

Hart, S., & Brassard, M. (1987). A major threat to children's mental health: Psychological maltreatment. *American Psychologist, 42*, 160–165.

Harter, S. (1998). The effects of child abuse on the self-system. *Journal of Aggression, Maltreatment & Trauma, 2*, 147–169.

Hoenigmann-Lion, N., & Whitehead, G. (2006). The relationship between codependency and borderline and dependent personality traits. *Alcoholism Treatment Quarterly, 24*, 55–77.

Horn, H., & Holzemer, W. (1991). Characteristics of Israeli women studying nursing compared with women studying education and engineering. *Journal of Nursing Education, 30*, 411–418.

Hughes-Hammer, C., Martsolf, D., & Zeller, R. (1998). Depression and codependency in women. *Archives of Psychiatric Nursing, 12*, 326–334.

Ichiyama, M., Colbert, D., Laramore, H., Heim, M., Carone, K., & Schmidt, J. (1993). Self-concealment and correlates of adjustment in college students. *Journal of College Student Psychotherapy, 7*, 55–68.

Irwin, H. (1995). Codependence, narcissism, and childhood trauma. *Journal of Clinical Psychology, 51*, 658–665.

Jack, D. (1991). *Silencing the self: Depression and women*. Cambridge, MA: Harvard University Press.

Jack, D., & Dill, D. (1992). The Silencing the Self Scale: Schemas of intimacy associated with depression in women. *Psychology of Women Quarterly, 16*, 97–106.

Jenkins, S., Buboltz, W., Schwartz, J., & Johnson, P. (2005). Differentiation of the self and psychosocial development. *Contemporary Family Therapy, 27*, 251–261.

Kent, A., & Waller, G. (2000). Childhood emotional abuse and eating psychopathology. *Clinical Psychology Review, 20*, 887–903.

Kim, J., & Cicchetti, D. (2006). Longitudinal trajectories of self-system processes and depressive symptoms among maltreated and nonmaltreated children. *Child Development, 77*, 624–639.

Larson, D., & Chastain, R. (1990). Self-concealment: Conceptualization, measurement, and health implications. *Journal of Social and Clinical Psychology, 9*, 439–455.

Lindley, N., Giordano, P., & Hammer, E. (1999). Codependency: Predictors and psychometric issues. *Journal of Clinical Psychology, 55*, 59–64.

MacKinnon, D. P., Fritz, M. S., Williams, J., & Lockwood, C. M. (2007). Distribution of the product confidence limits for the indirect effect: Program PRODCLIN. *Behavior Research Methods, 39*, 384–389.

McGee, R., & Wolfe, D. (1991). Psychological maltreatment: Toward an operational definition. *Development and Psychopathology, 3*, 3–18.

Mellody, P., Miller, A., & Miller, J. (1989). *Facing codependency: What it is, where it comes from, how it sabotages our lives*. New York: Harper & Row.

Messman-Moore, T., & Coates, A. (2007). Impact of childhood psychological abuse on adult interpersonal conflict: The role of early maladaptive schemas and patterns of interpersonal behavior. *Journal of Emotional Abuse, 7*, 75–92.

Moran, P., Vuchinich, S., & Hall, N. (2004). Associations between types of maltreatment and substance use during adolescence. *Child Abuse and Neglect, 28*, 565–574.

Page, J., Stevens, H., & Galvin, S. (1996). Relationships between depression, self-esteem, and self-silencing behavior. *Journal of Social and Clinical Psychology, 15*, 381–396.

Paradis, A., & Boucher, S. (2010). Child maltreatment history and interpersonal problems in adult couple relationships. *Journal of Aggression, Maltreatment and Trauma, 19*(2), 138–158.

Perry, A., DiLillo, D., & Peugh, J. (2007). Childhood psychological maltreatment and quality of marriage: The mediating role of psychological distress. *Journal of Emotional Abuse, 7*, 117–142.

Riggs, S. A. (2010). Childhood emotional abuse and the attachment system across the life cycle: What theory and research tell us. *Journal of Aggression, Maltreatment and Trauma, 19*(1), 5–51.

Riggs, S. A., & Kaminski, P. (2010). Childhood emotional abuse, adult attachment, and depression as predictors of relational adjustment and psychological aggression. *Journal of Aggression, Maltreatment and Trauma, 19*(1), 75–104.

Robinson, J., Shaver, P., & Wrightsman, L. (Eds.). (1991). *Measures of personality and social psychological attitudes*. New York: Academic.

Rosenberg, M. (1965). *Society and the adolescent self-image*. Princeton, NJ: Princeton University Press.

Sachs-Ericsson, N., Verona, E., Joiner, T., & Preacher, K. (2006). Parental verbal abuse and the mediating role of self-criticism in adult internalizing disorders. *Journal of Affective Disorders, 93*, 71–78.

Scaturo, D., Hayes, T., Sagula, D., & Walter, T. (2000). The concept of codependency of its context within family systems theory. *Family Therapy, 27*, 64–70.

Scher, C., Stein, M., Asmundson, G., McCreary, D., & Forde, D. (2001). The Childhood Trauma Questionnaire in a community sample: Psychometric properties and normative data. *Journal of Traumatic Stress, 14*, 843–857.

Schneider, M., Rosa, A., Graham, C., & Zielinski, A. (2005). Do allegations of emotional maltreatment predict developmental outcomes beyond that of other forms of maltreatment. *Child Abuse and Neglect, 29*, 513–532.

Showers, C., Zeigler-Hill, V., & Limke, A. (2006). Self-structure and childhood maltreatment: Successful compartmentalization and the struggle for integration. *Journal of Social and Clinical Psychology, 25*, 473–507.

Silber, E., & Tippet, J. (1965). Self-esteem: Clinical assessment and measurement validation. *Psychological Reports, 16*, 1017–1071.

Silcox, P., & Cummings, A. (1999). A comparison of women in nontraditional and traditional science majors: Implications for career counselors. *Canadian Journal of Counseling, 33*, 264–276.

Skowron, E., & Friedlander, M. (1998). The Differentiation of Self Inventory: Development and initial validation. *Journal of Counseling Psychology, 45*, 235–246.

Skowron, E., Wester, S., & Azen, R. (2004). Differentiation of the self mediates college stress and adjustment. *Journal of Counseling and Development, 82*, 69–78.

Sobel, M. E. (1982). Asymptotic confidence intervals for indirect effects in structural equation models. In S. Leinhardt (Ed.), *Sociological methodology 1982* (pp. 290–312). Washington, DC: American Sociological Association.

Spertus, I., Yehuda, R., Wong, C., Halligan, S., & Seremetis, S. (2003). Childhood emotional abuse and neglect as predictors of psychological and physical symptoms of women presenting to a primary care practice. *Child Abuse and Neglect, 27*, 1247–1258.

Springer, C., Britt, T., & Schlenker, B. (1998). Codependency: Clarifying the construct. *Journal of Mental Health Counseling, 20*, 141–158.

Swift, E., & Gayton, W. (1996). Further validation of the Psychological Maltreatment Inventory. *Journal of Clinical Psychology, 52*, 325–327.

Teicher, M., Samson, J., Polcari, A., & McGreenery, C. (2006). Sticks, stones and hurtful words: Relative effects of various forms of childhood maltreatment. *American Journal of Psychiatry, 163*, 993–1000.

Thompson, J. (1995). Silencing the self: Depressive symptomatology and close relationships. *Psychology of Women Quarterly, 19*, 337–353.

Thompson, M., Kingree, J., & Desai, S. (2004). Gender differences in the long term health consequences of physical abuse in children: Data from a nationally representative survey. *American Journal of Public Health, 94*, 599–604.

Uhrlass, D., & Gibb, B. (2007). Childhood emotional maltreatment and the stress generation model of depression. *Journal of Social and Clinical Psychology, 26*, 119–130.

Webb, M., Heisler, D., Call, S.,Chickering, S., & Colburn, T. (2007). Shame, guilt, symptoms of depression, and reported history of psychological maltreatment. *Child Abuse and Neglect, 31*, 1143–1153.

Wells, M., Glickauf-Hughes, C., & Bruss, K. (1998). The relationship of codependency to enduring personality characteristics. *Journal of College Student Psychotherapy, 12*, 25–38.

Wells, M., Glickauf-Hughes, C., & Jones, R. (1999). Codependency: A grass roots construct's relationship to shame-proneness, low self-esteem, and childhood parentification. *The American Journal of Family Therapy, 27*, 63–71.

Wells, M., Hill, M., Brack, G., Brack, C., & Firestone, E. (2006). Codependency's relationship to defining characteristics in college students. *Journal of College Student Psychotherapy, 20*, 71–84.

Widom, C., & Morris, S. (1997). Accuracy of adult recollections of childhood victimization: Part 2: Childhood sexual victimization. *Psychological Assessment, 8*, 412–421.

Widom, C., & Shepard, R. (1996). Accuracy of adult recollections of childhood victimization: Part 1. Childhood physical abuse. *Psychological Assessment, 9*, 34–46.

Witkiewitz, K., & Dodge Reyome, N. (2000). Recollections of childhood psychological maltreatment and self-reported eating disordered behaviors in undergraduate college females. *Journal of Emotional Abuse, 2*, 15–29.

Witte, T., Sherman, M., & Flynn, L. (2001). Silencing the self and the big five: A personological profile of silent women. *Psychological Reports, 88*, 655–663.

Zurbriggen, E. L., Gobin, R., & Freyd, J. J. (2010). Childhood emotional abuse and late adolescent sexual aggression perpetration and victimization. *Journal of Aggression, Maltreatment and Trauma, 19*(2), 204–223.

RESEARCH ON INTIMATE PARTNER VIOLENCE

A Developmental Process Analysis of the Contribution of Childhood Emotional Abuse to Relationship Violence

SARA R. BERZENSKI and TUPPETT M. YATES
University of California, Riverside, Riverside, California, USA

Despite indications that emotional abuse might be the core factor underlying the negative effects of child maltreatment, it has received little attention, particularly with respect to its impact on interpersonal relationships in adulthood. This study conducted a developmental process analysis of the contribution of childhood emotional abuse to relationship violence in a sample of undergraduates. Results indicated that emotional abuse was a stronger predictor of relationship violence than other maltreatment subtypes. Emotion dysregulation partially mediated this relationship, driven by its behavioral component, impulsivity. Gender and ethnicity effects were examined. Findings point to the need for increased attention to adult outcomes of emotional abuse and increased clinical awareness of emotion regulation as a key developmental mechanism of adaptation in adulthood.

Preparation of this work was supported by a University of California Chancellor's Graduate Research Fellowship awarded to the first author. This research was supported by an Academic Senate Research Grant awarded to the second author by the University of California, Riverside.

Child maltreatment undermines the development and maintenance of adaptive relationships in childhood and beyond (Colman & Widom, 2004; Dodge Reyome, 2010; Ehrensaft et al., 2003; Mueller & Silverman, 1989; Riggs, 2010; Swan & Snow, 2006; Taussig & Culhane, 2010). Moreover, evidence suggests that different kinds of maltreatment contribute to relational difficulties to varying degrees and via unique developmental processes (Kaplan, Pelcovitz, & Labruna, 1999; Mullen, Martin, Anderson, Romans, & Herbison, 1996; Wekerle et al., 2001; Widom, Schuck, & White, 2006). Amidst increasing efforts to clarify these specific effects and processes, childhood emotional abuse consistently emerges as central to understanding the insidious effects of child maltreatment.

Initially overlooked in the field of child maltreatment research, childhood emotional abuse has shown itself to be an especially pernicious influence on development, with predictive power surpassing physical and sexual abuse across varied outcomes, including psychopathology, subjective distress, interpersonal functioning, and destructive behavior (Briere & Runtz, 1988; Dodge Reyome, 2010; Gross & Keller, 1992; Hart, Binggeli, & Brassard, 1997; Kent, Waller, & Dagnan, 1999; McGee, Wolfe, & Wilson, 1997; Paradis & Boucher, 2010; Spertus, Yehuda, Wong, Halligan, & Seremetis, 2003; Vissing, Straus, Gelles, & Harrop, 1991). Characterized by rejecting, degrading, threatening, isolating, or exploiting caregiving (Hart et al., 1997), emotional abuse can occur in isolation, but also frequently accompanies other types of abuse, making it the most common type of maltreatment (Briere & Runtz, 1990; Claussen & Crittenden, 1991). Further, emotional abuse exacerbates the harmful consequences of physical or sexual abuse, which are at their most potent when an emotional component is present (Briere & Runtz, 1990; Hart et al., 1997; McGee et al., 1997; Ney, Fung, & Wickett, 1994; Vissing et al., 1991), suggesting that emotional abuse might be the core factor underlying the deleterious effects of child maltreatment (Hart et al., 1997).

Although this foundation of evidence has sparked a recent increase in clinical and empirical investigations of childhood emotional abuse (Wright, 2007; Yates & Wekerle, 2009), there remains a need to quantify and explain the long-term consequences of childhood emotional abuse with respect to relational outcomes (see Dodge Reyome, 2010). The connection between emotional abuse in childhood and future adult relationships is essential to understanding the intergenerational cycle of maltreatment. Adult relationships form the foundation on which the emotional context of the family is built, thereby influencing every aspect of the child's development. Therefore, it is important to examine childhood emotional abuse, not only for its short-term impact on children, but for its long-term consequences as well, particularly with respect to intimate relationships.

In childhood, emotional abuse has specific documented connections to internalizing problems, cognitive deficits, physiological impairments, aggression, delinquency, and interpersonal difficulties (Erickson, Egeland, & Pianta, 1989; McGee et al., 1997; Vissing et al., 1991; Yates, 2007). However, despite the obvious short-term problems these outcomes present, the most detrimental consequences of many of these childhood deficits are their contribution to later difficulties in adulthood, such as disordered eating, low self-esteem, revictimization, and suicidality (Briere & Runtz, 1990; Kaplan et al., 1999; Kent et al., 1999; Spertus et al., 2003). Thus, it is particularly important to examine adult interpersonal outcomes of childhood emotional abuse as a function of developmental processes, which might themselves have been influenced by childhood emotional abuse. These early effects can serve as mechanisms by which later outcomes emerge, and toward which effective intervention efforts should be targeted (Shirk & Eltz, 1998).

Although some research suggests that victims of childhood emotional abuse experience more difficulty and dissatisfaction in their adult intimate relationships (Dodge Reyome, 2010; Messman-Moore & Coates, 2007; Mullen et al., 1996; Paradis & Boucher, 2010; Perry, DiLillo, & Peugh, 2007; Varia, Abidin, & Dass, 1996), little is known about the developmental processes underlying such effects. Further, only a few studies have identified relationship violence as a specific outcome of childhood emotional abuse (Bender, Cook, & Kaslow, 2003; Crawford & Wright, 2007; Dodge Reyome, 2010; Simonelli, Mullis, Elliott, & Pierce, 2002; Wekerle et al., 2009; Zurbriggen, Gobin, & Freyd, 2010), whereas others have argued that relationship violence is a product of cooccurring maltreatment subtypes (i.e., emotional and physical abuse together; Paterson, Fairbairn-Dunlop, Cowley-Malcolm, & Schluter, 2007; Wekerle et al., 2001). Therefore, this study employed a developmental process perspective to explore the unique contribution of child emotional abuse to relationship violence in young adulthood.

One important early consequence of childhood emotional abuse that might be especially salient in the area of intimate relationships involves its interference with the ability to develop adaptive coping styles, particularly with respect to emotionally charged situations or contexts. Childhood emotional abuse is associated with maladaptive attributional styles, avoidant coping, inhibited emotional responses, and limited access to coping strategies (Gibb, Benas, Crossett, & Uhrlass, 2007; Gross & Keller, 1992; Hardy, Power, & Jaedicke, 1993; Krause, Mendelson, & Lynch, 2003; Rosenthal, Polusny, & Follette, 2006; Shipman et al., 2007). Given that the capacity to cope with emotionally straining situations is critical for successful intimate relationships, emotion regulation (i.e., the ability to accurately identify and respond to emotions) is central to adaptive coping in relational settings. Maltreatment-induced impairment in emotion regulation could be at the root of negative relational health, and in extreme cases, violence. Intimate partner violence represents the most dramatic negative consequence of poor coping and impaired social cognition on relationships, with the emotionally pressured context implicating emotion regulation as a likely mechanism by which these capabilities are disrupted. A few researchers have identified poor coping strategies as mechanisms by which maltreatment can lead to relationship violence (Ponce, Williams, & Allen, 2004; Swan & Snow, 2006), whereas Taft, Schumm, Marshall, Panuzio, and Holtzworth-Munroe (2008) suggested that social cognition deficits explain this relation. However, this study is the first to evaluate the role of emotion dysregulation as a specific explanatory mechanism underlying the relation between childhood emotional maltreatment and relationship violence. Further, this investigation explored both the global construct of emotion regulation and specific cognitive and behavioral dimensions of regulation in an effort to refine the understanding of emotion regulation and its implications for development.

Several studies have documented emotion regulation deficits in children who are victims of emotional abuse or neglect (Chang, Schwartz, Dodge, & McBride-Chang, 2003; Eisenberg et al., 2001; Shipman et al., 2007). It remains to be determined, however, whether emotional abuse has particular salience for certain dimensions of the emotion regulation construct. Because emotion regulation is a multidimensional construct, research that exclusively focuses on abilities to control and suppress emotional responses might be misleading (Gratz & Roemer, 2004). Therefore, this investigation explored the cognitive capacities to accurately identify and express emotions as potentially distinct from the behavioral capacities to moderate one's response to emotions. For an individual to produce an appropriate emotional response in a given situation, awareness and processing of the situation and possible responses take place, followed by enactment of a chosen response. This conceptualization of emotion regulation mirrors Crick and Dodge's (1994) model of social information processing, which was modified by Lemerise and Arsenio (2000) to include emotional responses. Following Lemerise and Arsenio, the model used in this study explored relations among childhood emotional abuse, a cognitive emotion regulation deficit (i.e., lack of awareness of emotions or alexithymia), a behavioral emotion regulation deficit (i.e., impulsivity), and relationship violence.

Some research suggests that deficits in different aspects of emotion regulation might follow from different types of maltreatment (Cicchetti & Toth, 2005). Although research links both alexithymia (Berenbaum, 1996; Hund & Espelage, 2006; Mazzeo & Espelage, 2002) and impulsivity (Corstorphine, Waller, Lawson, & Ganis, 2007; Roy, 2005) to childhood emotional abuse, these constructs have not been examined in the same sample. Similarly, these dimensions of emotion regulation have not been directly explored in connection to relationship violence, although both alexithymia (Dabkowska, 2007; Gortner, Gollan, & Jacobson, 1997) and impulsivity (often through reactive anger; Cohen et al., 2003; Gortner et al., 1997; Stuart & Holtzworth-Munroe, 2005) have been identified as correlates of violence.

This investigation examined cognitive and behavioral components of the emotion regulation construct as they might follow from child emotional abuse and contribute to relationship violence. First, it was expected that emotional abuse would predict poor relational health, as evidenced by relationship violence victimization or perpetration, above and beyond the contribution of physical abuse, sexual abuse, and childhood exposure to domestic violence. Further, it was expected that emotional abuse would have the strongest association with relationship violence, based on the theory that emotional abuse is the driving force behind child maltreatment consequences (Hart et al., 1997). Second, it was predicted that emotion dysregulation would mediate the relation between childhood emotional abuse and relationship violence in adulthood. Consistent with a developmental process approach and the documented impact of emotional abuse on coping capabilities, emotion regulation was hypothesized to be an important link between emotional abuse in childhood and relationship violence in adulthood. Third, this study examined if and how cognitive and behavioral elements of emotion dysregulation, as indicated by alexithymia and impulsivity, would differentially explain pathways to relationship violence perpetration versus victimization. Specifically, consistent with research suggesting that perpetration and victimization might have different early antecedents (Ehrensaft et al., 2003; Swan & Snow, 2006), it was hypothesized that impulsivity would mediate the link between emotional abuse and relationship violence perpetration, and alexithymia would explain pathways between emotional abuse and relationship violence victimization. Emotional abuse has been related to both types of emotion regulation deficits, and it was expected that it would be in this model as well. However, because violence perpetration has a behavioral component that victimization does not, impulsivity was expected to be related to perpetration. Although global emotion regulation was expected to play a significant role in relationship violence victimization as well, on a component level, it seems victimization has a less behavioral and more cognitive basis. For example, awareness and understanding of one's emotions might be related to recognizing the reality of relationship violence and the emotional toll it takes on oneself. Therefore, it was hypothesized that alexithymia, rather than impulsivity, would be related to victimization. Finally, exploratory analyses were conducted to evaluate if and how the mediation models already specified might be influenced by gender and ethnicity. Although it is clear that the mechanisms by which relationship violence occurs might be different for women and men (Widom et al., 2006), as well as for different ethnic groups (Swan & Snow, 2006), results regarding the experience of relationship violence in different populations have been varied and inconclusive (Wilt & Olson, 1996). Using a large and diverse sample, the unique opportunity to probe these questions was seized in this study.

METHOD

Participants

Participants were 2,169 (63.8% female) undergraduate students at a large West Coast university. The sample was 46.2% Asian, 27.1% Hispanic, 16.7%

Caucasian, 6.5% black, and 3.5% multiracial or other. Black, multiracial, and other categories were combined for analyses due to the small percentage of the sample each represented. The full sample reflects all participants who were able to complete the study during the first year of data collection, and was used to examine the relation between emotional abuse and emotion regulation. A subsample of 1,175 participants (68.6% female), who reported that they had been in a romantic relationship of 2 months or longer, was used to examine the process model predicting relationship violence. Compared to participants who had not been in a relationship, participants who endorsed having a romantic relationship of 2 months or longer were slightly older (*M* age of the dating group = 19.22, *SD* = 1.64; *M* age of the not dating group = 19.06, *SD* = 1.35), $t(2,121) = 2.33$, $p = .020$; more likely to be female (68.6% females in the dating group, 58.2% females in the not dating group), $t(2,186) = 5.06$, $p < .001$; and less likely to be Asian (42.2% Asian in the dating group, 50.1% Asian in the not dating group), $t(2,194) = 3.73$, $p < .001$.

Procedure

Participants completed a 2-hour computerized survey in small, supervised groups of up to 14 students at a time. Participants were recruited from introductory psychology courses and received class credit in exchange for their participation. Password-protected surveys were administered through a computerized survey management company. Responses were carefully monitored for completeness and the entered information was encrypted (until download) and was identified only by a code number to further ensure the security of the data. Participants completed the survey in private cubicles in a laboratory setting under the supervision of a trained research assistant. Participants were informed that the purpose of the study was to examine relations between adaptation in young adults and various experiences in childhood and adolescence. They were assured that their participation was anonymous and no personal identifying information was requested. Participants were required to stay for the full 2-hour survey block to minimize the incentive to rush through the questionnaires. All procedures were reviewed and approved by the Human Research Review Board of the university.

Measures

Maltreatment

The Childhood Maltreatment Interview Schedule (Briere, 1992) was used to assess the frequency of emotional maltreatment, physical abuse, and childhood exposure to interparental violence. Participants reported on the form and frequency of these maltreatment experiences using objective behavioral descriptors. This measure has demonstrated effectiveness at discriminating among long-term outcomes of various maltreatment subtypes (Briere & Runtz, 1990) and is often shortened and modified for use in ways similar to this investigation (Babcock, Miller, & Siard, 2003; McNutt, Carlson, Persaud, & Postmus, 2002). Emotional abuse was assessed with 14 items that captured how often the individual was yelled at, insulted, criticized, and humiliated by each caregiver during a typical childhood year. Each item was rated on a 7-point scale ranging from 0 (*never*) to 7 (*more than 20 times*) yielding two scores reflecting frequency of emotional maltreatment by mother (seven items, α = .91) and frequency of emotional maltreatment by father (seven items, α = .91). Emotional maltreatment scores were averaged across parents, if both were rated, to create a total emotional abuse frequency variable. Analyses were initially conducted separately for emotional abuse by mothers, emotional abuse by fathers, and emotional abuse averaged across both parents. No differences were found between perpetration by mothers and by fathers, so the variable representing abuse averaged across parents was used for all reported results. Physical abuse was defined as a caregiver doing something to the child on purpose (e.g., hitting, punching, cutting, or pushing the child) that made the child bleed, gave her or him bruises or scratches, or broke bones or teeth. Participants endorsing child physical abuse rated the frequency of such events with a single item ranging from 1 (*1 time*) to 7 (*more than 50 times*). Exposure to domestic violence was defined as the participant having seen or heard one parent hit or beat up the other parent. Frequency of exposure was rated with a single item ranging from 1 (*1 time*) to 7 (*more than 50 times*).

The Child Abuse and Trauma Scale (CATS; Sanders & Becker-Lausen, 1995), was used to assess the frequency of childhood sexual abuse. The sexual abuse subscale of the CATS consists of six items (e.g., "Did your relationship with your parents ever involve a sexual experience," α = .76), each rated on a 5-point scale from 0 (*never*) to 4 (*always*). The CATS has documented concurrent validity with objective measures of childhood sexual abuse and strong internal consistency and reliability in college student populations (Sanders & Becker-Lausen, 1995).

Emotion regulation

Emotion regulation was assessed with the Difficulties in Emotion Regulation Scale (DERS; Gratz & Roemer, 2004), a 36-item measure with six subscales including impulse control difficulties (e.g., "When I'm upset, I lose control over my behaviors") and lack of emotional awareness (e.g., "When I'm upset, I acknowledge my emotions"), which were used in this study, as well as a total score. Items were rated on a 5-point scale, measuring how often each descriptor applied to the participant, with scores ranging from 1 (*almost never or 0–10% of the time*) to 5 (*almost always or 91–100% of the time*). The measure demonstrated adequate reliability in this sample (36-item total score α = .94, 6-item impulse control difficulties α = .87, and 6-item lack of emotional awareness α = .83). The DERS shows strong internal consistency in other college student populations and good construct validity (Sloan & Kring, 2007).

Specific dimensions of the emotion regulation construct were assessed further with the Reactive Anger scale of the State–Trait Anger Scale (STAXI; Spielberger, Jacobs, Russell, & Crane, 1983) and the Toronto Alexithymia Scale–20 (TAS–20; Bagby, Parker, & Taylor, 1994). The STAXI Reactive Anger Scale assesses the tendency toward anger in response to environmental triggers (e.g., "I generally feel furious when criticized in front of others"), with six items rated on a 4-point scale ranging from 1 (*almost never*) to 4 (*almost always;* α = .80). The TAS–20 assesses alexithymia, or difficulty in recognizing and describing one's emotions, on a 5-point scale ranging from 1 (*strongly disagree*) to 5 (*strongly agree;* α = .85). Both scales have demonstrated good internal consistency and reliability in previous work (Bagby et al., 1994; Spielberger et al., 1983). For the mediation analyses, impulse control difficulties on the DERS and the Reactivity Anger Scale of the STAXI were used to create a composite variable impulsivity, and lack of emotional awareness on the DERS and the total score on the TAS–20 were composited to form the variable alexithymia.

Relationship violence

The Conflict Tactics Scale (CTS; Straus, 1979) consists of 29 specific descriptions of partner violence perpetration and victimization events (58 items total) rated on a 7-point scale from 0 (*never*) to 6 (*more than 21 times*). No differences were found among subscale scores representing types of relationship violence (i.e., psychological, physical, sexual) in relations with other variables. Therefore, total relationship violence victimization (23 items; α = .83) and perpetration (23 items; α = .85) were used here. The negotiation subscale, representing nonviolent conflict resolution, was not used in this analysis. The CTS has demonstrated good reliability and validity, especially among the psychological, physical, and sexual violence subscales used here (Straus, 1979).

Data Preparation

All data were examined for nonnormality (i.e., skewness > 2, kurtosis > 7; Curran, West, & Finch, 1996). A natural logarithm was used to transform select variables to render parametric statistics valid. Maltreatment scores for domestic violence (skew = 2.74 and kurtosis = 7.66 before transformation; skew = 1.64 and kurtosis = .775 after transformation), physical abuse (skew = 3.24 and kurtosis = 10.04 before transformation; skew = 2.32 and kurtosis = 3.46 after transformation), and sexual abuse (skew = 3.37 and kurtosis = 13.72

before transformation; skew = 2.21 and kurtosis = 4.15 after two transformations) were transformed. In addition, both relationship violence perpetration (skew = 2.25 and kurtosis = 6.41 before transformation; skew = 1.29 and kurtosis = 1.26 after transformation) and victimization (skew = 2.73 and kurtosis = 10.14 before transformation; skew = 1.48 and kurtosis = 2.00 after transformation) were transformed.

RESULTS

Descriptive Statistics and Bivariate Correlations

As shown in Table 1, participant reports of childhood emotional abuse were positively related to difficulties in emotion regulation ($r = .335$, $p < .001$) and increased relationship violence perpetration ($r = .208$, $p < .001$) and victimization ($r = .170$, $p < .001$). Similar relations were evident for these outcomes with childhood sexual abuse ($r = .203$, $p < .001$; $r = .142$, $p < .001$; $r = .132$, $p < .001$), physical abuse ($r = .071$, $p < .001$; $r = .097$, $p < .001$; $r = .063$, $p = .032$) and domestic violence exposure ($r = .115$, $p < .001$; $r = .095$, $p = .001$; $r = .067$, $p = .024$). However, relative to emotional abuse, the magnitude of these relations was considerably smaller for the other types of maltreatment, with the relation between physical abuse and alexithymia being nonsignificant ($r = .019$, $p = .376$). Participants endorsing difficulties with emotion regulation, particularly in the domain of impulsivity, reported higher levels of relationship violence perpetration ($r = .256$, $p < .001$ for impulsivity) and victimization ($r = .227$, $p < .001$ for impulsivity).

Table 1 also displays descriptive statistics and bivariate correlations for the study variables by gender. Emotional abuse generally had stronger effects for females, whereas other types of maltreatment had similar effects for both genders. In addition, the relation between difficulties in emotion regulation and relationship violence was stronger for females than males.

A two-way multivariate analysis of variance (MANOVA; Gender × Ethnicity) revealed significant main effects for gender (Wilks's $\lambda = .95$), $F(9, 1052) = 6.77$, $p < .001$, and ethnicity (Wilks's $\lambda = .91$), $F(27, 3073) = 3.18$, $p < .001$, but not their interaction. Females reported higher levels of sexual abuse ($F = 20.94$, $p < .001$), difficulties in emotion regulation ($F[1, 1055] = 10.69$, $p = .001$), relationship violence perpetration ($F[1, 1055] = 6.14$, $p = .013$), and marginally higher levels of relationship violence victimization ($F[1, 1055] = 2.93$, $p = .087$) than males. Bonferroni corrected post-hoc comparisons confirmed that Asians and others reported more emotional abuse than Hispanics ($p < .001$ and $p = .001$, respectively). Asians also reported significantly more difficulties in emotion regulation than Hispanics ($p = .045$) and Whites ($p = .008$). Whites reported fewer difficulties with emotional awareness than Hispanics and Asians ($p = .012$ and $p < .001$, respectively), whereas Asians reported more impulsivity than Hispanics ($p = .003$) and Whites ($p = .016$).

TABLE 1 Descriptive Statistics and Bivariate Correlations Among Study Variables

	1	2	3	4	5	6	7	8	9	*n*	*M*	*SD*
Maltreatment history												
1. Emotional abuse	—	.301***	.202***	.231***	.335***	.366***	.187***	.208***	.170***	2,169	41.29	19.62
2. Physical abuse	.206***	—	.114***	.238***	.071***	.127***	.019	.097***	.063*	2,134	.41	1.24
	.348***											
3. Sexual abuse	.178***	.038	—	.149***	.203***	.212***	.148***	.142***	.132***	2,061	7.00	2.45
	.211***	.147***										
4. Domestic violence	.201***	.178***	.089*	—	.115***	.129***	.062**	.095**	.067*	2,124	.48	1.18
	.243***	.260***	.171***									
Emotion regulation												
5. Total difficulties in	.267***	.070#	.262***	.127***	—	.729***	.617***	.150***	.156***	2,165	84.21	22.17
emotion regulation												
	.370***	.071**	.172***	.106***								
6. Impulsivity	.332***	.147***	.267***	.121**	.712***	—	.322***	.256***	.227***	2,169	.001	.85
	.393***	.121***	.195***	.137***	.742***							
7. Alexithymia	.178***	.010	.226***	.077*	.648***	.284***	—	.065*	.082**	2,169	.000	.87
	.195***	.029	.121***	.063*	.560***	.339***						
Relationship violence												
8. Perpetration	.187***	.096#	.079	.088#	.063	.162**	.007	—	.815***	1,175	31.74	11.99
	.214***	.095**	.151***	.090*	.174***	.302***	.095**					
9. Victimization	.178***	.034	.052	.027	.068	.140**	.060	.876***	—	1,174	31.85	13.48
	.165***	.074*	.154***	.075*	.188***	.270***	.096**	.793***				
n	788	780	754	775	788	789	789	368	367			
	1,375	1,351	1,301	1,343	1,372	1,374	1,375	803	803			
M	40.54	.35	6.77	.36	83.32	.05	.08	30.45	31.07			
	41.69	.45	7.14	.56	84.76	-.03	-.04	32.34	32.21			
SD	19.15	1.13	2.46	.99	20.39	.85	.82	10.74	13.56			
	19.86	1.30	2.44	1.27	23.13	.85	.90	12.50	13.44			

Note: Statistics for the total sample above the diagonal; split by gender below the diagonal: males above females.
#$p < .10$. *$p < .05$. **$p < .01$. ***$p < .001$.

No differences in relationship violence were found across ethnic groups. Because Asians differed from each of the other ethnic groups on several key variables (emotional abuse and emotion regulation), remaining analyses were done comparing Asians to all non-Asians.

Relationship Violence Predicted by Maltreatment History

Linear regressions predicted each relationship violence outcome from all types of child maltreatment (see Table 2). Results confirmed that child maltreatment significantly predicted both violence perpetration (R^2 = .046, p < .001) and violence victimization (R^2 = .035, p < .001), with emotional abuse emerging as the strongest predictor among all types of maltreatment (β = .145, p < .001 for perpetration and β = .134, p < .001 for victimization). Physical abuse did not significantly predict either relationship violence outcome after controlling for the other types of maltreatment. Sexual abuse predicted both relationship violence perpetration (β = .087, p = .005) and victimization (β = .089, p = .004). Domestic violence exposure contributed significantly to explaining violence perpetration (β = .065, p = .04), but not victimization (β = .045, p = .155).

The Mediating Role of Emotion Regulation

Mediation analyses were conducted to determine the mechanism by which emotional abuse predicted relationship violence, following Baron and Kenny's (1986) procedures. Regression analyses evaluated each step of mediation, with physical abuse, sexual abuse, and exposure to domestic violence included as covariates. Analyses confirmed that emotional abuse predicted both violence perpetration (β = .145, p < .001) and victimization (β = .134, p < .001), as well as global difficulties in emotion regulation (β = .340, p < .001). Further, emotion regulation difficulties predicted violence perpetration (β = .067, p = .041) and victimization (β = .090, p = .006). After controlling for emotion regulation difficulties, emotional abuse was a

TABLE 2 Simultaneous Regression Models Predicting Relationship Violence From Maltreatment History

	Violence perpetration		Violence victimization	
	β	p	β	p
Emotional abuse	.145	< .001	.134	< .001
Physical abuse	.009	.773	−.016	.618
Sexual abuse	.087	.005	.089	.004
Domestic violence exposure	.065	.036	.045	.155
Total model R^2, Adjusted R^2, F	.046, .042, 12.749*		.035, .032, 9.723*	

*p < .001.

weaker predictor of relationship violence perpetration (β = .123, p < .001) and victimization (β = .104, p = .003). The Sobel test (Sobel, 1982) confirmed the presence of partial mediation for both perpetration (z = 2.205, p = .027) and victimization (z = 2.533, p = .011). Both models were significant (F[5, 1067] = 11.036, p < .001, R^2 = .049 for perpetration, F[5, 1066] = 9.293, p < .001, R^2 = .042 for victimization).

Multiple Mediation by Emotion Regulation

Analyses were conducted to test the hypothesis that emotion regulation is a multidimensional construct, with diverging aspects of emotion regulation explaining the relation between emotional abuse and relationship violence to differing degrees. Following Preacher and Hayes (2008), multiple mediation models evaluated the differential strength of alexithymia and impulsivity as possible mediators underlying observed relations between childhood emotional abuse and relationship violence, and capturing cognitive and behavioral elements of emotion regulation. As in the unidimensional model, childhood physical abuse, sexual abuse, and exposure to domestic violence were included as covariates. The model revealed significant mediation, with the effect of emotional abuse on relationship violence decreasing to β = .079, p = .020 for perpetration (R^2 total model = .080, p < .001) and β = .072, p = .037 for victimization (R^2 total model = .061, p < .001). Impulsivity emerged as a stronger mediator in both models, with the indirect effect of emotional abuse on violence perpetration through impulsivity emerging as β = .074, p = .011 compared to the indirect effect of β = –.008, p = .394 through alexithymia. Results were similar for the victimization model, with a significant indirect effect through impulsivity (β = .064, p = .014), but not through alexithymia (β = –.002, p = .472).

Moderation of Multiple Mediation Model by Gender and Ethnicity

Finally, the multiple mediation model was tested to see if findings differed between males and females as well as between Asians and non-Asians. Models were run separately for each subgroup (see Figures 1 and 2). Moderation was confirmed for gender, with mediation results holding for females but not for males. In males, emotion regulation did not predict violence perpetration or victimization, and therefore mediation by emotion regulation was not present. However, the mediation model was significant for females, with the direct effect of emotional abuse on relationship violence dropping to β = .041, p = .320, for violence perpetration and β = .019, p = .660, for violence victimization, after controlling for impulsivity and alexithymia. Modest ethnic differences emerged as well, with the multiple mediation model most effective for non-Asians, although mediation remained significant for both groups. Post-hoc exploratory analyses further

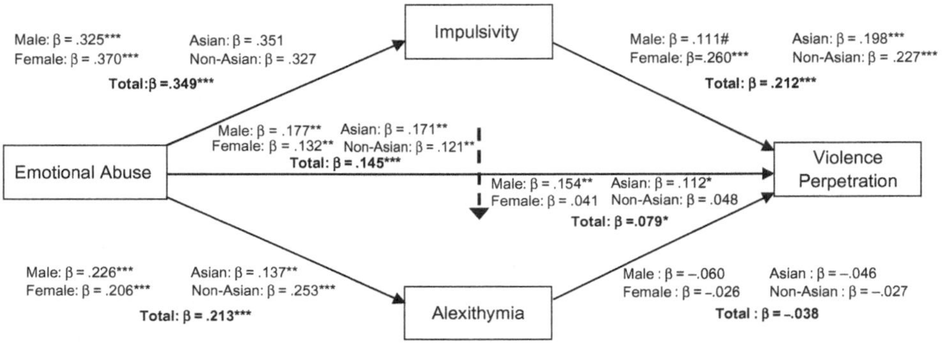

FIGURE 1 Relation Between Emotional Abuse and Relationship Violence Perpetration Mediated by Impulsivity and Lack of Emotion Awareness: Moderated by Gender and Ethnicity.

Note: Childhood physical abuse, sexual abuse and domestic violence exposure were included as covariates; statistics in bold type represent the total sample.

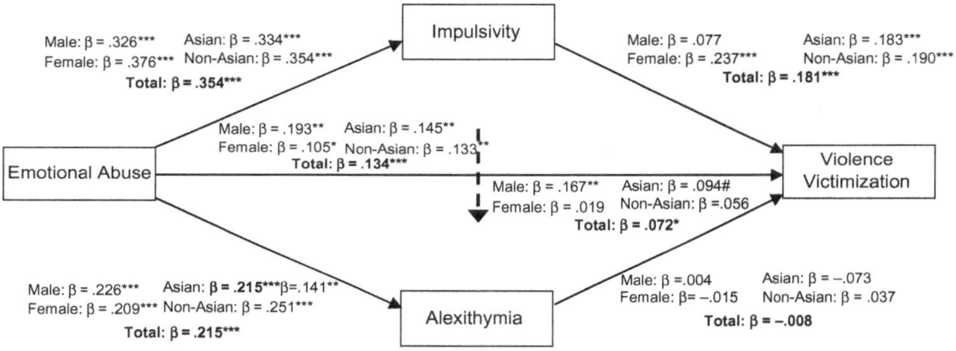

FIGURE 2 Relation Between Emotional Abuse and Relationship Violence Victimization Mediated by Impulsivity and Lack of Emotion Awareness: Moderated by Gender and Ethnicity.

Note: Childhood physical abuse, sexual abuse, and domestic violence exposure were included as covariates; statistics in bold type represent the total sample.

probed the Asian subgroup as a function of their immigrant status (29.6% of this group was born outside the United States). Within Asians, the model remained significant for those born in the United States, but mediation by impulsivity dropped to nonsignificant levels (p = .134 for perpetration, p = .145 for victimization) for those born outside the United States.

DISCUSSION

As the foundation of future generations, adult intimate relationships are an especially salient domain for understanding the long-term impact of child emotional maltreatment and preventing its transmission to subsequent generations. This investigation examined the relation between childhood emotional maltreatment and relationship violence in young adulthood among a large, ethnically diverse, college student sample. Adopting a developmental process perspective, this study examined global emotion regulation as a potential explanatory mechanism underlying this pathway, as well as the contribution of specific cognitive and behavioral components of emotion regulation to the explanation of relationship violence.

The findings reported here support prior indications of unique relations between childhood emotional abuse and relationship violence in adulthood (Bender et al., 2003; Crawford & Wright, 2007; Dodge Reyome, 2010; Simonelli et al., 2002; Wekerle et al., 2009). Childhood emotional abuse predicted both relationship violence victimization and perpetration above and beyond the contributions of childhood physical abuse, sexual abuse, and domestic violence exposure. This finding extends the extant literature on emotional maltreatment and relational health to highlight partner violence as an indicator of maladaptive relational outcomes. Moreover, childhood emotional abuse was by far the most robust predictor of relationship violence, compared to other types of maltreatment. This finding supports the growing body of work suggesting that emotional abuse is an especially pernicious form of maltreatment that warrants greater research and clinical attention.

Clinical efforts to address the deleterious effects of emotional abuse will be furthered to the extent that empirical investigations clarify the specific developmental processes by which emotional abuse eventuates in maladaptive outcomes. In this study, emotion regulation emerged as a significant mediator of the observed relation between childhood emotional abuse and relationship violence. Consistent with the broader literature on emotion regulation and positive development (Durbin & Shafir, 2008; Parke, McDowell, Cladis, & Leidy, 2006; Silk, Shaw, Forbes, Lane, & Kovacs, 2006), these findings point to the need for efforts to protect and support core emotion regulation capacities in all children, particularly in those who have been exposed to emotional maltreatment. Recent reviews point to the promise of interventions that promote emotional competence through teacher training in modeling or reward-based programs, home-based parenting programs, or multipronged home- and school-based interventions (Izard, 2002; Raver, 2002). For example, children attending Head Start and receiving the Emotion Based Program evidence significant improvements in emotional competence, as well as subsequent indirect improvements in social competence (Izard et al., 2008). The findings reported here also extend the literature on maltreatment and coping deficits, suggesting that emotion regulation might be a particularly important influence on coping when it comes to intimate relationships, perhaps via its influence on the ability to engage in positive, goal-directed behavior in emotionally charged situations.

The data further suggest that effective efforts to support adaptive emotion regulation might be tailored to target specific behavioral and cognitive deficits in emotion regulation. Emotion regulation emerged as a multifaceted construct with important cognitive and behavioral elements that evidenced differential salience for understanding the long-term effects of emotional abuse on relationship violence. Specifically, the multiple mediation model examining cognitive and behavioral components of emotion regulation revealed that impulsivity was a stronger mediator than alexithymia of the relation between childhood emotional abuse and relationship violence. Although alexithymia was related to emotional abuse, as previous research has suggested (Berenbaum, 1996; Hund & Espelage, 2006; Mazzeo & Espelage, 2002), it was not related to either violence perpetration or victimization after controlling for impulsivity.

These findings suggest that emotion regulation significantly explains the relation between emotional abuse and relationship violence; however, this relation is driven by behavioral components of emotion regulation more so than by cognitive ones. Although victims of childhood emotional abuse do evidence deficits in emotional awareness and processing (the first step to regulating emotions in a stressful situation), deficits in the second part of that process (the behavioral or response enactment phase), appear to drive the outcome of relationship violence. These data are consistent with prior research documenting risk factors for violence perpetration, including a general tendency toward anger, lack of coping strategies, acceptance of violent coping strategies, and the propensity to choose reactive anger as a coping strategy (Riggs, Caulfield, & Street, 2000). Furthermore, the greater explanatory power of the multiple mediation model supports previous assertions that emotion regulation is a multidimensional construct, and that its developmental significance is best understood in consideration of that complexity (Gratz & Roemer, 2004). However, the data suggest that such models can also vary across gender and ethnic groups.

The mediation model explained observed pathways for females and for non-Asians to a greater degree than for male or Asian participants. The model was unsuccessful in explaining the link between childhood emotional abuse and relationship violence of either type for males. The absence of a mediating relation between emotion regulation and relationship violence among males is surprising given that the bulk of the literature on the role of anger and coping deficits in violence perpetration has been done exclusively with males (Cohen et al., 2003; Riggs et al., 2000). The data reported here suggest that other mechanisms (e.g., substance use, stress; Anderson, 2002; Riggs et al., 2000) might account for observed relations between emotional abuse and relationship violence among males, or perhaps specifically among male college students. Indeed, the presence of only partial mediation indicates that other mechanisms in addition to emotion regulation are involved in pathways from emotional maltreatment to relationship violence, and this might be particularly true for males and for Asians. Little research has been done on domestic violence in the Asian population. Research is similarly lacking on maltreatment among Asian ethnic groups, although preliminary data suggest that maltreatment and its sequelae might differ in meaningful ways within and across Asian ethnic groups and warrant further attention (Kim, Lau, & Chang, 2007). Although information about the specific ethnic makeup of the Asian population in the sample was unavailable, exploratory analyses suggested that the diminished ability of the model to explain the relation between childhood emotional abuse and relationship violence for Asians might reflect differences in immigrant status, with the model failing to explain these patterns for Asians who were not born in the United States.

These data are among the first to clarify specific pathways among child emotional abuse, cognitive and behavioral elements of emotion regulation, and relationship violence. However, as noted previously, the presence of partial mediation suggests that other developmental systems (e.g., the self-system; Briere & Runtz, 1990; Gross & Keller, 1992) might also be important in understanding the long-term effects of emotional abuse. Alternately, emotion regulation could contribute to relational outcomes via indirect pathways not explored here. For example, maltreated children are often victims of peer rejection due to difficulties in emotion regulation that manifest during the early school years (Feiring & Furman, 2000). This rejection might lead to identification with deviant peer groups. If continued into adulthood, this pathway could explain why victims of emotional maltreatment end up with romantic partners who also might have been rejected by peers, and perhaps are more aggressive (Ehrensaft et al., 2003). Further, these processes might vary in explaining relationship violence perpetration versus victimization.

Although not apparent in this study, some evidence suggests that pathways to violence perpetration are distinct from those toward victimization. Research has identified numerous risk factors for relationship violence victimization that hinge on cognitive and emotional characteristics of the victim, including depression, traumatic stress, and substance abuse (Anderson, 2002; Riggs et al., 2000). In addition, cognitive variables such as self-concept and lack of personal control have been examined for their role in victimization (Anderson, 2002; Gelles, 1985; Umberson, Anderson, Glick, & Shapiro, 1998). However, it is often difficult to ascertain whether these are risk factors for victimization, outcomes of victimization, or cooccurring consequences of a common risk factor such as child maltreatment. Although individual studies of perpetration or victimization have identified unique predictors for each, most of these studies have not examined perpetration and victimization in the same sample. High levels of comorbidity between perpetration and victimization might complicate efforts to elucidate specific predictors of each (Ehrensaft et al., 2003).

The sample reported here evidenced significant violence overlap, with 80% of respondents endorsing nearly equal amounts of perpetration and victimization. Indeed, some have posited that the reciprocity of relationship violence is such that relationship violence perpetration and victimization might explain one another to a greater extent than outside factors (Swan & Snow, 2006). In support of this assertion, Anderson (2002) found that victimization actually mediated the relation between risk factors and perpetration. Comorbidity both obscures potential contributing factors and complicates interpretation of the findings. For example, it is interesting that impulsivity partially mediated the relation between emotional abuse and relationship violence victimization in this sample, because impulsivity has not yet been associated with victimization. It might be that the behavioral component of an emotion regulation deficit prevents the victim from enacting a goal-directed response to violence (i.e., leaving the situation), even when cognitively he or she recognizes it as an appropriate option. However, it might also be that impulsivity was an explanatory mechanism for underlying perpetration, and only emerged in this sample as connected with victimization because of the overlap in endorsements and the reciprocal nature of the phenomena. Similarly, although the hypothesis that alexithymia would be uniquely related to victimization was not supported in this investigation, this relation might emerge in future studies that focus on victimization occurring independently of perpetration.

This study contributes to the extant literature in several ways. First, the findings stress the importance of childhood emotional abuse as a critical predictor of later adjustment difficulties, particularly in intimate relationships, above and beyond other types of child maltreatment. Second, this study provides evidence for the emerging conceptualization of emotion regulation as a multidimensional construct, highlighting specific cognitive and behavioral deficits. Third, this study demonstrates that a developmental process perspective is imperative when examining the pathways from childhood abuse to adult outcomes, especially when considering clinical applications. Finally, the findings point to a specific mechanism that is new to the emerging literature on maltreatment and relationship violence: emotion regulation.

Nevertheless, the significance of these findings must be considered in light of limitations in the study design. First, although this sample is notable for its size and ethnic diversity, the representativeness of a college student sample to the broader population is limited. Yet, although limited in age range, the sample represented an age range that is characterized by marked risk for dating violence (Capaldi, Shortt, & Kim, 2005; Wilt & Olson, 1996), and perhaps was more clinically relevant than a sample of varied ages. However, as noted previously, the absence of significant mediation findings among males might reflect a misspecified model for males, or, perhaps more likely, for males attending college and particularly male psychology students, a group that consistently evidences meaningful differences with males not in college (Smart, 1966).

Second, the cross-sectional design of this study constrains the ability to evaluate directional hypotheses regarding cause and effect. In light of this design, it cannot be surmised that emotional abuse causes emotion regulation difficulties that, in turn, contribute to relationship violence. Rather, one is limited to saying that the observed findings are consistent with an overall model wherein these relations hold. Although emotion regulation difficulties might follow from relationship violence, emotion regulation was selected as a process variable that is conceptually likely to cause developmental change because it relates to a coping process rather than a state of mind (e.g., depression), which is more likely to follow from relationship violence.

Third, the obtained data were acquired through self-report measures exclusively. As such, interrelations among variables could be elevated as a function of shared method variance. Further, self-report has particular limitations where maltreatment is concerned because of its retrospective nature. However, a recent review of the literature on retrospective reports of adverse childhood experiences indicates that errors of omission (i.e., failure to report negative events) are more common than false positive reporting. These authors conclude that the use of retrospective reports is appropriate in a research context unless detailed information is necessary (Hardt & Rutter, 2004). Despite these limitations, however, it is clear that these findings have significance for ongoing empirical investigations of childhood emotional abuse and efforts to ameliorate its negative effects.

Childhood emotional abuse is a tangible, quantifiable risk to healthy development. The data reported here suggest that recurrent experiences of rejection, humiliation, and isolation by caregivers exact a powerful and enduring toll on adaptation with effects evident well into young adulthood. Emotion regulation appears to be a promising target for understanding such pathways, and for correcting pathological developmental trajectories toward interpersonal difficulties. Although emotion regulation has garnered increasing attention as a central mechanism of psychopathology (Cicchetti, Ackerman, & Izard, 1995; Gross & Munoz, 1995), less attention has been directed to the added value of attending to specific aspects of the emotion regulation construct in understanding particular forms of pathological functioning. These findings suggest that emotion regulation globally, and particularly behavioral aspects of such regulation, are critically important for fostering adaptive relationship skills among children exposed to emotional abuse. Further, evidence of gender and ethnic differences in these processes and pathways bolster calls for socioculturally sensitive prevention and intervention efforts. Although these findings warrant replication using diverse samples and longitudinal research designs, the data provide convincing support for the enduring and damaging effects of child emotional maltreatment through more proximal developmental processes. As in previous studies, emotional abuse emerged as the most salient predictor of later difficulties, and yet it remains the most difficult to detect and identify (O'Hagan, 1995). These findings and the arguments they support confirm the need for increased funding for treatment, child welfare, and research efforts focused on childhood emotional maltreatment.

REFERENCES

Anderson, K. L. (2002). Perpetrator or victim? Relationships between intimate partner violence and well-being. *Journal of Marriage and Family, 64*, 851–863.

Babcock, J., Miller, S., & Siard, C. (2003). Toward a typology of abusive women: Differences between partner-only and generally violent women in the use of violence. *Psychology of Women Quarterly, 27*, 153–161.

Bagby, R. M., Parker, J. D. A., & Taylor, G. J. (1994). The twenty-item Toronto Alexithymia Scale: I. Item selection and cross-validation of the factor structure. *Journal of Psychosomatic Research, 38*, 23–32.

Baron, R. M., & Kenny, D. A. (1986). The moderator–mediator variable distinction in social psychological research: Conceptual, strategic, and statistical considerations. *Journal of Personality and Social Psychology, 51*, 1173–1182.

Bender, M., Cook, S., & Kaslow, N. (2003). Social support as a mediator of revictimization of low-income African American women. *Violence and Victims, 18*, 419–431.

Berenbaum, H. (1996). Childhood abuse, alexithymia and personality disorder. *Journal of Psychosomatic Research, 41*, 585–595.

Briere, J. (1992). *Child abuse trauma: Theory and treatment of the lasting effects.* Thousand Oaks, CA: Sage.

Briere, J., & Runtz, M. (1988). Multivariate correlates of childhood psychological and physical maltreatment among university women. *Child Abuse & Neglect, 12*, 331–341.

Briere, J., & Runtz, M. (1990). Differential adult symptomatology associated with three types of child abuse histories. *Child Abuse & Neglect, 14*, 357–364.

Capaldi, D. M., Shortt, J. W., & Kim, H. K. (2005). A life span developmental systems perspective on aggression toward a partner. In W. Pinsof & J. Lebow (Eds.), *Family psychology: The art of the science* (pp. 141–167). New York: Oxford University Press.

Chang, L., Schwartz, D., Dodge, K. A., & McBride-Chang, C. (2003). Harsh parenting in relation to child emotion regulation and aggression. *Journal of Family Psychology, 17*, 598–606.

Cicchetti, D., Ackerman, B. P., & Izard, C. E. (1995). Emotions and emotion regulation in developmental psychopathology. *Development and Psychopathology, 7*(1), 1–10.

Cicchetti, D., & Toth, S. L. (2005). Child maltreatment. *Annual Review of Clinical Psychology, 1*(1), 409–438.

Claussen, A. H., & Crittenden, P. M. (1991). Physical and psychological maltreatment: Relations among types of maltreatment. *Child Abuse & Neglect, 15*, 5–18.

Cohen, R. A., Brumm, V., Zawacki, T. M., Paul, R., Sweet, L., & Rosenbaum, A. (2003). Impulsivity and verbal deficits associated with domestic violence. *Journal of the International Neuropsychological Society, 9*, 760–770.

Colman, R. A., & Widom, C. S. (2004). Childhood abuse and neglect and adult intimate relationships: A prospective study. *Child Abuse & Neglect, 28*, 1133–1151.

Corstorphine, E., Waller, G., Lawson, R., & Ganis, C. (2007). Trauma and multi-impulsivity in the eating disorders. *Eating Behaviors, 8*(1), 23–30.

Crawford, E., & Wright, M. O. D. (2007). The impact of childhood psychological maltreatment on interpersonal schemas and subsequent experiences of relationship aggression. *Journal of Emotional Abuse, 7*(2), 93–116.

Crick, N. R., & Dodge, K. A. (1994). A review and reformulation of social information-processing mechanisms in children's social adjustment. *Psychological Bulletin, 115*(1), 74–101.

Curran, P. J., West, S. G., & Finch, J. F. (1996). The robustness of test statistics to nonnormality and specification error in confirmatory factor analysis. *Psychological Methods, 1*(1), 16–29.

Dabkowska, M. (2007). Relationships between the emotional and cognitive components of alexythymia and PTSD in victims of domestic violence. *Psychiatria Polska, 41*, 851–862.

Dodge Reyome, N. (2010). Childhood emotional maltreatment and later Intimate relationships: Themes from the empirical literature *Journal of Aggression, Maltreatment and Trauma, 19*(2), 224–242.

Durbin, C. E., & Shafir, D. M. (2008). Emotion regulation and risk for depression. In J. Abela & B. Hankin (Eds.), *Handbook of depression in children and adolescents* (pp. 149–176). New York: Guilford.

Ehrensaft, M. K., Cohen, P., Brown, J., Smailes, E., Chen, H., & Johnson, J. G. (2003). Intergenerational transmission of partner violence: A 20-year prospective study. *Journal of Consulting and Clinical Psychology, 71*, 741–753.

Eisenberg, N., Gershoff, E. T., Fabes, R. A., Shepard, S. A., Cumberland, A. J., Losoya, S. H., et al. (2001). Mother's emotional expressivity and children's behavior problems and social competence: Mediation through children's regulation. *Developmental Psychology, 37*, 475–490.

Erickson, M. F., Egeland, B., & Pianta, R. (1989). The effects of maltreatment on the development of young children. In D. Cicchetti & V. Carlson (Eds.), *Child maltreatment: Theory and research on the causes and consequences of child abuse and neglect* (pp. 647–684). New York: Cambridge University Press.

Feiring, C., & Furman, W. C. (2000). When love is just a four-letter word: Victimization and romantic relationships in adolescence. *Child Maltreatment, 5*, 293–298.

Gelles, R. J. (1985). Family violence. *Annual Review of Sociology, 11*(1), 347–367.

Gibb, B. E., Benas, J. S., Crossett, S. E., & Uhrlass, D. J. (2007). Emotional maltreatment and verbal victimization in childhood: Relation to adults' depressive cognitions and symptoms. *Journal of Emotional Abuse, 7*(2), 59–73.

Gortner, E. T., Gollan, J. K., & Jacobson, N. S. (1997). Psychological aspects of perpetrators of domestic violence and their relationships with the victims. *Psychiatric Clinics of North America, 20*, 337–352.

Gratz, K. L., & Roemer, L. (2004). Multidimensional assessment of emotion regulation and dysregulation: Development, factor structure, and initial validation of the difficulties in emotion regulation scale. *Journal of Psychopathology and Behavioral Assessment, 26*(1), 41–54.

Gross, A. B., & Keller, H. R. (1992). Long-term consequences on childhood physical and psychological maltreatment. *Aggressive Behavior, 18*, 171–185.

Gross, J., & Munoz, R. (1995). Emotion regulation and mental health. *Clinical Psychology: Science and Practice, 2*, 151–164.

Hardt, J., & Rutter, M. (2004). Validity of adult retrospective reports of adverse childhood experiences: Review of the evidence. *Journal of Child Psychology and Psychiatry, 45*, 260–273.

Hardy, D. F., Power, T. G., & Jaedicke, S. (1993). Examining the relation of parenting to children's coping with everyday stress. *Child Development, 64*, 1829–1841.

Hart, S. N., Binggeli, N. J., & Brassard, M. R. (1997). Evidence for the effects of psychological maltreatment. *Journal of Emotional Abuse, 1*(1), 27–58.

Hund, A. R., & Espelage, D. L. (2006). Childhood emotional abuse and disordered eating among undergraduate females: Mediating influence of alexithymia and distress. *Child Abuse & Neglect, 30*, 393–407.

Izard, C. E. (2002). Translating emotion theory and research into preventive interventions. *Psychological Bulletin, 128*, 796–824.

Izard, C. E., King, K. A., Trentacosta, C. J., Morgan, J. K., Laurenceau, J.-P., Krauthamer-Ewing, E. S., et al. (2008). Accelerating the development of emotion competence in Head Start children: Effects on adaptive and maladaptive behavior. *Development and Psychopathology, 20*(1), 369–397.

Kaplan, S. J., Pelcovitz, D., & Labruna, V. (1999). Child and adolescent abuse and neglect research: A review of the past 10 years. Part I: Physical and emotional abuse and neglect. *Journal of the American Academy of Child & Adolescent Psychiatry, 38*, 1214–1222.

Kent, A., Waller, G., & Dagnan, D. (1999). A greater role of emotional than physical or sexual abuse in predicting disordered eating attitudes: The role of mediating variables. *International Journal of Eating Disorders, 25*, 159–167.

Kim, I. J., Lau, A. S., & Chang, D. F. (2007). Family violence among Asian Americans. In F. T. L. Leong, A. G. Inman, A. Ebreo, L. H. Yang, L. M. Kinoshita, & M. Fu (Eds.), *Handbook of Asian American psychology* (pp. 363–378). Thousand Oaks, CA: Sage.

Krause, E. D., Mendelson, T., & Lynch, T. R. (2003). Childhood emotional invalidation and adult psychological distress: The mediating role of emotional inhibition. *Child Abuse & Neglect, 27*, 199–213.

Lemerise, E. A., & Arsenio, W. F. (2000). An integrated model of emotion processes and cognition in social information processing. *Child Development, 71*, 107–118.

Mazzeo, S. E., & Espelage, D. L. (2002). Association between childhood physical and emotional abuse and disordered eating behaviors in female undergraduates: An investigation of the mediating role of alexithymia and depression. *Journal of Counseling Psychology, 49*, 86–100.

McGee, R. A., Wolfe, D. A., & Wilson, S. K. (1997). Multiple maltreatment experiences and adolescent behavior problems: Adolescents' perspectives. *Development and Psychopathology, 9*, 131–149.

McNutt, L.-A., Carlson, B. E., Persaud, M., & Postmus, J. (2002). Cumulative abuse experiences, physical health and health behaviors. *Annals of Epidemiology, 12*, 123–130.

Messman-Moore, T. L., & Coates, A. A. (2007). The impact of childhood psychological abuse on adult interpersonal conflict: The role of early maladaptive schemas and patterns of interpersonal behavior. *Journal of Emotional Abuse, 7*(2), 75–92.

Mueller, E., & Silverman, N. (1989). Peer relations in maltreated children. In D. Cicchetti & V. Carlson (Eds.), *Child maltreatment: Theory and research on the causes and consequences of child abuse and neglect* (pp. 529–578). New York: Cambridge University Press.

Mullen, P. E., Martin, J. L., Anderson, J. C., Romans, S. E., & Herbison, G. P. (1996). The long-term impact of the physical, emotional, and sexual abuse of children: A community study. *Child Abuse & Neglect, 20*, 7–21.

Ney, P. G., Fung, T., & Wickett, A. R. (1994). The worst combinations of child abuse and neglect. *Child Abuse & Neglect, 18*, 705–714.

O'Hagan, K. P. (1995). Emotional and psychological abuse: Problems of definition. *Child Abuse & Neglect, 19*, 449–461.

Paradis, A., & Boucher, S. (2010). Child maltreatment history and interpersonal problems in adult couple relationships. *Journal of Aggression, Maltreatment and Trauma, 19*(2), 138–158.

Parke, R. D., McDowell, D. J., Cladis, M., & Leidy, M. S. (2006). Family and peer relationships: The role of emotion regulatory processes. In D. K. Snyder, J. S. Simpson, & J. N. Hughes (Eds.), *Emotion regulation in couples and families: Pathways to dysfunction and health* (pp. 143–162). Washington, DC: American Psychological Association.

Paterson, J., Fairbairn-Dunlop, P., Cowley-Malcolm, E. T., & Schluter, P. J. (2007). Maternal childhood parental abuse history and current intimate partner violence: Data from the Pacific Islands Families Study. *Violence and Victims, 22*, 474–488.

Perry, A. R., DiLillo, D., & Peugh, J. (2007). Childhood psychological maltreatment and quality of marriage: The mediating role of psychological distress. *Journal of Emotional Abuse, 7*, 117–142.

Ponce, A. N., Williams, M. K., & Allen, G. J. (2004). Experience of maltreatment as a child and acceptance of violence in adult intimate relationships: Mediating effects of distortions in cognitive schemas. *Violence and Victims, 19*(1), 97–108.

Preacher, K. J., & Hayes, A. F. (2008). Asymptotic and resampling strategies for assessing and comparing indirect effects in multiple mediator models. *Behavioral Research Methods, 40*, 879–891.

Raver, C. C. (2002). Emotions matter: Making the case for the role of young children's emotional development for early school readiness. *Social Policy Report, 16*, 3–19.

Riggs, S. A. (2010). Childhood emotional abuse and the attachment system across the life cycle: What theory and research tell us. *Journal of Aggression, Maltreatment and Trauma, 19(1)*, 5–51.

Riggs, D. S., Caulfield, M. B., & Street, A. E. (2000). Risk for domestic violence: Factors associated with perpetration and victimization. *Journal of Clinical Psychology, 56*, 1289–1316.

Rosenthal, M. Z., Polusny, M. A., & Follette, V. M. (2006). Avoidance mediates the relationship between perceived criticism in the family of origin and psychological distress in adulthood. *Journal of Emotional Abuse, 6*(1), 87–102.

Roy, A. (2005). Childhood trauma and impulsivity: Possible relevance to suicidal behavior. *Archives of Suicide Research, 9*, 147–151.

Sanders, B., & Becker-Lausen, E. (1995). The measurement of psychological maltreatment: Early data on the Child Abuse and Trauma Scale. *Child Abuse & Neglect, 19*, 315–323.

Shipman, K. L., Schneider, R., Fitzgerald, M. M., Sims, C., Swisher, L., & Edwards, A. (2007). Maternal emotion socialization in maltreating and non-maltreating families: Implications for children's emotion regulation. *Social Development, 16*, 268–285.

Shirk, S. R., & Eltz, M. (1998). Multiple victimization and the process and outcome of child psychotherapy. *Journal of Aggression, Maltreatment & Trauma, 2*, 233–251.

Silk, J. S., Shaw, D. S., Forbes, E. E., Lane, T. L., & Kovacs, M. (2006). Maternal depression and child internalizing: The moderating role of child emotion regulation. *Journal of Clinical Child and Adolescent Psychology, 35*(1), 116–126.

Simonelli, C. J., Mullis, T., Elliott, A. N., & Pierce, T. W. (2002). Abuse by siblings and subsequent experiences of violence within the dating relationship. *Journal of Interpersonal Violence, 17*, 103–121.

Sloan, D. M., & Kring, A. M. (2007). Measuring changes in emotion during psychotherapy: Conceptual and methodological issues. *Clinical Psychology: Science and Practice, 14*, 307–322.

Smart, R. G. (1966). Subject selection bias in psychological research. *Canadian Psychologist/Psychologie canadienne, 7*, 115–121.

Sobel, M. S. (1982). Asymptotic confidence intervals for indirect effects in structural equation models. *Sociological Methodology, 13*, 290–312.

Spertus, I. L., Yehuda, R., Wong, C. M., Halligan, S., & Seremetis, S. V. (2003). Childhood emotional abuse and neglect as predictors of psychological and physical symptoms in women presenting to a primary care practice. *Child Abuse & Neglect, 27*, 1247–1258.

Spielberger, C. D., Jacobs, G., Russell, S., & Crane, R. S. (1983). Assessment of anger: The State-Trait Anger Scale. In J. N. Butcher & C. D. Spielberger (Eds.), *Advances in personality assessment* (pp. 159–187). Hillsdale, NJ: Lawrence Erlbaum Associates.

Straus, M. A. (1979). Measuring intrafamily conflict and violence: The Conflict Tactics (CT) Scales. *Journal of Marriage & the Family, 41*(1), 75–88.

Stuart, G. L., & Holtzworth-Munroe, A. (2005). Testing a theoretical model of the relationship between impulsivity, mediating variables, and husband violence. *Journal of Family Violence, 20*, 291–303.

Swan, S. C., & Snow, D. L. (2006). The development of a theory of women's use of violence in intimate relationships. *Violence Against Women, 12*, 1026–1045.

Taft, C. T., Schumm, J. A., Marshall, A. D., Panuzio, J., & Holtzworth-Munroe, A. (2008). Family-of-origin maltreatment, posttraumatic stress disorder symptoms, social information processing deficits, and relationship abuse perpetration. *Journal of Abnormal Psychology, 117*, 637–646.

Taussig, H. N., & Culhane, S. E. (2010). Emotional maltreatment and psychosocial functioning in preadolescent youth placed in out-of-home care. *Journal of Aggression, Maltreatment and Trauma, 19(1)*, 52–74.

Umberson, D., Anderson, K., Glick, J., & Shapiro, A. (1998). Domestic violence, personal control, and gender. *Journal of Marriage & the Family, 60*, 442–452.

Varia, R., Abidin, R. R., & Dass, P. (1996). Perceptions of abuse: Effects on adult psychological and social adjustment. *Child Abuse & Neglect, 20*, 511–526.

Vissing, Y. M., Straus, M. A., Gelles, R. J., & Harrop, J. W. (1991). Verbal aggression by parents and psychosocial problems of children. *Child Abuse & Neglect, 15*, 223–238.

Wekerle, C., Leung, E., Wall, A., MacMillan, H., Boyle, M., Trocme, N., et al. (2009). The contribution of childhood emotional abuse to teen dating violence among child protective services-involved youth. *Child Abuse & Neglect, 33*, 45–58.

Wekerle, C., Wolfe, D. A., Hawkins, D. L., Pittman, A.-L., Glickman, A., & Lovald, B. E. (2001). Childhood maltreatment, posttraumatic stress symptomatology, and adolescent dating violence: Considering the value of adolescent perceptions of abuse and a trauma mediational model. *Development and Psychopathology, 13*, 847–871.

Widom, C. S., Schuck, A. M., & White, H. R. (2006). An examination of pathways from childhood victimization to violence: The role of early aggression and problematic alcohol use. *Violence and Victims, 21*, 675–690.

Wilt, S., & Olson, S. (1996). Prevalence of domestic violence in the United States. *Journal of the American Medical Women's Association, 51*(3), 77–82.

Wright, M. O. (Ed.). (2007). Childhood emotional abuse: Mediating and moderating processes affecting long-term impact [Special issue]. *Journal of Emotional Abuse, 7*(2).

Yates, T. M. (2007). The developmental consequences of child emotional abuse: A neurodevelopmental perspective. *Journal of Emotional Abuse, 7*(2), 19–34.

Yates, T. M., & Wekerle, C. (2009). The long-term consequences of childhood emotional maltreatment on development: (Mal)adaptation in adolescence and young adulthood. *Child Abuse & Neglect, 33*, 19–21.

Zurbriggen, E. L., Gobin, R., & Freyd, J. J. (2010). Childhood emotional abuse and late adolescent sexual aggression perpetration and victimization. *Journal of Aggression, Maltreatment and Trauma, 19*(2), 204–223.

Childhood Emotional Abuse Predicts Late Adolescent Sexual Aggression Perpetration and Victimization

EILEEN L. ZURBRIGGEN
University of California, Santa Cruz, Santa Cruz, California, USA

ROBYN L. GOBIN and JENNIFER J. FREYD
University of Oregon, Eugene, Oregon, USA

Childhood physical and sexual abuse are known risk factors for adult sexual aggression perpetration and victimization, but less is known about the role played by childhood emotional abuse. College sophomores were surveyed regarding their childhood physical, sexual, and emotional abuse victimization and their late-adolescent experiences of sexual aggression victimization and perpetration. Controlling for social desirability and childhood physical and sexual abuse, childhood emotional abuse was the strongest predictor of adolescent sexual perpetration for women and the strongest predictor of adolescent sexual victimization for men. Emotional abuse was a marginally reliable predictor of adolescent sexual victimization in women. These results show the importance of childhood emotional abuse victimization as a risk factor for sexual victimization and perpetration in adolescent intimate relationships.

Two decades ago, Hart and Brassard (1987) argued that psychological maltreatment "is the core issue in child maltreatment" (p. 161). Since that time,

---

Data collection was supported by a grant from the National Institute of Mental Health (MH071334) to Eileen L. Zurbriggen.

there has been a growing interest in understanding the effects of childhood psychological and emotional abuse. Although emotional abuse is less well studied than physical or sexual abuse, it is consistently found to be a predictor of negative outcomes in adulthood, including anger and irritability (Teicher, Samson, Polcari, & McGreenery, 2006), depression (Gibb, Chelminski, & Zimmerman, 2007), dissociation (Teicher et al., 2006), eating disorders (Kennedy, Ip, Samra, & Gorzalka, 2007; Witkiewitz & Dodge-Reyome, 2001), marital dissatisfaction (Perry, DiLillo, & Peugh, 2007), and social phobias (Gibb et al., 2007). Moreover, studies that look at multiple types of abuse simultaneously often find that the effects of emotional abuse remain reliable even when controlling for physical and sexual abuse. For example, Spertus, Yehuda, Wong, Halligan, and Seremetis (2003) found that emotional abuse and neglect (jointly) predicted anxiety, depression, posttraumatic stress symptoms, and physical symptoms even when controlling for physical and sexual abuse and lifetime trauma exposure. Some studies have also found that the effect sizes for emotional abuse are as large as, or larger than, the effect sizes for physical or sexual abuse. For example, Gibb et al. (2007) found stronger associations between childhood emotional abuse and later depression than between childhood physical and sexual abuse and depression. Clearly, it is important to consider all forms of childhood maltreatment to fully understand the long-term impact of abuse.

Recently, researchers have noted the importance of taking this broader approach when examining participants' victimization profiles. Failure to account for all types of abuse a participant has experienced might lead to inaccurate conclusions about the unique contribution of specific types of abuse to mental health outcomes and social functioning (Finkelhor, Ormrod, & Turner, 2007). Such information could enhance interventions aimed at reducing revictimization risk. The following review summarizes the many findings that confirm a relationship between childhood physical and sexual abuse and subsequent victimization and perpetration. Then, those studies that specifically addressed the role of emotional abuse are described, while highlighting the emotional components of abusive experiences that might create vulnerability for later victimization and perpetration.

PHYSICAL AND SEXUAL ABUSE PREDICT AGGRESSION PERPETRATION

Childhood physical and sexual abuse have consistently been associated with aggression perpetration in adolescents and adults. Childhood physical abuse has been associated with criminality and violence (Widom, 2000), intimate partner violence (Graves, Sechrist, White, & Paradise, 2005; White & Widom, 2003), and sexual assault perpetration (White & Smith, 2004). Similarly, childhood sexual abuse has been associated with sexual assault perpetration (Glasser et al., 2001; White & Smith, 2004) and criminality (Freyd et al., 2005).

Given the elevated rates of childhood sexual and physical victimization among pedophiles and child abusers, some theorists have posited a developmental progression from victim to perpetrator (Finkelhor & Araji, 1986). According to this theory, perpetration of abuse develops out of a need for victims to gain mastery over their childhood victimization experiences by adopting the role of the powerful aggressor (Finkelhor & Araji, 1986; Irwin, 1999). More recent theories have become increasing complex, including multiple mediating and moderating variables as well as protective factors that might buffer victims from the negative consequences of childhood maltreatment (Arata, 2002). Dissociation, in particular, has received empirical support as a potential mediator. For example, Becker-Blease and Freyd (2007) studied a sample of convicted sex offenders and reported that high levels of dissociation in response to victimization were related to dissociation during perpetration. The role of emotions might also be important. Lisak, Hopper, and Song (1996) examined several factors that might increase risk for perpetration of abuse among men who report childhood sexual abuse, physical abuse, or both. Results indicated that high levels of gender rigidity and emotional constriction were associated with increased risk for perpetration. Although Lisak et al. did not measure emotional abuse, Goldsmith and Freyd (2005) found that emotional abuse was strongly related to difficulty identifying feelings, suggesting that emotional abuse might be an important underlying factor in emotional constriction that is related to perpetration.

Other findings also support the idea that emotions might play an important role in the cycle of violence. Many studies have demonstrated a connection between childhood abusive experiences and emotional distress such as increased rates of depression, anxiety, and anger (for a review, see Briere & Elliott, 1994). Emotional distress resulting from abusive childhood experiences might be directed inwardly and result in depression, self-hatred, and low self-esteem (Briere & Elliott, 1994). Conversely, emotional distress can be manifested externally in the form of physical, sexual, and emotional aggression (Briere & Elliott, 1994).

In addition to emotional consequences, abusive experiences often result in cognitive distortions. Many researchers have posited that the development of the self is intrinsically tied to social interactions (Roche, Runtz, & Hunter, 1999). It is in the context of interpersonal relationships (especially early attachment relationships with caregivers) that children develop a sense of self (see Riggs, 2010). The experience of childhood sexual abuse is one type of interpersonal interaction that might have deleterious effects on a child's schema of relationship models and thus lead to interpersonal problems in the future (Classen, Field, Kooperman, Nevill-Manning, & Spiegel, 2001). Theorists have proposed that childhood sexual abuse disrupts a developing child's "basic beliefs about safety and trust" in interpersonal relationships thus resulting in a false understanding of elements of satisfying healthy relationships in adolescence and adulthood (Cole & Putnam, 1992). In the instance of perpetration of abuse, victims might have developed a cognitive schema of relationships in which violence is seen as an appropriate method of emotional expression. According to social learning theory, the cycle of violence occurs as physical aggression is modeled by parents and influential members of society (Widom, 1989). Consequently children learn that aggression is an acceptable vehicle through which to express emotions or achieve needs and desires (Bandura, 1973; Widom, 1989).

PHYSICAL AND SEXUAL ABUSE PREDICT AGGRESSION VICTIMIZATION

Revictimization has also been extensively studied and theorized. A particular focus has been the path from childhood sexual abuse victimization to adult sexual assault victimization, although physical abuse has been studied as well. Hosser, Raddatz, and Windzio (2007) found that childhood physical abuse victimization predicted adult physical assault and crime victimization. Studies have consistently found that childhood sexual abuse victimization increased the risk of adult sexual assault victimization (Gidycz, Hanson, & Layman, 1995; Humphrey & White, 2000; Koss & Dinero, 1989; Messman-Moore & Long, 2003; Siegel & Williams, 2003). This finding has been confirmed in at least two meta-analyses (Neumann, Houskamp, Pollock, & Briere, 1996; Roodman & Clum, 2001). As with the "cycle of violence," in which childhood victimization can lead to adult perpetration, dissociation is one of the likely mediational pathways between childhood victimization and adult victimization (Hall, 2003; Svedin, Nilsson, & Lindell, 2004).

Another set of pathways might involve impairment in the ability to recognize risky situations (Wilson, Calhoun, & Bernat, 1999) and betrayal (Gobin & Freyd, 2009). Gobin and Freyd (2009) found an association between the experience of traumas high in betrayal (such as childhood sexual, physical, or emotional abuse by someone emotionally close to the child) and subsequent awareness for betrayals in interpersonal contexts. Specifically, they found that survivors of high betrayal traumas reported lower levels of awareness for infidelity in their romantic partnerships when compared to participants without high betrayal trauma histories. Moreover, there was an association between high betrayal trauma history and response to interpersonal betrayals in adulthood such that high betrayal trauma survivors were more likely to report remaining in a relationship following a betrayal of trust. Decreased awareness for betrayals and remaining in relationships with disloyal partners might heighten revictimization risk.

EMOTIONAL ABUSE AS A PREDICTOR OF AGGRESSION PERPETRATION AND VICTIMIZATION

The theoretical and empirical work discussed previously links childhood physical and sexual abuse with aggression perpetration and victimization as an adult. It is reasonable to ask whether childhood emotional abuse is similarly a risk factor for aggression perpetration or victimization as an adult, especially given the demonstrated importance of emotions as outcomes, mediators, or moderators in many of the studies on physical and sexual abuse. A handful of studies related to this question have been conducted (see Berzenski & Yates, 2010). Their findings suggest that both victimization and perpetration might be more likely among emotional abuse survivors.

The most directly relevant studies measure childhood emotional abuse (along with other types of abuse) and use these childhood trauma variables to predict aggression perpetration or victimization as an adult or adolescent (e.g., see Dodge Reyome, 2010, for a discussion of childhood emotional maltreatment and intimate partner violence). In one study (Crawford & Wright, 2007), childhood emotional abuse and neglect (jointly) predicted relationship aggression (predominantly a measure of general physical aggression, with a few items concerning sexual aggression) in college students. This relationship held, even when controlling for gender, income, parental alcoholism, child sexual abuse, child physical abuse, and neglect (see Riggs & Kaminski, 2010, for a discussion of childhood emotional maltreatment and relational aggression). In another study (Linder & Collins, 2005), researchers found that boundary violations between adolescents and their parents predicted physical victimization and perpetration in later dating relationships (at ages 21 and 23). Boundary violations included behaviors such as being casually seductive and reversing roles. Although this construct has important differences from emotional abuse as conceived by most researchers who study it, it seems related to emotional abuse.

Two studies have looked specifically at sexual assault victimization as the outcome variable. Recruiting from a sample of women receiving outpatient services at a Canadian hospital, Stermac, Reist, Addison, and Millar (2002) found that childhood neglect by mother or father and psychological maltreatment by mother predicted adult sexual assault victimization. Similarly, Messman-Moore and Brown (2004) found more cases of adult rape victimization among participants who had experienced childhood emotional abuse than among those who had not. This finding was still marginally (p = .07) reliable when physical abuse, sexual abuse, and family functioning were statistically controlled.

THIS STUDY

This study was designed to test the hypotheses that childhood emotional abuse would be positively associated with late adolescent sexual aggression victimization as well as perpetration, and that this would be true for both genders. In addition, it assessed whether these results will still hold when controlling for childhood physical and sexual abuse, which are often positively correlated with emotional and psychological abuse. Because self-reports of violence perpetration or victimization might be contaminated by self-presentation response biases (Saunders, 1991), a measure of social desirability was included in data collection and analysis.

METHOD

Participants

Participants were 79 male and 105 female college sophomores attending a large state university on the West Coast. They were part of a larger two-wave longitudinal study on sex and dating that was begun the year before (when participants were incoming first-year college students). At the time of original recruitment, all participants were between the ages of 18 and 20, were beginning their first year of college (i.e., not transfer students), and had learned English before the age of 5. At the time of this data collection, most (87%) of the participants were 19 years old (M = 19.04, SD = 0.36, range = 18–20). Just under two thirds (n = 119, 64.7%) of participants identified as European American. The sample also included 25 (13.6%) Asian American, 14 (7.6%) Latina or Latino, 6 (3.3%) African American, and 15 (8.2%) biracial or multiracial participants. Five participants indicated another ethnicity or did not respond to the question.

Measures

Childhood abuse

A 12-item version of the Brief Betrayal Trauma Survey (BBTS; Goldberg & Freyd, 2006) was used to assess retrospective self-reports of childhood physical, sexual, and emotional abuse before the age of 18. The BBTS includes behaviorally specific questions about exposure to a variety of traumas including noninterpersonal trauma, witnessing violence, and direct interpersonal trauma. For each item, the participant indicated how many times the event had happened to him or her: never (coded as 0), 1 or 2 times (coded as 1), or 3 or more times (coded as 2). For this study, responses to six items were analyzed: emotional abuse ("You were emotionally or psychologically mistreated over a significant period of time by someone with whom you were very close [such as a parent or lover]"), physical abuse by someone close ("You were deliberately attacked that severely [so severely as to result in marks, bruises, blood, broken bones, or broken teeth] by someone with whom you were very close"), physical abuse by someone not close ("You were deliberately attacked that severely by someone with whom you were not close"), sexual abuse by someone close ("You were made to have some form of sexual contact, such as touching or penetration, by someone with whom you were very close [such as a parent or lover]"), and sexual abuse by someone not close ("You were made to have such sexual contact by someone with whom you were not close"). In previous research, good construct validity has been reported for the BBTS and its test–retest reliability has been high (83% for events that occurred during childhood and 75% for adult experiences; Goldberg & Freyd, 2006). Further evidence for the construct validity of the BBTS was provided by DePrince (2001), who found high agreement between scores on the BBTS and responses to a much more extensive trauma questionnaire, the Betrayal Trauma Inventory, which was derived from the well-validated Abuse and Perpetration Inventory (Lisak et al., 2000).

Adolescent sexual aggression perpetration and victimization

Adolescent sexual aggression experiences were measured using a modified version of the Sexual Experiences Survey (SES; Koss, Gidycz, & Wisniewski, 1987). Reliability and validity data for the SES were reported in Koss and Gidycz (1985) and Testa, VanZile-Tamsen, Livingston, and Koss (2004). For this study, a superset of the items in the modified version of the SES described by Testa et al. and the original SES (Koss & Oros, 1982) was used. All items were rewritten to be gender neutral. For example, "Have you had sexual intercourse when you didn't want to because a man threatened or used some degree of physical force (twisting your arm, holding you down, etc.) to make you?" was rewritten as, "Have you had sexual intercourse with someone when you didn't want to because they threatened or used some degree of physical force (twisting your arm, holding you down, etc.) to make you?" and "Have you had a man attempt to insert his penis (but intercourse did not occur)" was rewritten as, "Have you been in a situation where someone attempted to have sexual intercourse with you when you didn't want to (but intercourse did not occur)." Participants first answered a version of the SES (SES–V) that measured sexual aggression victimization and then a second version (SES–P) that measured sexual aggression perpetration. For both versions, participants indicated on a scale from 0 (*not at all*) to 5 (*5 or more times*) how often they had engaged in behaviorally specific acts of sexual aggression perpetration or victimization. Additional examples of items include "How many times have you fondled, kissed, or touched someone sexually when they didn't want to because you threatened or used some degree of physical force (twisting their arm, holding them down, etc.) to make them?" and "How many times have you had sexual intercourse with someone when you didn't want to because they used their position of authority (boss, teacher, camp counselor, supervisor) to make you?" Responses were summed to create the final outcome variables.

Social desirability

The Impression Management subscale of the Balanced Inventory of Desirable Responding (Paulhus, 1991) was used to assess social desirability. Construct validity of this scale has been demonstrated by Paulhus (1991). Sample items include "I sometimes drive faster than the speed limit," and "I never swear." Responses were on a scale ranging from 1 (*disagree strongly*) to 7 (*agree strongly*). Coefficient alpha for this scale was .74. In accordance with Paulhus's recommendations for scoring, responses were dichotomized such that the two most socially desirable responses (e.g., *disagree strongly* and *disagree moderately* for the item "I sometimes drive faster than the speed limit") were coded as a one and the other five responses were coded as a zero; these recoded responses were then summed to create the final score.

Procedure

All participants were taking part in the second wave of a two-wave longitudinal study in which they were assessed once in the fall of their first year of college and again in the fall of their second year of college. All measures previously described were included as part of a larger questionnaire packet (with additional measures not analyzed for this study) that participants completed individually in a quiet, private room. The full procedure for this wave of the study included a timed, individually administered computer task and a semistructured one-to-one interview, both of which preceded the administration of the questionnaire. Total administration time was approximately 2 to 3 hours; participants were given snacks, beverages, and breaks throughout the procedure. Participants were paid $25 plus a bonus based on their performance on the computer task and an additional "scheduling bonus" (for those who arrived on time for their originally scheduled appointment); total compensation was capped at $40.

RESULTS

Descriptive Statistics and Tests for Gender Differences

Means and standard deviations for all variables are presented in Table 1. Means for social desirability were similar to those previously reported by Paulhus (1991) for a college sample. There were no statistically reliable gender differences in mean levels of social desirability, childhood physical or sexual abuse by someone close, or adolescent sexual aggression perpetration.

TABLE 1 Descriptive Statistics and Tests of Gender Differences

	Men		Women		
Variable	*M*	*SD*	*M*	*SD*	*T*
Social desirability	4.00	3.09	4.04	2.63	0.08
Childhood emotional abuse (close)	0.18	0.50	0.44	0.75	2.83**
Childhood physical abuse (close)	0.15	0.49	0.11	0.40	−0.60
Childhood physical abuse (not close)	0.17	0.41	0.03	0.22	−2.72**
Childhood sexual abuse (close)	0.08	0.32	0.16	0.48	1.41
Childhood sexual abuse (not close)	0.05	0.22	0.12	0.36	1.68†
Adolescent sexual aggression perpetration	0.62	1.83	0.32	1.09	−1.31
Adolescent sexual aggression victimization	1.29	3.55	2.68	4.12	2.44*

*Note: N*s for men ranged from 76 to 79. *N*s for women ranged from 104 to 105. Social desirability could range from 0 to 20. Individual abuse items could range from 0 to 2. The possible range for aggression perpetration and victimization was 0 to 75. The *t* statistics provide tests of the gender differences in means. †$p < .10$. *$p < .05$. **$p < .01$.

Women reported more childhood emotional abuse, more adolescent sexual aggression victimization, and (marginally) more childhood sexual abuse from someone they were not close to than did men. Men reported more childhood physical abuse from someone they were not close to than did women.

Social Desirability, Childhood Abuse, and Adolescent Sexual Aggression: Zero-Order Correlations

Zero-order correlations for all variables are presented in Table 2. For women, childhood emotional abuse was positively correlated with both types of physical abuse and with sexual abuse by someone close. For men, childhood emotional abuse was correlated with both types of physical abuse, but was not correlated with either type of sexual abuse (both *p*s > .50). The difference in the size of the men's correlation between emotional abuse and sexual abuse by someone close (r = .07) was reliably different than the size of the women's correlation between these two variables (r = .39), tested via Fisher's r-to-z transformation, z = 2.18, p = .03.

Childhood emotional abuse was positively correlated with adolescent sexual aggression victimization and perpetration, and this was true for both men and women. The correlation between adolescent sexual aggression victimization and perpetration was stronger in men (r = .68) than in women (r = .22), z = 4.01, $p < .001$.

Women's social desirability scores were negatively correlated with adolescent sexual aggression perpetration and positively correlated with childhood physical abuse victimization. Men's social desirability scores were (marginally)

TABLE 2 Intercorrelations of All Variables for Women (Above Diagonal) and Men (Below Diagonal)

	1	2	3	4	5	6	7	8
1. Social desirability		.06	.17†	.22*	.05	−.07	−.28**	−.06
2. Childhood emotional abuse (close)	−.14		.44***	.22*	.39***	.01	.19*	.38***
3. Childhood physical abuse (close)	−.10	.58***		.40***	.15	.10	.07	.20*
4. Childhood physical abuse (not close)	−.00	.55***	.52***		.05	.20*	−.04	.12
5. Childhood sexual abuse (close)	.13	.07	.09	−.00		.16	.02	.46***
6. Childhood sexual abuse (not close)	−.15	.03	−.07	−.10	−.06		.10	.11
7. Adolescent sexual aggression perpetration	−.20†	.35**	.18	.46***	−.06	−.08		.22*
8. Adolescent sexual aggression victimization	−.15	.49***	.15	.34**	.04	−.04	.68***	

Note: *N*s for men range from 75 to 79. *N*s for women range from 103 to 105.
$^{\dagger}p < .10$. $^{*}p < .05$. $^{**}p < .01$. $^{***}p < .001$.

negatively correlated with adolescent sexual aggression perpetration. Therefore, social desirability was included in the multivariate analyses reported here, to adjust for the possible effects of self-presentation response bias.

Childhood Abuse and Adolescent Sexual Aggression: Regression Analyses

To further explore the zero-order correlations between childhood emotional abuse and adolescent sexual aggression experiences, and to control for correlated variables, four hierarchical multiple regression analyses were conducted. These results are presented in Table 3. Analyses were conducted separately for men and women, first with sexual aggression perpetration and then sexual aggression victimization used as the outcome variable. For all analyses, social desirability and childhood emotional abuse were entered in the first block, with the four childhood physical abuse and sexual abuse variables entered in the second block.

The overall percentage of variance predicted by the final models ranged from 13.8% (regression predicting women's experiences of sexual aggression perpetration) to 31.2% (regression predicting men's experiences of sexual aggression victimization). For each of the four analyses the total variance explained was large enough to be statistically reliable (all *p*s $< .05$). In general, social desirability was not an important predictor; it was, however, statistically reliable for the prediction of women's reports of their sexual aggression perpetration.

As in the zero-order correlational analyses, childhood emotional abuse was an important predictor of sexual aggression perpetration and victimization, and this was true for both men and women. In general, the relationship between childhood emotional abuse and adolescent sexual aggression was not affected by the addition of childhood physical and sexual abuse into the regression model. In other words, emotional abuse was predictive of adolescent sexual aggression perpetration and victimization, even after controlling for the possible effects of childhood physical and sexual abuse (which were not, in general, predictive of sexual aggression). An exception was the case of men's sexual aggression perpetration. In this model, childhood emotional abuse was a moderately strong predictor of perpetration ($B = 1.245$, $\beta = .34$, $t = 3.15$, $p = .002$). Once sexual abuse (and physical abuse) were added to the model, the standardized partial regression coefficient for childhood emotional abuse decreased (from $\beta = .34$ to $\beta = .20$) and was, in the final model, not a statistically reliable predictor ($p = .13$).

TABLE 3 Hierarchical Regressions Predicting Adolescent Sexual Aggression Perpetration and Victimization From Social Desirability and Childhood Physical, Sexual, and Emotional Abuse

	Men				Women			
	Sexual aggression perpetration[a]		Sexual aggression victimization[b]		Sexual aggression perpetration[c]		Sexual aggression victimization[c]	
Predictor	Step 1	Step 2	Step 1	Step 2	Step 1	Step 2	Step 1	Step 2
Social desirability	−.13	−.17	−.06	−.10	−.30**	−.28**	−.06	−.11
Child emotional abuse (close)	.34**	.20	.49***	.54***	.21*	.23*	.39***	.18†
Child physical abuse (close)		−.19		−.28*		.04		.10
Child physical abuse (not close)		.45***		.19		−.06		.06
Child sexual abuse (close)		−.04		.04		−.07		.37***
Child sexual abuse (not close)		−.08		−.07		.09		.05
ΔR^2		.146*		.058		.012		.133**
Total R^2	.148**	.294***	.254***	.312***	.125**	.138*	.150***	.283***

Note: Social desirability and childhood emotional abuse were entered in the first block; childhood physical and sexual abuse variables were entered in the second block. Standardized partial regression coefficients (βs) are reported.

[a]$n = 76$. [b]$n = 75$. [c]$n = 103$.

†$p < .10$. *$p < .05$. **$p < .01$. ***$p < .001$.

DISCUSSION

Previous work has emphasized the deleterious consequences of childhood sexual and physical abuse on adolescent and adult interpersonal functioning, and less attention has been paid to the relative contribution of childhood emotional abuse. This study examined the relationship between childhood emotional abuse and late adolescent sexual aggression victimization and perpetration. As predicted, for both men and women, childhood emotional abuse was positively correlated with adolescent sexual aggression victimization and perpetration. This effect was robust and, in most cases, held even after controlling for childhood sexual and physical abuse and social desirability.

This investigation highlights the importance of emotional abuse as a risk factor for later sexual victimization and perpetration among survivors of childhood maltreatment. The associations between child maltreatment and sexual and physical revictimization have been well substantiated by the literature. However, an overwhelming majority of previous studies have focused on child physical or sexual abuse, while excluding childhood emotional abuse from consideration. Similarly, emotional abuse is rarely measured in cycle of violence investigations that seek to predict adult or adolescent perpetration from childhood victimization (see Berzenski & Yates, 2010). Our findings suggest that childhood emotional abuse is related to both late adolescent sexual aggression perpetration and victimization. Therefore, to adequately assess risk for adolescent sexual aggression, the presence and extent of childhood emotional abuse must be known.

A failure to include emotional abuse in research on the sequelae of child maltreatment could also lead to false conclusions about the relationship between other types of childhood abuse and subsequent perpetration and victimization. For example, interpretation of results might be adversely affected when researchers fail to control for covarying types of abuse, such that difficulties experienced by the survivor might be mistakenly attributed to one type of abuse as opposed to another (Simeon, Guralnik, Schmeidler, Sirof, & Knutelska, 2001). In the data reported above, zero-order correlations suggested that men's physical abuse by someone they were not close to could lead to adolescent sexual aggression victimization. However, this correlation was no longer reliable in the multiple regression analysis, suggesting that risk of revictimization was instead due to (covarying) emotional abuse. Similarly, the pattern of zero-order correlations in women between physical abuse by someone close, sexual abuse by someone close, and adolescent sexual aggression victimization suggested that either of these types of childhood abuse could lead to later revictimization. However, the multiple regression analyses revealed that physical abuse was no longer a reliable predictor, once other types of abuse were controlled for. The important predictors were sexual abuse by someone close and (to a lesser extent) emotional abuse.

Possible Mediating Mechanisms

This study did not include a direct investigation of mechanisms that mediate between childhood maltreatment and adolescent outcomes, but several such mechanisms are possible candidates. One mechanism that has frequently been proposed to increase revictimization risk is dissociation (Becker-Blease & Freyd, 2007; Hall, 2003). Dissociation often develops as a coping mechanism that allows survivors to dismiss information from conscious awareness that is perceived as overwhelming (Kluft, 1990). Although dissociation is successful, in that it defends the survivor from incorporating overwhelming information into his or her conscious awareness, it is dangerous in that it can become adaptive for the survivor and generalize to other dangerous situations in adolescence and adulthood (Noll, Horowitz, Bonanno, Trickett, & Putnam, 2003). This can result in an inability to detect dangerous situations in the future (e.g., Cloitre, 1998). Dissociation might also be a mediator between childhood emotional abuse and sexual aggression perpetration. Adult perpetrators who dissociated during their childhood victimization experiences are more likely to dissociate when perpetrating (Becker-Blease & Freyd, 2007). It could be that their perpetration is facilitated by the dissociated state, which allows for an unawareness of the harmful nature of the abusive actions.

Other cognitive mediators might also play a role. Zurbriggen and Freyd (2004) posited that childhood sexual abuse leads to changes in schemas about relationships and damaged "consensual sex decision mechanisms," resulting in impaired sexual decision making. For example, healthy decision rules such as "If I don't want to have sex, say no" might be absent or damaged in sexual abuse survivors. Emotional abuse might similarly be expected to result in damage to schemas and decision rules related to sexuality and romantic relationships. Such damage could lead to increased risk for sexual aggression perpetration and victimization.

In addition to cognitive mediators, the possibility that emotional mediators could be important in understanding the sequelae of childhood emotional abuse is intriguing. Emotional abuse has been found to predict a variety of emotions, including anger and irritability (Teicher et al., 2006), anxiety and phobias (Gibb et al., 2007; Spertus et al., 2003), and depression (Gibb et al., 2007; Spertus et al., 2003). Emotional disorders such as depression and anxiety might make it difficult for survivors to appreciate risky situations or to stand up for themselves, thus increasing revictimization risk. If emotional abuse interferes with healthy emotional development it might lead to deficits in important emotional skills such as the ability to empathize with others. Because low empathy is a risk factor for sexual aggression perpetration (Dean & Malamuth, 1997; Seto & Barbaree, 1993), such deficits could partially explain the increased levels of sexual aggression perpetration that were found in survivors of emotional abuse. Impaired facility in emotion regulation is another possible mediator. Without the ability to self-regulate and appropriately moderate one's irritation, frustration can lead to anger and aggression toward the person who is the perceived cause of the frustration. It is easy to imagine a situation in a budding romantic relationship in which a frustrated desire for sexual fulfillment, combined with inadequate skills in managing frustration, could lead someone to commit sexual assault. These speculations about possible emotional mediators deserve further thought and study. It could be that, especially for emotional abuse, it would be fruitful to move away from a reliance on cognitive mediators and focus more intently on emotions in developing treatment and intervention protocols.

Limitations and Future Directions

Despite the support found for the connection between childhood emotional abuse and adult sexual aggression perpetration and victimization, limitations of the study must be acknowledged. Rates of childhood sexual, physical, and emotional abuse were obtained via retrospective self-reports. Because memories can fade or change over time, reliance on retrospective reports of childhood traumatic experiences highlights concerns regarding false negatives. Thus, a possible limitation of this study is underreporting of childhood abuse.

Self-reports have additional limitations, including their sensitivity to demand characteristics such as social desirability bias. The inclusion of social desirability as a control variable in the multiple regression analyses helps to mitigate against this bias, but is not guaranteed to adjust for it completely. In addition, because all three types of abuse were measured via self-report, it is possible that the associations between abuse types might be artificially high due to shared method variance. Again, this becomes less of a problem in the multiple regression analyses because all shared method variance is partialed out. However, it would be wise to interpret the zero-order correlations between abuse types with some caution. Future research that directly compares retrospective self-reports of abuse history with information obtained using other methodologies (e.g., reports from other family members, archival court or child protective services reports, self-reports at the time of the abuse, implicit measures such as physiological or emotional reactivity to abuse-related stimuli) would be welcome. Of course, because of the secrecy that often surrounds childhood abuse (especially childhood sexual abuse), the fact that abuse often goes unreported, and the memory impairment that can accompany trauma (Freyd, 1996), such research is likely to be difficult to conduct.

The use of a college sample limits the generalizability of results. College students have a tendency to display higher levels of functioning than might be observed in community and clinical samples. Thus, it will be important to replicate these findings outside of college samples. It should be noted, however, that other researchers have found support for the detrimental effects of emotional abuse in clinical samples (e.g., Gibb et al., 2007; Simeon et al., 2001; Spertus et al., 2003).

The 12-item BBTS used in this study asked only about emotional abuse committed by someone close to the child. In contrast, for both physical and sexual abuse, separate questions were asked concerning abuse perpetrated by someone close to and not close to the child. It is possible that associations between variables might change if emotional abuse by someone not close was measured and included in analyses. The most recent (14-item) version of the BBTS (available at http://dynamic.uoregon.edu/~jjf/bbts/) includes this additional question about emotional abuse; for future research it would be best to use this expanded instrument.

Emotional abuse might be different from sexual and physical abuse in regards to the likelihood that it can be perpetrated by someone not close to the child. For sexual and physical abuse, potential perpetrators who are not close to the child might not have much access to him or her; however, if they do gain access their abusive actions (e.g., hitting, beating, raping) would presumably inflict the same damage as would identical actions perpetrated by someone close to the child. In contrast, abusive language and harsh criticism conceivably might hurt much less when coming from a stranger than when coming from a beloved caregiver. In addition, emotional abuse might take its heavy toll in part because of the frequency with which it is delivered. Parents and other individuals close to a child can (and often do) inflict emotional abuse day after day for years on end, to an extent that would simply not be possible for strangers or acquaintances. Indeed, researchers have found that the majority of perpetrators of childhood emotional abuse are parents (e.g., Simeon et al., 2001). Future research can continue to explore the association between frequency of emotional abuse and the relationship between the child and the perpetrator. In addition, such research can investigate the effect of emotional abuse "dosage." It could be that part of the damage caused by emotional abuse can be attributed to the massive amounts of it that many maltreated children receive.

One might also speculate that the high level of betrayal inherent in emotional abuse perpetrated by someone close to the victim could contribute to the toxicity of emotional abuse. According to betrayal trauma theory (Freyd, 1996), memory for, awareness of, and processing of traumatic experiences will be impaired depending on the level of betrayal inherent in the event. It is possible that emotional abuse perpetrated by someone close to the victim could increase risk for subsequent victimization and perpetration through the mediating mechanism of memory impairment. Future research should explore the relative contribution of closeness of perpetrator of emotional abuse to outcomes such as adult sexual aggression victimization and perpetration.

This study has provided further evidence that childhood emotional abuse is an important predictor of later problems, at least as important as other types of abuse (such as childhood physical or sexual abuse) that are often considered more serious. These results support the assessment of other researchers (e.g., Finkelhor et al., 2007; Hart & Brassard, 1987) who have advocated for a fuller investigation of this hurtful and damaging form of child maltreatment.

REFERENCES

Arata, C. M. (2002). Child sexual abuse and sexual revictimization. *Clinical Psychology, 9*, 135–164.

Bandura, A. (1973). *Aggression: A social learning analysis.* Englewood Cliffs, NJ: Prentice-Hall.

Becker-Blease, K. A., & Freyd, J. J. (2007). Dissociation and memory for perpetration among convicted sex offenders. *Journal of Trauma and Dissociation, 8*(2), 69–80.

Berzenski, S. R., & Yates, T. M. (2010). A developmental process analysis of the contribution of childhood emotional abuse to relationship violence. *Journal of Aggression, Maltreatment and Trauma, 19*(2), 180–203.

Briere, J. N., & Elliott, D. M. (1994). Immediate and long term impacts of child sexual abuse. *The Future of Children, 4*, 54–69.

Classen, C., Field, N., Kooperman, C., Nevill-Manning, K., & Spiegel, D. (2001). Interpersonal problems and their relationship to sexual revictimization among women abused in childhood. *Journal of Interpersonal Violence, 16*, 495–509.

Cloitre, M. (1998). Sexual revictimization: Risk factors and prevention. In V. M. Follette, J. I. Ruzek, & F. R. Abueg (Eds.), *Cognitive-behavioral therapies for trauma* (pp. 278–304). New York: Guilford.

Cole, P. C., & Putnam, F. W. (1992). Effect of incest on self and social functioning: A developmental psychopathology perspective. *Journal of Consulting and Clinical Psychology, 60*, 174–184.

Crawford, E., & Wright, M. O. (2007). The impact of childhood psychological maltreatment on interpersonal schemas and subsequent experiences of relationship aggression. *Journal of Emotional Abuse, 7*(2), 93–116.

Dean, K., & Malamuth, N. M. (1997). Characteristics of men who aggress sexually and of men who imagine aggressing: Risk and moderating variables. *Journal of Personality and Social Psychology, 72*, 449–455.

DePrince, A. P. (2001). *Trauma and posttraumatic responses: An examination of fear and betrayal.* Unpublished doctoral dissertation, University of Oregon, Eugene, OR.

Dodge Reyome, N. (2010). Childhood emotional maltreatment and later intimate relationships: Themes from the empirical literature. *Journal of Aggression, Maltreatment and Trauma, 19*(2), 224–242.

Finkelhor, D., & Araji, S. (1986). Explanations of pedophilia: A four factor model. *The Journal of Sex Research, 22*, 145–161.

Finkelhor, D., Ormrod, R. K., & Turner, H. A. (2007). Poly-victimization: A neglected component in child victimization. *Child Abuse and Neglect, 31*, 7–26.

Freyd, J. J. (1996). *Betrayal trauma: The logic of forgetting childhood abuse*. Cambridge, MA: Harvard University Press.

Freyd, J. J., Putnam, F. W., Lyon, T. D., Becker-Blease, K. A., Cheit, R. E., Siegel, N. B., et al. (2005). The science of child sexual abuse. *Science, 308*, 501.

Gibb, B. E., Chelminski, I., & Zimmerman, M. (2007). Childhood emotional, physical, and sexual abuse, and diagnoses of depressive and anxiety disorders in adult psychiatric outpatients. *Depression and Anxiety, 24*, 256–263.

Gidycz, C. A., Hanson, K., & Layman, M. J. (1995). A prospective analysis of the relationships among sexual assault experiences: An extension of previous findings. *Psychology of Women Quarterly, 19*, 5–29.

Glasser, M., Kolvin, I., Campbell, D., Glasser, A., Leitch, I., & Farrelly, S. (2001). Cycle of child sexual abuse: Links between being a victim and becoming a perpetrator. *British Journal of Psychiatry, 179*, 482–494.

Gobin, R. L., & Freyd, J. J. (2009). Betrayal and revictimization: Preliminary findings. *Psychological Trauma: Theory, Research, Practice, and Policy, 1*, 242–257.

Goldberg, L. R., & Freyd, J. J. (2006). Self-reports of potentially traumatic experiences in an adult community sample: Gender differences and test–retest stabilities of the items in a Brief Betrayal-Trauma Survey. *Journal of Trauma and Dissociation, 7*(3), 39–63.

Goldsmith, R., & Freyd, J. J. (2005). Awareness for emotional abuse. *Journal of Emotional Abuse, 5*(1), 95–123.

Graves, K. N., Sechrist, S. M., White, J. W., & Paradise, M. J. (2005). Intimate partner violence perpetrated by college women within the context of a history of victimization. *Psychology of Women Quarterly, 29*, 278–289.

Hall, J. M. (2003). Dissociative experiences of women child abuse survivors: A selective constructivist review. *Trauma, Violence, and Abuse, 4*, 283–308.

Hart, S. N., & Brassard, M. R. (1987). A major threat to children's mental health: Psychological maltreatment. *American Psychologist, 42*, 160–165.

Hosser, D., Raddatz, S., & Windzio, M. (2007). Child maltreatment, revictimization, and violent behavior. *Violence and Victims, 22*, 318–333.

Humphrey, J. A., & White, J. W. (2000). Women's vulnerability to sexual assault from adolescence to young adulthood. *Journal of Adolescent Health, 27*, 419–424.

Irwin, H. J. (1999). Violent and nonviolent revictimization of women abused in childhood. *Journal of Interpersonal Violence, 14*, 1095–1110.

Kennedy, M. A., Ip, K., Samra, J., & Gorzalka, B. B. (2007). The role of childhood emotional abuse in disordered eating. *Journal of Emotional Abuse, 7*(1), 17–36.

Kluft, R. P. (1990). Dissociation and subsequent vulnerability: A preliminary study. *Dissociation, 3*, 167–173.

Koss, M. P., & Dinero, T. E. (1989). Discriminant analysis of risk factors for sexual victimization among a national sample of college women. *Journal of Consulting and Clinical Psychology, 57*, 242–250.

Koss, M. P., & Gidycz, C. A. (1985). Sexual Experiences Survey: Reliability and validity. *Journal of Consulting and Clinical Psychology, 53*, 422–423.

Koss, M. P., Gidycz, C. A., & Wisniewski, N. (1987). The scope of rape: Incidence and prevalence of sexual aggression and victimization in a national sample of higher education students. *Journal of Consulting and Clinical Psychology, 55*, 162–170.

Koss, M. P., & Oros, C. J. (1982). Sexual Experiences Survey: A research instrument investigating sexual aggression and victimization. *Journal of Consulting and Clinical Psychology, 50*, 455–457.

Linder, J. R., & Collins, W. A. (2005). Parent and peer predictors of physical aggression and conflict management in romantic relationships in early adulthood. *Journal of Family Psychology, 19*, 252–262.

Lisak, D., Conklin, A., Hopper, J., Miller, P., Altschuler, L., & Smith, B. M. (2000). The Abuse-Perpetration Inventory: Development of an assessment instrument for research on the cycle of violence. *Family Violence and Sexual Assault Bulletin, 16*, 21–30.

Lisak, D., Hopper, J., & Song, P. (1996). Factors in the cycle of violence: Gender rigidity and emotional constriction. *Journal of Traumatic Stress, 9*, 721–743.

Messman-Moore, T. L., & Brown, A. L. (2004). Child maltreatment and perceived family environment as risk factors for adult rape: Is child sexual abuse the most salient experience? *Child Abuse and Neglect, 28*, 1019–1034.

Messman-Moore, T. L., & Long, P. J. (2003). The role of childhood sexual abuse sequelae in the sexual revictimization of women: An empirical review and theoretical reformulation. *Clinical Psychology Review, 23*, 537–571.

Neumann, D. A., Houskamp, B. M., Pollock, V. E., & Briere, J. (1996). The long-term sequelae of childhood sexual abuse in women: A meta-analytic review. *Child Maltreatment, 1*, 6–16.

Noll, J. G., Horowitz, L. A., Bonanno, G. A., Trickett, P. K., & Putnam, F. W. (2003). Revictimization and self-harm in females who experienced childhood sexual abuse: Results from a prospective study. *Journal of Interpersonal Violence, 18*, 1452–1471.

Paulhus, D. R. (1991). Measurement and control of response bias. In J. P. Robinson, P. R. Shaver, & L. S. Wrightsman (Eds.), *Measures of personality and social psychological attitudes* (pp. 17–59). San Diego, CA: Academic.

Perry, A. R., DiLillo, D., & Peugh, J. (2007). Childhood psychological maltreatment and quality of marriage: The mediating role of psychological distress. *Journal of Emotional Abuse, 7*(2), 117–142.

Riggs, S. A. (2010). Childhood emotional abuse and the attachment system across the life cycle: What theory and research tell us. *Journal of Aggression, Maltreatment and Trauma, 19*(1), 5–51.

Riggs, S. A., & Kaminski, P. (2010). Childhood emotional abuse, adult attachment, and depression as predictors of relational adjustment and psychological aggression. *Journal of Aggression, Maltreatment and Trauma, 19*(1), 75–104.

Roche, D. N., Runtz, M. G., & Hunter, M. A. (1999). Adult attachment: A mediator between child sexual abuse and later psychological adjustment. *Journal of Interpersonal Violence, 14*, 184–207.

Roodman, A. A., & Clum, G. A. (2001). Revictimization rates and method variance: A meta- analysis. *Clinical Psychology Review, 21*, 183–204.

Saunders, D. G. (1991). Procedures for adjusting self-reports of violence for social desirability bias. *Journal of Interpersonal Violence, 6*, 336–344.

Seto, M. K., & Barbaree, H. E. (1993). Victim blame and sexual arousal to rape cues in rapists and nonoffenders. *Annals of Sex Research, 6*, 167–183.

Siegel, J. A., & Williams, L. M. (2003). Risk factors for sexual victimization of women: Results from a prospective study. *Violence Against Women, 9*, 902–930.

Simeon, D., Guralnik, O., Schmeidler, J., Sirof, B., & Knutelska, M. (2001). The role of childhood interpersonal trauma in depersonalization disorder. *American Journal of Psychiatry, 158*, 1027–1033.

Spertus, I. L., Yehuda, R., Wong, C. M., Halligan, S., & Seremetis, S. V. (2003). Childhood emotional abuse and neglect as predictors of psychological and physical symptoms in women presenting to a primary care practice. *Child Abuse and Neglect, 27*, 1247–1258.

Stermac, L., Reist, D., Addison, M., & Millar, G. M. (2002). Childhood risk factors for women's sexual victimization. *Journal of Interpersonal Violence, 17*, 647–670.

Svedin, C. G., Nilsson, D., & Lindell, C. (2004). Traumatic experiences and dissociative symptoms among Swedish adolescents: A pilot study using Dis-Q-Sweden. *Nordic Journal of Psychiatry, 58*, 349–355.

Teicher, M. H., Samson, J. A., Polcari, A., & McGreenery, C. E. (2006). Sticks, stones, and hurtful words: Relative effects of various forms of childhood maltreatment. *American Journal of Psychiatry, 163*, 993–1000.

Testa, M., VanZile-Tamsen, C., Livingston, J. A., & Koss, M. P. (2004). Assessing women's experiences of sexual aggression using the Sexual Experiences Survey: Evidence for validity and implications for research. *Psychology of Women Quarterly, 28*, 256–265.

White, H. R., & Widom, C. S. (2003). Intimate partner violence among abused and neglected children in young adulthood: The mediating effects of early aggression, antisocial personality, hostility, and alcohol problems. *Aggressive Behavior, 29*, 332–345.

White, J. W., & Smith, P. H. (2004). Sexual assault perpetration and reperpetration: From adolescence to young adulthood. *Criminal Justice and Behavior, 31*, 182–202.

Widom, C. S. (1989). Does violence beget violence? A critical examination of the literature. *Psychological Bulletin, 106*, 3–28.

Widom, C. S. (2000). Motivation and mechanisms in the "cycle of violence." In D. J. Hansen (Ed.), *Motivation and child maltreatment: Nebraska Symposium on Motivation* (Vol. 46, pp. 1–37). Lincoln: University of Nebraska Press.

Wilson, A., Calhoun, K., & Bernat, J. (1999). Risk recognition and trauma related symptoms among sexually revictimized women. *Journal of Consulting and Clinical Psychology, 67*, 705–710.

Witkiewitz, K., & Dodge-Reyome, N. (2001). Recollections of childhood psychological maltreatment and self-reported eating disordered behaviors in undergraduate college females. *Journal of Emotional Abuse, 2*(1), 15–29.

Zurbriggen, E. L., & Freyd, J. J. (2004). The link between child sexual abuse and risky sexual behavior: The role of dissociative tendencies, information-processing effects, and consensual sex decision mechanisms. In L. J. Koenig, A. O'Leary, L. S. Doll, & W. Pequegnat (Eds.), *From child sexual abuse to adult sexual risk: Trauma revictimization and intervention* (pp. 117–134). Washington, DC: American Psychological Association.

LITERATURE REVIEW

Childhood Emotional Maltreatment and Later Intimate Relationships: Themes from the Empirical Literature

NANCY DODGE REYOME
State University of New York at Potsdam, Potsdam, New York, USA

Within the last three decades, researchers have begun to investigate the long-term consequences of childhood emotional maltreatment on interpersonal and intrapersonal functioning. These investigations have led to the realization that survivors of childhood emotional maltreatment suffer from myriad psychological and social difficulties. These difficulties influence the quality and nature of intimate relationships formed by emotional abuse survivors. The empirical literature looking at the effect of childhood emotional maltreatment on intimate relationships is summarized and discussed. Implications of the current body of research for future research and clinical practice are addressed.

Emotional maltreatment is a commonly occurring form of child maltreatment. In a recent comprehensive national telephone survey conducted in the United States, 2,030 children and adolescents were asked questions regarding the types of victimization they had experienced. Finkelhor, Ormrod, Turner, and Hamby (2005) found that of the different forms of child maltreatment assessed, psychological and emotional forms of maltreatment were the most frequently reported by the children and youth surveyed.

Scher, Forde, McQuaid, and Stein (2004) found similar results after conducting a telephone survey of 967 men and women in a major metropolitan area in Tennessee. In their study, emotional abuse was one of the most common forms of childhood trauma reported by the adult participants. Although emotional maltreatment has been recognized and documented as a commonly occurring form of childhood maltreatment, research on the short- and long-term effects has lagged behind other forms of child maltreatment.

Garbarino, Eckenrode, and Bolger (1997) considered emotional maltreatment to be "an elusive crime." In their estimation, it is too often overlooked, difficult to demonstrate, and is clearly not studied as frequently as other forms of maltreatment. Emotional maltreatment is comprised of parental behaviors that often ignore a child's emotional and psychological needs (Garbarino et al., 1997; Hart & Brassard, 1987; McGee & Wolfe, 1991). These actions might involve isolation, rejection, exploitation, terrorization, or outright neglect of the child who is the target of these parental actions. Glaser (2002) proposed a framework comprised of five categories to encompass parental behaviors that constitute emotional maltreatment: (a) emotional unavailability, unresponsiveness, and neglect; (b) negative attributions or misattributions to the child; (c) developmentally inappropriate or inconsistent interactions with the child; (d) failure to recognize or acknowledge the child's individuality and psychological boundary; and (e) failing to promote the child's social adaptation. As with other forms of maltreatment, an isolated incident of emotional maltreatment is not thought to have lasting developmental implications, however, a repeated and chronic pattern of exposure to psychologically and emotionally abusive actions is considered to be especially deleterious to the growing child's psychological, social, and emotional well-being (Hart & Brassard, 1987; McGee & Wolfe, 1991; Teicher, Samson, Polcari, & McGreenery, 2006).

Harter (1998) argued that child abuse in general and emotionally abusive parenting in particular has a harmful effect on the child's emerging sense of self. She explains that child abuse leads to multiple self-system impairments including impairments in self-awareness, agency, self-continuity, and self-coherence. According to Harter, children who experience child abuse struggle with low self-esteem and a "profound sense of inner badness," which often leads the child to engage in behavior that is not congruent with the true self. Harter pointed out that guilt, depression, shame, and anger are among the negative emotional problems experienced by abused children.

Consistent with Harter's concerns, a childhood history of emotional maltreatment has been linked with myriad psychosocial problems. Repeatedly, empirical investigations have discovered that survivors of childhood emotional abuse suffer from both internalizing and externalizing symptoms. A childhood history of emotional maltreatment has been found to be associated with low self-worth, anxiety, depression, anger, dissociation, somatization, heightened self-criticism, and intense feelings of shame (Briere & Runtz,

1988; Chapman et al., 2004; Dodge Reyome, Ward, & Witkiewitz, 2010; Kim & Cicchetti, 2006; Sachs-Ericsson, Verona, Joiner, & Preacher, 2006; Schneider, Rosa, Graham, & Zielinski, 2005; Showers, Ziegler-Hill, & Limke, 2006; Spertus, Yehuda, Wong, Halligan, & Seremetis, 2003; Teicher et al., 2006; Uhrlass & Gibb, 2007; Webb, Heisler, Call, Chickering, & Colburn, 2007). Given the psychological and emotional problems reported by survivors of emotional maltreatment, it is not surprising that research indicates that individuals with childhood histories of emotional maltreatment often report suffering from eating disorders, substance abuse, and posttraumatic stress disorder (Moran, Vuchinich, & Hall, 2004; Schneider, Baumrind, & Kimberling, 2007; Witkiewitz & Dodge Reyome, 2000).

These early impairments in self-development and the resulting psychosocial aftereffects often translate into poor interpersonal relationships as the individual grows and develops (Berzenski & Yates, 2010; Dodge Reyome et al., 2010; Riggs, 2010; Taussig & Culhane, 2010). In fact, the experience of any form of maltreatment has been shown to set off a vulnerability toward poor peer relationships. In an early influential study of maltreated toddlers' social interactions with other toddlers and adults, George and Main (1979) found that the young maltreated children in their study were more likely to verbally and physically assault peers and adults than the children who had not experienced maltreatment. These researchers also found that the maltreated toddlers were more likely to respond to positive social interactions with avoidance or a mixture of approach-avoidance behaviors. By the preschool and elementary school years, maltreated children have been found to be rated as more disliked, more physically and verbally aggressive, and more socially withdrawn than nonmaltreated children (Anthonysamy & Zimmer-Gembeck, 2007; Bolger & Patterson, 2001; Darwish, Esquivel, Houtz, & Alfonso, 2001; Shonk & Cicchetti, 2001). Duncan (1999) found that children who have experienced parental maltreatment are not only more likely to bully others, but are also likely to be the victims of peer bullying. Although these studies did not focus exclusively on emotional maltreatment, researchers have identified similar developmental outcomes regarding peer relationships in emotionally maltreated children (Egeland, 2009).

Although many studies have documented the long-term effects of physical and sexual abuse (or childhood maltreatment in general) on peer and intimate relationships, the emerging literature has only begun to examine the nature and quality of intimate relationships for adolescents and adults who have a history of childhood emotional maltreatment. This article intends to review the current literature that has been published on the long-term consequences of childhood emotional maltreatment for intimate relationships in adolescence and adulthood. The studies considered in the review fall into three areas or themes of relationship functioning and difficulties: (a) intimacy and relationship quality, (b) codependency, and (c) intimate partner violence. This review is not intended to be exhaustive of the published literature in each area, but is meant to be illustrative of the current state of knowledge regarding this expanding topic of inquiry in the field of child maltreatment. Following this review, suggestions are made for future research on the connection between childhood emotional maltreatment and relationship functioning. Brief remarks on the practice implications of these research findings are made as well.

As mentioned previously, emotional maltreatment can include a multitude of emotionally abusive and neglectful behaviors and because of this, it has been not been clearly defined in the literature and researchers often use different criteria in defining emotional maltreatment across studies. Due to the lack of consistency in the research, this review uses a broad definition for emotional maltreatment and considers a range of studies to summarize the research that has been conducted on this specific area of study. To provide clarification of what emotionally abusive behaviors are being classified as emotional maltreatment in each study, the assessment tool used to measure emotional maltreatment is presented for each study reviewed. Finally, because emotional maltreatment and psychological maltreatment are terms that are both used to describe the emotional abusive behaviors that are intended to be captured in this review, they are both considered to be interchangeable in this article.

CHILDHOOD EMOTIONAL MALTREATMENT, INTIMACY, AND RELATIONSHIP QUALITY

Given the chronic nature of emotional maltreatment and the effect this form of trauma has on self-development and psychosocial well-being, researchers have sought to understand the influence of childhood emotional maltreatment on beliefs about relationships, relationship quality, and satisfaction. Repeatedly, investigators have arrived at the conclusion that a history of childhood emotional maltreatment is strongly associated with serious difficulties in interpersonal relationships in adolescence and adulthood.

Childhood psychological maltreatment has been found to be significantly associated with lower relationship quality, greater fear of intimacy, and distance in interpersonal relationships. Davis, Petretic-Jackson, and Ting (2001) conducted a study looking at the impact of various child abuse experiences on functioning in partner relationships. Davis and his colleagues measured psychological maltreatment using a scale that incorporated Briere and Runtz's (1990) Scale of Psychological Maltreatment and items reflecting Hart and Brassard's (1987) definition of psychological abuse. In this study, a childhood history of psychological maltreatment accounted for more variance in predicting quality of current interpersonal relationships than either a history of childhood sexual abuse or physical abuse. Of the child abuse variables measured in their study, only a history of psychological abuse or multiple abuse experiences were related to a greater fear of intimacy (see Paradis & Boucher, 2010).

Similarly, Drapeau and Perry (2004) looked at how different forms of childhood trauma influence adult relationship patterns. These researchers used vignettes to elicit narratives concerning wishes, needs, motivations, and intentions in interpersonal relationships. Childhood trauma history was measured using a modified version of the Traumatic Antecedents Interview Scale (Herman, Perry, & Van der Kolk, 1989). They found that those participants with a history of verbal abuse during childhood reported "more desire to be distant from others" than those who had not experienced trauma. They also experienced others as "less strong," and they were more likely to react by "not being open" in interpersonal interactions. Those with a history of emotional neglect had "less desire to avoid conflicts" and "more of a wish to be distant from others" than those who had not experienced trauma. In a study looking at the long-term effects of parental physical abuse, verbal abuse (as measured by Straus's [1979] Conflict Tactics Scale), and emotional neglect (as measured by Parker's [1979] Caring Subscale of the Parental Bonding Instrument), Loos and Alexander (1997) found that undergraduates who reported a history of emotional neglect had the highest rates of loneliness and social isolation in their sample. The researchers underscore this finding by pointing out that the association between parental emotional neglect and high rates of loneliness and social isolation among their college student sample was the strongest relationship uncovered in their research. Finally, in a community sample, Mullen, Martin, Anderson, Romans, and Herbison (1996) found emotional abuse survivors, as determined by scores on Parker's (1979) Parental Bonding Instrument, were more likely to report their current partner as uncaring and overintrusive and more frequently reported marital dissolution than a nonabused comparison group.

The extent to which a childhood history of emotional maltreatment is recognized and acknowledged also appears to be associated with the quality of later intimate relationships. Varia and Abidin (1999) discovered that psychological maltreatment survivors who minimize their maltreatment history report higher quality relationships than those who actively acknowledge their abuse history. Using the Psychological Maltreatment Scale (Briere & Runtz, 1988), they identified three groups of participants in their study: those who had no history of psychological abuse (nonabused), those who reported a history of psychological abuse and acknowledged the abuse (acknowledgers), and those who reported a history of psychological abuse experiences but did not label themselves as psychologically abused as a child (minimizers). They found the acknowledgers had the lowest quality of adult relationships and the nonabused group had the highest quality relationships. The minimizers fell in between these two groups on measures of relationship quality. Acknowledgers reported less spousal support and more spousal conflict than either of the other two groups and were least likely to report having securely attached adult relationships. Interestingly, minimizers tended to report higher levels of overall maternal care than acknowledgers and the researchers reported that it was possible that this level of maternal care moderated the effects of childhood emotional and psychological maltreatment on the quality of adult interpersonal relationships.

Related to the findings that individuals with a childhood history of emotional maltreatment report lower quality relationships marred by loneliness, isolation, and mistrust, survivors of childhood emotional maltreatment also report higher rates of interpersonal conflict in intimate relationships than individuals without a history of emotional maltreatment. Using the psychological abuse scale from the Computer Assisted Maltreatment Inventory (DiLillo et al., 2006), Messman-Moore and Coates (2007) found that a childhood history of psychological abuse was directly correlated with adult interpersonal conflict. They also discovered that the relationship between a history of childhood emotional abuse and adult interpersonal conflict is mediated by an individual's beliefs about the self and interpersonal relationships. Messman-Moore and Coates referred to these beliefs as *early maladaptive schemas*. According to these researchers, the early maladaptive schemas, which guide the interpersonal relationships of psychological abuse survivors, involve mistrust, abandonment, deprivation, and defectiveness (see Riggs, 2010, for a discussion of the development of internal working models in emotional abuse survivors). In their research, they found that the relationship between childhood history of psychological abuse and adult interpersonal conflict was fully mediated by the mistrust or abuse and abandonment schema and partially mediated by the defectiveness or shame schema. The demonstration of mediation indicates that certain rigid interpersonal beliefs about the self in relation to others accounted for the connection between a childhood history of psychological maltreatment and interpersonal conflict in adulthood.

As time unfolds, the interpersonal difficulties of childhood emotional abuse survivors can impact marital relationship quality and satisfaction. Belt and Abidin (1996) looked at quality of parenting history and the nature of childhood abuse experiences in a sample of married couples with children. In this study, verbal abuse was measured using a verbal maltreatment scale adapted from Berger and Knutson (1984) and Briere and Runtz (1988). Belt and Abidin discovered that the quality of family-of-origin functioning and childhood abuse experiences (physical and sexual maltreatment were also measured) were more consistently associated with the quality of the marital relationship for women than men. For men, neither the quality of childhood parenting nor the extent of childhood abuse predicted the depth or the level of supportiveness of their current marital relationship. The extent of childhood care was a significant predictor of the depth of women's marital relationships. Also for women, verbal abuse during childhood significantly predicted conflict in the marital relationship.

In a recent prospective study that also considered gender differences in childhood maltreatment and marital functioning, DiLillo et al. (2009) assessed marital functioning at three points over a 2-year period in 202 recently married couples. They measured childhood history of psychological maltreatment using the Computer Assisted Maltreatment Inventory (DiLillo et al., 2006) and the Childhood Trauma Questionnaire (Bernstein & Fink, 1998). In contrast to Belt and Abidin (1996), DiLillo and his colleagues found that a history of childhood psychological abuse was related to lower marital satisfaction at the first point of measurement for husbands but not for wives. Husbands with histories of psychological maltreatment had declining marital satisfaction throughout the study. Overall, these researchers found that husbands with psychological maltreatment histories reported far more problems with marital relationships than did wives with similar histories.

Finally, Perry, DiLillo, and Peugh (2007) investigated the role of psychological difficulties as possible mediators of the relationship between childhood history of psychological maltreatment and marital satisfaction in a sample of newly married couples. The Childhood Trauma Questionnaire was employed in this study to measure both history of emotional abuse and history of emotional neglect (Bernstein & Fink, 1998). As with previous studies, Perry et al. (2007) found a significant negative association between having a history of childhood emotional maltreatment and marital satisfaction for the entire sample. Furthermore, for the entire sample of male and female participants, these researchers found the association between a childhood history of emotional abuse and emotional neglect and marital satisfaction and quality was completely mediated by psychological distress, hostility, and depression (see Riggs & Kaminski, 2010, for a discussion of the connection between childhood emotional abuse and depression). When looking at gender differences in mediation, Perry et al. found the association between childhood emotional abuse and marital quality in males was mediated by psychological distress and paranoia. In females, psychological distress, hostility, and obsessive-compulsive tendencies served to mediate the relationship between childhood emotional abuse and emotional neglect and marital satisfaction and quality.

In summary, childhood emotional abuse survivors report a greater fear of intimacy, a need for interpersonal distance in relationships, and a general lack of trust in others. At the same time, they report feeling lonely, disconnected, and socially isolated. Many individuals who have experienced emotional abuse during childhood possess maladaptive beliefs about themselves and others (e.g., "other people can't be trusted") that negatively influence their interpersonal relationships. A history of childhood emotional abuse tends to be related to lower quality marital relationships, lower marital satisfaction, and marital dissolution. A few researchers have found that there are gender differences in the impact of childhood emotional maltreatment on marital relationships, however, these findings are mixed and warrant further investigation. Finally, there is emerging evidence that particular psychological and social variables such as psychological distress and depression can account for the connection between childhood emotional abuse and the quality of later relationships.

CHILDHOOD EMOTIONAL MALTREATMENT AND CODEPENDENCY

The literature linking childhood emotional maltreatment with codependency in later relationships is conceptually similar to the Messman-Moore and Coates (2007) study that found maladaptive schemas of self-sacrifice and mistrust underlie the connection between childhood emotional maltreatment and later relationship problems. Noriega, Ramos, Medina-Mora, and Villa (2008) referred to codependency as a "relational problem" characterized by a tendency to remain within stressful, abusive, and unhealthy relationships. Codependents tend to engage in self-sacrificing, self-defeating, controlling, and rigid behavior in an attempt to control and change their partner (Dear, Roberts, & Lange, 2005; Dodge Reyome & Ward, 2007; Dodge Reyome et al., 2010). Originally, codependency was believed to emerge from a family context of substance abuse, especially alcoholism (Beattie, 1987; Mellody, Miller, & Miller, 1989). As investigations into the link between substance abuse and codependency progressed and only a weak relationship between familial substance abuse and codependency emerged, researchers broadened their focus to look at the influence of different family and parenting environments and the influence of other forms of childhood trauma on the development of codependent tendencies in intimate relationships. Eventually, investigators began to consider child abuse and neglect history as a possible precursor of codependency in adulthood.

Early studies examining the link between childhood abuse history and codependency focused on physical and sexual abuse. These studies are mixed in regard to whether or not there is a relationship between childhood physical abuse or sexual abuse and codependency in adulthood. For instance, in a study looking at the relationship between different forms of childhood trauma, Irwin (1995) found that codependency in adulthood was not predicted by either childhood sexual abuse or physical abuse. Similarly, Cullen and Carr (1999) found that individuals labeled as high codependency were no more likely to have childhood histories of physical abuse or sexual abuse than those in the low codependency group. However, F. Parker, Faulk, and LoBello (2003) did find a positive association between codependency and both childhood physical abuse and sexual abuse.

Unlike physical abuse and sexual abuse, researchers have consistently found a direct relationship between childhood emotional abuse and codependency in late adolescence and adulthood. Carson and Baker (1994) were perhaps the earliest researchers to report on the strong connection between emotional and psychological forms of abuse and codependency. They found that individuals in their sample with histories of emotional abuse tended to score high in codependency. Although Cullen and Carr (1999) focused their study on other forms of maltreatment, they did note that family environments that lacked warmth and appropriate emotional expression tended to be associated with codependency. Investigations into parenting styles and practices and codependency tend to support this overall conclusion that emotional maltreatment is linked with codependency. Crothers and Warren (1996) found that codependency was positively associated with coercive, controlling, and nonnurturing forms of parenting. Related to this finding, Fischer and Crawford (1992) found paternal authoritarian parenting was linked with high codependency scores.

Dodge Reyome and Ward (2007) conducted a comprehensive study to investigate the link between childhood abuse history and codependency by looking at all five major forms of childhood maltreatment and looking at the association of each form with codependency. Childhood abuse history was measured using the Childhood Trauma Questionnaire (Bernstein et al., 1994), which has emotional abuse and emotional neglect subscales. Additionally, childhood psychological maltreatment was assessed using the Psychological Maltreatment Inventory (Engels & Moisan, 1994). They found that although all forms of child abuse and neglect measured in the study were significantly positively associated with codependency, the most robust relationships were between emotional abuse and emotional neglect and codependency (see Dodge Reyome et al., 2010, for further exploration of the link between childhood emotional maltreatment and codependency). In a sample of young women seeking primary health care in Mexico, Noriega et al. (2008) found that women who reported a history of familial emotional maltreatment (measured by a three-item scale) were more than two times more likely to be codependent than other young women without a childhood history of emotional abuse and neglect. Interestingly, in this same study, neither childhood physical nor sexual abuse was found to be significantly associated with codependence in this sample of young women.

In summary, for some time, researchers and theoreticians believed that family-of-origin alcohol and substance abuse was the primary familial context of codependency in adult relationships. However, investigations looking at the relationship between exposure to substance and alcohol abuse and codependency found only a weak association. Studies looking at other forms of childhood trauma and codependency in adulthood have consistently found a moderate to strong relationship between childhood emotional maltreatment and codependency. Further research is needed to look at explanatory mechanisms for the connection between emotional maltreatment and codependency.

CHILDHOOD EMOTIONAL MALTREATMENT AND INTIMATE PARTNER VIOLENCE

Initially, researchers looking at the association between child maltreatment and intimate partner violence focused on a history of physical child abuse or witnessing domestic violence as possible antecedents of relationship violence in adulthood (Rich, Gidycz, Warkentin, Loh, & Weiland, 2005). Some investigators also linked child sexual abuse with a high likelihood of sexual victimization in adult relationships (Arata & Lindman, 2002). Only recently have researchers turned their attention to the role of childhood emotional maltreatment in the experience of intimate violence in partner relationships during late adolescence and adulthood (see Berzenki & Yates, 2010; Zurbriggen, Gobin, & Freyd, 2010).

Childhood emotional maltreatment has been found to be associated with intimate partner violence in marital relationships. In an early study looking at childhood emotional maltreatment among battered married women, Cascardi, O'Leary, Lawrence, and Schlee (1995) compared three groups of women on a variety of psychosocial and family history measures. Child abuse history including childhood history of emotional abuse was measured using the Child Abuse Assessment (Neidig, 1989). Cascardi et al. (1995) utilized three groups of women in their study: abused women, unhappily married nonabused women, and martially content women. They found that rates of childhood physical abuse and sexual abuse did not differ significantly across groups. However, the abused women and the unhappily married women reported significantly higher rates of childhood emotional abuse than did the women who were content in their marriage. Further, the abused women reported the highest rate of childhood emotional maltreatment of all three groups in the study.

In a telephone survey of 637 women in the Memphis, Tennessee area, Seedat, Stein, and Ford (2005) examined the association between childhood maltreatment history (as measured by the Childhood Trauma Questionnaire), substance misuse, posttraumatic stress disorder (PTSD), suicidal behavior, and intimate partner violence victimization. Approximately half of the women surveyed in their study were married or cohabitating and the average age of the participants was 37 years for those who reported intimate partner violence and 40 years for those reporting no history of intimate partner violence. Using a simultaneous regression model, childhood emotional abuse (among other variables) significantly predicted experiencing intimate partner violence. Stepwise regression analysis revealed that childhood emotional abuse along with childhood sexual abuse and low educational attainment were the only significant predictors of intimate partner violence victimization in their study.

Studies also indicate that a history of childhood emotional abuse is strongly associated with dating violence. Sappington, Pharr, Tunstall, and Rickert (1997) looked at the relationship among a history of child abuse, dating violence, and psychological problems in a sample of 133 female undergraduates. Verbal abuse was assessed in this study using a measure designed by the researchers called the Experiences Questionnaire. These researchers found that a reported history of parental verbal abuse was strongly associated with being forced to have sex on a date, being physically abused by a date, being verbally abused by a date, and verbally abusing a date. In essence, Sappington et al. found a strong association between having a history of parental verbal abuse and reported dating violence victimization and perpetration. Similarly, in a college student sample, Rich et al. (2005) looked at the link between childhood victimization experiences and college-age victimization experiences, including dating violence. In this study, verbal aggression between parent and child was measured using Straus's (1979) Conflict Tactics Scale. Sixty-seven percent of the college-age women in this study reported a history of paternal verbal abuse with close to 50% reporting severe paternal verbal abuse. Eighty percent reported maternal verbal abuse and almost 54% of the sample reported severe verbal abuse from their mothers. In this sample, a reported history of maternal and paternal verbal abuse was significantly related to dating violence victimization during late adolescence. In fact, the only forms of childhood victimization (physical abuse and sexual abuse were also measured) that predicted experiencing dating violence during adolescence were maternal and paternal verbal abuse during childhood.

Recently, investigators have begun to look at potential mediators of the relationship between a history of childhood emotional abuse and intimate partner violence victimization and perpetration. As with the connection between childhood emotional maltreatment and interpersonal conflict in adult relationships, early maladaptive schemas have been found to be one of the possible links explaining the association between having a history of childhood emotional abuse and later experiencing intimate violence in adolescence and adulthood. Using a sample of college males and females, Crawford and Wright (2007) studied the relationship between childhood emotional maltreatment and intimate partner violence and the role of early maladaptive schemas in this connection. These researchers utilized the Lifetime Experiences Questionnaire to measure childhood emotional abuse and childhood emotional neglect. Similar to other researchers, Crawford and Wright found that childhood emotional maltreatment emerged as a significant predictor of both victimization and perpetration of intimate partner violence. In addition, they found different schemas mediated the relationship between a history of emotional maltreatment and intimate violence victimization and emotional maltreatment and intimate violence perpetration. The schemas of mistrust, self-sacrifice, and emotional inhibition all emerged as full mediators of the relationship between childhood emotional abuse and intimate partner victimization. The schemas of entitlement, emotional inhibition, and insufficient self-control emerged as partial mediators of the relationship between the perpetration of intimate partner violence and a childhood history of emotional abuse.

Other psychological and social mechanisms have been investigated as possible explanatory mechanisms for the established relationship between childhood emotional maltreatment and intimate partner violence. Taft, Schumm, Marshall, Pamuzio, and Holzworth-Munroe (2008) considered PTSD and social information processing deficits as potential mediators of the association between a history of childhood maltreatment and intimate partner violence in a sample of adult couples who were married or living together. Of the forms of childhood maltreatment (childhood exposure to parental violence and childhood physical abuse were also measured) assessed in the Taft et al. study, only parental rejection emerged as being significantly related to the perpetration of physical and psychological forms of relationship violence. Parental rejection in childhood, as measured by the Rejection subscale of the EMBU (Perris, Jacobsson, Lindstrom, von Knorring, & Perris, 1980), was also strongly correlated with posttraumatic stress symptoms and social information processing deficits. Finally, Taft et al. found the association of parental rejection with the perpetration of intimate partner violence was mediated by posttraumatic stress symptoms and social information processing deficits.

In a recent study, Wekerle et al. (2009) also looked at PTSD as a mediator of the relationship between a childhood history of emotional maltreatment and dating violence in a sample of adolescents involved with protective services. These researchers gathered information from 402 teenagers receiving child protective services. Most of the teens in their sample had begun dating and between half and two thirds reported some form of dating violence. Two instruments were utilized to measure childhood emotional maltreatment in this study: the Childhood Trauma Questionnaire (Bernstein et al., 1994) and the Childhood Experiences of Victimization Questionnaire (Walsh, MacMillan, Trocme, Jamieson, & Boyle, 2008). Similar to Taft et al. (2008), these researchers found childhood emotional maltreatment was a significant predictor of PTSD symptoms and intimate partner violence. Interestingly, they found childhood emotional abuse was a significant predictor of both perpetration of violence and victimization in dating relationships among males. In females, only being a victim of dating violence was significantly predicted by a history of childhood emotional abuse. Also, posttraumatic stress symptoms were found to be a significant mediator of childhood emotional abuse and dating violence perpetration in males and dating violence victimization in females.

In summary, although not as frequently studied as physical abuse, emotional forms of child abuse have been found to be linked with intimate partner violence in adolescent and adult populations in dating and marital relationships. Those individuals with a history of emotional maltreatment are far more likely than those without such a history to be involved in relationship violence perpetration and victimization. Recent studies have begun to look at possible explanations for the link between a history of emotional maltreatment and intimate partner violence in both dating and marital relationships. Some promising explanatory mechanisms for this connection are

PTSD, maladaptive schemas about the self and others, and social information processing deficits.

IMPLICATIONS FOR FUTURE RESEARCH AND CLINICAL PRACTICE

Although the research literature on the long-term consequences of childhood emotional maltreatment is growing, the sheer volume of studies lags behind the amount of empirical research that has been carried out on other forms of child maltreatment. It is especially important that child maltreatment researchers continue to shine a light on the effect of childhood emotional maltreatment on adolescent and adult interpersonal functioning. Future investigations looking at aspects of adult interpersonal functioning associated with childhood emotional maltreatment could advance this field of inquiry by utilizing diverse samples, exploring protective factors, studying mediators of the relationship, and employing prospective designs.

Studies looking at relationship functioning have tended to focus on female participants and overlook male participants. This tendency has been especially true in intimate violence studies seeking to understand the background and psychosocial history of victims of intimate violence. The importance of conducting studies that include male and female participants is exemplified by studies where gendered relationship patterns have been uncovered. For instance, DiLillo et al. (2009) found that husbands with a history of childhood emotional abuse and emotional neglect reported declining marital satisfaction, whereas wives with similar histories did not. Similarly, Wekerle et al. (2009) found that a history of childhood emotional abuse was predictive of dating violence victimization in females and dating violence perpetration in males.

Whereas the connection between a history of childhood emotional maltreatment and deleterious intimate relationships is clear, it is much less clear what conditions could or do serve as protective factors in this connection. In their research, Varia and Abidin (1999) discovered that individuals with a history of childhood psychological maltreatment who minimize their history report higher quality relationships than individuals who have similar histories of childhood psychological abuse who label themselves as being childhood victims of emotional maltreatment. Besides minimizing the importance of their history of parental psychological abuse, the only other factor Varia and Abidin could identify for ameliorating the effect of the abuse on their adult relationships was the higher level of maternal care that the individuals who minimized their history reported receiving. It will be important for future studies to begin to identify, explore, and understand other protective factors that soften the blow of parental emotional maltreatment on later intimate relationships.

Researchers have begun to identify explanatory mechanisms for the connection between a childhood history of emotional maltreatment and later problems in intimate relationships. In marital relationships, Perry et al. (2007) identified psychological distress as a mediator of the relationship between a childhood history of emotional abuse and neglect and marital satisfaction in males and females. Crawford and Wright (2007) found the early maladaptive schemas of mistrust, self-sacrifice, and emotional inhibition were full mediators of the association between childhood emotional abuse and intimate partner victimization. Both Wekerle et al. (2009) and Taft et al. (2008) identified PTSD as a mediator of the relationship between childhood emotional abuse and partner violence. It is likely that other psychological or contextual variables will be found to serve as pathways between a childhood history of emotional abuse and relationship difficulties in adolescence and adulthood (see Berzenski & Yates, 2010; Dodge Reyome et al., 2010).

The importance of employing prospective research designs in understanding the consequences of child maltreatment has been addressed in other venues (Widom, Raphael, & DuMont, 2004). One of the greatest advantages of using prospective, longitudinal research designs in looking at the long-term consequences of emotional abuse is the ability to avoid recall bias, which might artificially inflate the relationship between childhood emotional abuse and later relationship problems. At the present time, most of the studies looking at the relationship between childhood emotional maltreatment and later relationship functioning are retrospective in nature. Short-term prospective designs have been utilized in the research literature on the effect of childhood emotional maltreatment on intimate relationships. For instance, DiLillo et al. (2009) looked at childhood emotional abuse and marital functioning in newlyweds over a 2-year period. However, longer term prospective studies have been carried out looking at the effect of other forms of childhood maltreatment on interpersonal relationships in adolescence and adulthood (Colman & Widom, 2004). Similar studies are needed that follow individuals with a history of childhood emotional maltreatment over longer spans of time and measure stage-salient aspects of relationship functioning.

The findings of the current literature looking at the effect of childhood emotional maltreatment history on later intimate relationships hold considerable promise for clinical practice. Adult survivors of childhood emotional victimization clearly have lowered opinions of themselves in relationship to others and maladaptive beliefs and expectations of interpersonal relationships. These early maladaptive schemas serve to guide their behavior in intimate relationships and can result in mistrust, disconnection, and loneliness. Therapeutic approaches that explore and rework these negative self and relationship schemas will assist the individual in adopting new and more constructive ways of thinking about the self and other people (see Carbone, 2010, for further exploration of therapeutic interventions). This cognitive reworking should help the adult survivor form more meaningful, peaceful, and connected relationships with others.

Moreover, psychological distress and PTSD have been identified as pathways by which a childhood history of emotional maltreatment is linked with lower relationship satisfaction and quality as well as intimate violence in adolescence and adulthood. Exploring and addressing these possible avenues of relationship discord with adult survivors of emotional maltreatment and providing targeted therapeutic intervention for these difficulties should prove fruitful in assisting these individuals in finding ways to live more productive and satisfying lives.

REFERENCES

Anthonysamy, A., & Zimmer-Gembeck, M. (2007). Peer status and behaviors of maltreated children and their classmates in the early years of school. *Child Abuse and Neglect, 31*, 971–991.

Arata, C., & Lindman, L. (2002). Marriage, child abuse & sexual revictimization. *Journal of Interpersonal Violence, 17*, 953–971.

Beattie, M. (1987). *Codependent no more: How to stop controlling others and start caring for yourself.* Center City, MN: Hazelton Press.

Belt, W., & Abidin, R. (1996). The relation of childhood abuse and early parenting experiences to current marital quality in a non-clinical sample. *Child Abuse and Neglect, 20*, 1019–1030.

Berger, A., & Knutson, J. (1984). *The Assessing Environment III: A questionnaire for assessing punitive abuse-related childhood histories.* Unpublished manuscript.

Bernstein, D., & Fink, L. (1998). *Childhood Trauma Questionnaire: A retrospective self-report questionnaire and manual.* San Antonio, TX: Psychological Corporation.

Bernstein, D., Fink, L., Handelsman, L., Lovejoy, M., Wenzel, K., Saparento, E., et al. (1994). Initial reliability and validity of a new retrospective measure of child abuse and neglect. *American Journal of Psychiatry, 151*, 1132–1136.

Berzenski, S. R., & Yates, T. M. (2010). A developmental process analysis of the contribution of childhood emotional abuse to relationship violence. *Journal of Aggression, Maltreatment and Trauma, 19*(2), 180–203.

Bolger, K., & Patterson, C. (2001). Developmental pathways from child maltreatment to peer rejection. *Child Development, 72*, 549–568.

Briere, J., & Runtz, M. (1988). Multivariate correlates of childhood psychological and physical maltreatment among university women. *Child Abuse and Neglect, 12*, 331–341.

Briere, J., & Runtz, M. (1990). Differential adult symptomatology associated with three types of child abuse histories. *Child Abuse and Neglect, 14*, 357–364.

Carbone, D. J. (2010). Using cognitive therapies to treat unstable attachment patterns in adults with childhood histories of social rejection. *Journal of Aggression, Maltreatment and Trauma, 19*(*1*), 105–134.

Carson, A., & Baker, R. (1994). Psychological correlates of codependency in women. *The International Journal of Addictions, 29*, 395–407.

Cascardi, M., O'Leary, D., Lawrence, E., & Schlee, K. (1995). Characteristics of women physically abused by their spouses and who seek treatment regarding marital conflict. *Journal of Counseling and Clinical Psychology, 63*, 616–623.

Chapman, D., Whitfield, C., Felitti, V., Dube, S., Edwards, V., & Anda, R. (2004). Adverse childhood experiences and the risk of depressive disorders in adulthood. *Journal of Affective Disorders, 82*, 217–225.

Colman, R., & Widom, C. (2004). Child abuse and neglect and adult intimate relationships: A prospective study. *Child Abuse and Neglect, 28*, 1133–1151.

Crawford, E., & Wright, M. (2007). The impact of childhood psychological maltreatment on interpersonal schemas and subsequent experiences of relationship aggression. *Journal of Emotional Abuse, 7*, 93–116.

Crothers, M., & Warren, L. (1996). Parental antecedents of adult codependency. *Journal of Clinical Psychology, 52*, 231–239.

Cullen, J., & Carr, A. (1999). Codependency: An empirical study from a systemic perspective. *Contemporary Family Therapy, 21*, 505–526.

Darwish, D., Esquivel, G., Houtz, J., & Alfonso, V. (2001). Play and social skills in maltreated and non-maltreated preschoolers during peer interactions. *Child Abuse and Neglect, 25*, 13–31.

Davis, J., Petretic-Jackson, P., & Ting, L. (2001). Intimacy dysfunction and trauma symptomatology: Long-term correlates of different types of child abuse. *Journal of Traumatic Stress, 14*, 63–79.

Dear, G., Roberts, C., & Lange, L. (2005). Defining codependency: A thematic analysis of published definitions. In S. Shobov (Ed). *Advances in psychological research* (Vol. 34, pp. 189–205). Hauppage, NY: Nova Science.

DiLillo, D., Fortier, M., Hayes, S., Trask, E., Perry, A., Messman-Moore, T., et al. (2006). Retrospective assessment of childhood sexual and physical abuse: A comparison of scaled and behaviorally specific approaches. *Assessment, 13*, 297–312.

DiLillo, D., Peugh, J., Walsh, K., Panuzio, J., Trask, E., & Evans, S. (2009). Child maltreatment history among newlywed couples: A longitudinal study of marital outcomes and mediating pathways. *Journal of Consulting and Clinical Psychology, 77*, 680–692.

Dodge Reyome, N., & Ward, K. (2007). Self reported history of childhood maltreatment and codependency in undergraduate nursing students. *Journal of Emotional Abuse, 7*, 37–50.

Dodge Reyome, N., Ward, K. S., & Witkiewitz, K. (2010). Psychosocial variables as mediators of the relationship between childhood emotional maltreatment, codependency, and self silencing. *Journal of Aggression, Maltreatment and Trauma, 19*(2), 159–179.

Drapeau, M., & Perry, J. (2004). Childhood trauma and adult interpersonal functioning: A study using the Core Conflictual Relationship Theme Method (CCRT). *Child Abuse and Neglect, 28*, 1049–1066.

Duncan, R. (1999). Maltreatment by parents and peers: The relationship between child abuse, bully victimization, and psychological distress. *Child Maltreatment, 4*, 45–55.

Egeland, B. (2009). Taking stock: Childhood emotional maltreatment and developmental psychopathology. *Child Abuse and Neglect, 33*, 22–26.

Engels, M., & Moisan, D. (1994). The Psychological Maltreatment Inventory: Development of a measure of psychological maltreatment in childhood for use in adult clinical settings. *Psychological Reports, 74*, 595–604.

Finkelhor, D., Ormrod, R., Turner, H., & Hamby, S. (2005). The victimization of children and youth: A comprehensive, national survey. *Child Maltreatment, 10*, 5–25.

Fischer, J., & Crawford, D. (1992). Codependency and parenting styles. *Journal of Adolescent Research, 7*, 352–363.

Garbarino, J., Eckenrode, J., & Bolger, K. (1997). The elusive crime of psychological maltreatment. In J. Garbarino & J. Eckenrode (Eds.), *Understanding abusive families* (pp. 101–113). San Francisco: Jossey-Bass.

George, C., & Main, M. (1979). Social interactions of young abused children: Approach, avoidance and aggression. *Child Development, 50*, 306–318.

Glaser, D. (2002). Emotional abuse and neglect (psychological maltreatment): A conceptual framework. *Child Abuse and Neglect, 26*, 697–714.

Hart, S., & Brassard, M. (1987). A major threat to children's mental health: Psychological maltreatment. *American Psychologist, 42*, 160–165.

Harter, S. (1998). The effects of child abuse on the self system. *Journal of Aggression, Maltreatment and Trauma, 2*, 147–169.

Herman, J., Perry, J., & Van der Kolk, B. (1989). Childhood trauma in borderline personality disorder. *American Journal of Psychiatry, 146*, 490–495.

Irwin, H. (1995). Codependence, narcissism, and childhood trauma. *Journal of Clinical Psychology, 51*, 658–665.

Kim, J., & Cicchetti, D. (2006). Longitudinal trajectories of self system processes and depressive symptoms among maltreated and non-maltreated children. *Child Development, 77*, 624–639.

Loos, M., & Alexander, P. (1997). Differential effects associated with self-reported histories of abuse and neglect in a college sample. *Journal of Interpersonal Violence, 12*, 340–360.

McGee, R., & Wolfe, D. (1991). Psychological maltreatment: Toward an operational definition. *Development and Psychopathology, 3*, 3–18.

Mellody, P., Miller, A., & Miller, J. (1989). *Facing codependency: What it is, where it comes from, how it sabatoges our lives*. New York: Harper & Row.

Messman-Moore, T., & Coates, A. (2007). The impact of childhood psychological abuse on adult interpersonal conflict: The role of maladaptive schemas and patterns of interpersonal behavior. *Journal of Emotional Abuse, 7*, 75–92.

Moran, P., Vuchinich, S., & Hall, N. (2004). Associations between types of maltreatment and substance use during adolescence. *Child Abuse and Neglect, 28*, 565–574.

Mullen, P., Martin, J., Anderson, J., Romans, S., & Herbison, G. (1996). The long-term impact of physical, emotional, and sexual abuse of children: A community sample. *Child Abuse and Neglect, 20*, 7–21.

Neidig, P. (1989). *Family history assessment interview*. Stony Brook, NY: Behavioral Science Associates.

Noriega, G., Ramos, L., Medina-Mora, M., & Villa, A. (2008). Prevalence of codependence in young women seeking primary health care and associated risk factors. *American Journal of Orthopsychiatry, 78*, 199–210.

Paradis, A., & Boucher, S. (2010). Child maltreatment history and interpersonal problems in adult couple relationships. *Journal of Aggression, Maltreatment and Trauma, 19*(2), 138–158.

Parker, F., Faulk, D., & LoBello, S. (2003). Assessing codependency and family pathology in nursing students. *Journal of Addictions Nursing, 14*, 85–90.

Parker, G. (1979). Parental characteristics in relations to depressive disorders. *British Journal of Psychiatry, 134*, 138–147.

Perris, C., Jacobsson, L., Lindstrom, H., von Knorring, L., & Perris, H. (1980). Development of a new inventory for assessing memories of parental rearing behaviour. *Acta Psychiatrica Scandinavica, 61*, 265–274.

Perry, A., DiLillo, D., & Peugh, J. (2007). Childhood psychological maltreatment and quality of marriage: The mediating role of psychological distress. *Journal of Emotional Abuse, 7*, 117–142.

Rich, C., Gidycz, C., Warkentin, J., Loh, C., & Weiland, P. (2005). Child and adolescent abuse and subsequent victimization: A prospective study. *Child Abuse and Neglect, 29*, 1373–1394.

Riggs, S. A. (2010). Childhood emotional abuse and the attachment system across the life cycle: What theory and research tell us. *Journal of Aggression, Maltreatment and Trauma, 19*(*1*), 5–51.

Riggs, S. A., & Kaminski, P. (2010). Childhood emotional abuse, adult attachment, and depression as predictors of relational adjustment and psychological aggression. *Journal of Aggression, Maltreatment and Trauma, 19*(*1*), 75–104.

Sachs-Ericsson, N., Verona, E., Joiner, T., & Preacher, K. (2006). Parental verbal abuse and the mediating role of self criticism in adult internalizing disorders. *Journal of Affective Disorders, 93*, 71–78.

Sappington, A., Pharr, R., Tunstall, A., & Rickert, E. (1997). Relationships among child abuse, date abuse and psychological problems. *Journal of Clinical Psychology, 53*, 319–329.

Scher, C., Forde, D., McQuaid, J., & Stein, M. (2004). Prevalence and demographic correlates of childhood maltreatment in an adult community sample. *Child Abuse and Neglect, 28*, 167–180.

Schneider, M., Rosa, A., Graham, C., & Zielinski, A. (2005). Do allegations of emotional maltreatment predict developmental outcomes beyond that of other forms of maltreatment? *Child Abuse and Neglect, 29*, 513–532.

Schneider, R., Baumrind, N., & Kimberling, R. (2007). Exposure to child abuse and risk for mental health problems in women. *Violence and Victims, 22*, 620–631.

Seedat, S., Stein, M., & Forde, D. (2005). Association between physical partner violence, posttraumatic stress, childhood trauma, and suicide attempts in a community sample of women. *Violence and Victims, 20*, 87–98.

Shonk, S., & Cicchetti, D. (2001). Maltreatment, competency deficits, and risk for academic and behavioral adjustment. *Developmental Psychology, 37*, 3–17.

Showers, C., Ziegler-Hill, V., & Limke, A. (2006). Self-structure and childhood maltreatment: Successful compartmentalization and the struggle for integration. *Journal of Social and Clinical Psychology, 25*, 473–507.

Spertus, I., Yehuda, R., Wong, C., Halligan, S., & Seremetis, S. (2003). Childhood emotional abuse and neglect as predictors of psychological and physical symptoms of women presenting to a primary care practice. *Child Abuse and Neglect, 27*, 1247–1258.

Straus, M. (1979). Measuring intrafamily conflict and violence: The Conflict Tactics (CT) Scale. *Journal of Marriage and the Family, 41*, 75–88.

Taft, C., Schumm, J., Marshall, A., Pamuzio, J., & Holzworth-Munroe, A. (2008). Family-of-origin maltreatment, posttraumatic stress disorder symptoms, social information processing deficits, and relationship abuse perpetration. *Journal of Abnormal Psychology, 17*, 637–646.

Taussig, H. N., & Culhane, S. E. (2010). Emotional maltreatment and psychosocial functioning in preadolescent youth placed in out-of-home care. *Journal of Aggression, Maltreatment and Trauma, 19*,(1), 52–74.

Teicher, M., Samson, J., Polcari, A., & McGreenery, C. (2006). Sticks, stones, and hurtful words: Relative effects of various forms of childhood maltreatment. *American Journal of Psychiatry, 163*, 993–1000.

Uhrlass, D., & Gibb, B. (2007). Childhood emotional maltreatment and the stress generation model of depression. *Journal of Social and Clinical Psychology, 26*, 119–130.

Varia, R., & Abidin, R. (1999). The minimizing style: Perceptions of psychological abuse and quality of past and current relationships. *Child Abuse and Neglect, 23*, 1041–1055.

Walsh, C., MacMillan, H., Trocme, N., Jamieson, E., & Boyle, M. (2008). Measurement of victimization in adolescence: Development and validation of the childhood experiences of violence questionnaire. *Child Abuse and Neglect, 32*, 1037–1057.

Webb, M., Heisler, D., Call, S., Chickering, S., & Colburn, T. (2007). Shame, guilt, symptoms of depression and reported history of psychological maltreatment. *Child Abuse and Neglect, 31*, 1143–1153.

Wekerle, C., Leung, E., Wall, A., MacMillan, H., Boyle, M., Trocme, N., et al. (2009). The contribution of childhood emotional abuse to teen dating violence among child protective services-involved youth. *Child Abuse and Neglect, 33*, 45–58.

Widom, C., Raphael, K., & DuMont, K. (2004). The case for prospective, longitudinal studies in child maltreatment research: Commentary of Dube, Williamson, Thompson, Felliti, and Anda. *Child Abuse and Neglect, 28*, 715–722.

Witkiewitz, K., & Dodge Reyome, N. (2000). Recollections of childhood psychological maltreatment and self-reported eating disordered behaviors in undergraduate college females. *Journal of Emotional Abuse, 2*, 15–29.

Zurbriggen, E. L., Gobin, R., & Freyd, J. J. (2010). Childhood emotional abuse and late adolescent sexual aggression perpetration and victimization. *Journal of Aggression, Maltreatment and Trauma, 19*(2), 204–223.

Index

Page numbers in *Italics* represent tables.
Page numbers in **Bold** represent figures.

Index